Clinical Nurse Leader Certification Review

Cynthia R. King, PhD, MSN, NP, RN, CNL, FAAN, went into nursing after completing a BS in biology and psychology. Over several decades, Cyndy has worked as a clinician (staff nurse, CNS, NP), educator/faculty, administrator, and researcher. Additionally, she has had her own consulting business for 21 years and worked in hospice/home care and in the pharmaceutical/biotechnology industry.

She has published extensively, including completing a book with her father, Dr. John A. King, for patients and families called *100 Questions and Answers about Communicating with Your Healthcare Provider*. She has also published a book called *Advances in Oncology Nursing Research* and finished her third edition of a book on quality of life.

Dr. King is principal and consultant at Special Care Consultants in Charlotte, North Carolina and is editor in chief of the *Journal of Clinical Nursing*. Cyndy has been involved in developing and teaching in the clinical nurse leader (CNL) program. She is CNL certified and is a member of the Clinical Nurse Leader Association. Cyndy serves on many national advisory boards and grant review teams and consults on leadership, research/evidence-based practice, and shared governance. She has been involved in shared governance since 1987. Dr. King has spoken and consulted internationally, nationally, regionally, and locally.

Sally O'Toole Gerard, DNP, RN, CDE, CNL, is an assistant professor at Fairfield University School of Nursing. She has been in nursing for over 25 years and has a strong background in critical care nursing and hospital education. She specializes in diabetes and is a certified diabetes educator. Her publications and research focus on the improvement of patient-related outcomes related to diabetes and other topics. Dr. Gerard had been involved in a number of academic collaborations with local hospitals to introduce evidence-based practice and improve quality care in the acute setting. This strong link between practice and academia is consistent with her role as track coordinator for the clinical nurse leader graduate program. She has completed a national partnership of health care improvement practices with the Dartmouth Institute for Health Policy and the American Association of Colleges of Nursing. She is passionate about the role of CNL-prepared nurses leading change, making health care a safer environment for all persons.

Clinical Nurse Leader
Certification Review

Cynthia R. King, PhD, MSN, NP, RN, CNL, FAAN
Sally O'Toole Gerard, DNP, RN, CDE, CNL

Editors

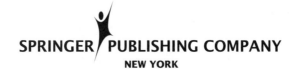
SPRINGER PUBLISHING COMPANY
NEW YORK

Springer Publishing Company, LLC
11 West 42nd Street
New York, NY 10036
www.springerpub.com

Acquisitions Editor: Allan Graubard
Composition: S4Carlisle

ISBN: 978-0-8261-7117-7
E-book ISBN: 978-0-8261-7118-4

13 14 15 / 5 4 3 2

The author and the publisher of this Work have made every effort to use sources believed to be reliable to provide information that is accurate and compatible with the standards generally accepted at the time of publication. Because medical science is continually advancing, our knowledge base continues to expand. Therefore, as new information becomes available, changes in procedures become necessary. We recommend that the reader always consult current research and specific institutional policies before performing any clinical procedure. The author and publisher shall not be liable for any special, consequential, or exemplary damages resulting, in whole or in part, from the readers' use of, or reliance on, the information contained in this book. The publisher has no responsibility for the persistence or accuracy of URLs for external or third-party Internet websites referred to in this publication and does not guarantee that any content on such websites is, or will remain, accurate or appropriate.

Library of Congress Cataloging-in-Publication Data
Clinical nurse leader certification review / Cynthia R. King, Sally O'Toole Gerard, editors.
  p.; cm.
Includes bibliographical references and index.
ISBN 978-0-8261-7117-7—ISBN 0-8261-7117-6—ISBN 978-0-8261-7118-4 (e-book)
I. King, Cynthia R. II. Gerard, Sally O'Toole.
[DNLM: 1. Nurse Clinicians—Outlines. 2. Certification—Outlines. 3. Leadership—Outlines. 4. Nurse's Role—Outlines. WY 18.2]
610.73076--dc23   2012033046

Printed in the United States of America by Bang Printing.

*To all the clinical nurse leaders and clinical nurse leader students who
are working hard to make all aspects of our health care system
a model that will exceed expectations of quality and safety
for all Americans. We gratefully recognize the dedication
of faculty and health care organizations who are working
collaboratively to support these master's-prepared nurses
to lead change in this important era of health care.*

Contents

Contributors

Jonathan P. Auld, MS, RN, CNL
Professional Practice Leader
Oregon Health and Science University
Portland, Oregon

Audrey Marie Beauvais, DNP, MSN, MBA, RN-BC
Assistant Professor
Sacred Heart University
College of Health Professions
Fairfield, Connecticut

Denise M. Bourassa, MSN, CNL, RN
Assistant Clinical Professor
University of Connecticut
School of Nursing
Storrs, Connecticut

Grace O. Buttriss, DNP, RN, FNP-BC
Assistant Professor
Queens University of Charlotte
Charlotte, North Carolina

Carol Fackler, DNSc, RN
Assistant Professor
University of Southern Maine
Portland, Maine

Sally O'Toole Gerard, DNP, RN, CDE, CNL
Assistant Professor
Fairfield University School of Nursing
Fairfield, Connecticut

Bonnie Haupt, MSN, RN, CNL-BC
Acute Care Clinical Nurse Leader
VA Connecticut Healthcare System
West Haven, Connecticut

Deborah C. Jackson, MSN, RN, CCRN, CNL
Clinical Assistant Professor
College of Health Professions
Sacred Heart University
Fairfield, Connecticut

Cynthia R. King, PhD, NP, MSN, RN, CNL, FAAN
Principal and Consultant
Special Care Consultants
Charlotte, North Carolina

Dawn Marie Nair, DNP, RN
Visiting Assistant Professor
Fairfield University School of Nursing
Fairfield, Connecticut

September T. Nelson, MS, RN, CNL
Instructor and Director, Learning Resource Center
University of Portland School of Nursing
Portland, Oregon

E. Carol Polifroni, EdD, CNE, NEA-BC, RN
Professor
University of Connecticut
Storrs, Connecticut

Kathryn B. Reid, PhD, RN
Coordinator, Clinical Nurse Leader Program
University of Virginia School of Nursing
Charlottesville, Virginia

Catherine Winkler, PhD, MPH, RN
Director of Cardiovascular Services
St. Vincent's Medical Center
Bridgeport, Connecticut

Teri Moser Woo, PhD, RN, CNL, CPNP, FAANP
Associate Professor
Director, Clinical Nurse Leader Program
University of Portland School of Nursing
Portland, Oregon

Post-Test Questions

Kimberlee-Ann Bridges, MSN, RN, CNL
Care Coordinator
Western Health Network
Danbury, Connecticut

Leah Ledford, MSN, RN, CNL, SANE
Clinical Nurse Leader
Carolinas Medical Center
Charlotte, North Carolina

Marie D. Litzelman, MSN, RN, CMSRN, CNL
Clinical Nurse Leader
Carolinas Medical Center
Charlotte, North Carolina

Danielle Morton, MSN, RN, CNL
Pediatric Nurse Educator
Yale New Haven Hospital
New Haven, Connecticut

Sara Pratt, MSN, RN, CNL
Clinical Nurse Leader
Carolinas Medical Center
Charlotte, North Carolina

Katarzyna A. Qutermous, MSN, RN, CNL
Clinical Nurse Leader
Carolinas Medical Center
Charlotte, North Carolina

Josephine Ritchie, MSN, RN, CNL
Performance Improvement Manager
Norwalk Hospital
Norwalk, Connecticut

Mary-Jo Smith, MSN, RN, CNL
Patient Services Manager
Yale-New Haven Children's Hospital
New Haven, Connecticut

Foreword

I am pleased to write the Foreword of the new *Clinical Nurse Leader Certification Review*. The authors have done excellent work, reinforcing major skills and responsibilities of this advanced generalist role. This will be a most useful textbook for students as they prepare for certification. The textbook is peppered with innumerable vignettes to reinforce concepts. Foundational work on test-taking skills is presented. The authors address concepts of horizontal leadership, interdisciplinary communication and collaboration skills, and health care advocacy. Care management, including lateral integration of care services, team coordination, illness/disease management, health promotion and disease prevention management, and advanced clinical assessment is also featured. Health care systems, including topics on finance, economics, policy, health care informatics, ethics, and evidence-based practice are called out and integrated into the clinical nurse leader's role and presented from a test-taking perspective. I believe that the authors can be assured that students preparing to take the certification exam can gain a broader view of the role as a result of their efforts.

Linda Roussel, DSN, RN, NEA-BC, CNL
Co-author of Initiating and
Sustaining the Clinical
Nurse Leader Role:
A Practical Guide

Preface

Clinical Nurse Leader Certification Review is written by experts in this new clinical nurse leader (CNL) role. The book is written for nurses who have completed a qualified CNL program and who are ready to take the certification examination. Because of the changes and additions to the "new" topics in the certification examination, this book may be especially helpful for faculty preparing the CNL curriculum and CNL review courses.

Chapters 1 and 2 provide information on the actual certification examination and how to prepare to take any test. The remaining chapters cover the key topics outlined in the new Examination Outline (Appendix A). Chapters 3 through 7 are grouped in the content outline under Nursing Leadership. Chapters 8 through 12 are grouped under Clinical Outcomes. The last chapters, 13 through 19, fall under Care Environment Management.

Of those chapters more specifically related to nursing leadership, Chapter 3 focuses on topics related to horizontal leadership, while Chapter 4 describes interdisciplinary collaboration and communication skills. Chapter 5 identifies key concepts related to health care advocacy and how CNLs serve as advocates. Chapter 6 outlines the specifics of how CNLs must integrate their new role in their health care setting. Chapter 7 is the last chapter related to nursing leadership in this section and describes the CNL's role in lateral integration of care services.

In the section devoted to clinical outcomes, Chapter 8 discusses management of illnesses and diseases, while Chapter 9 focuses more on knowledge management as a role for CNLs. Other areas of importance for CNLs are health promotion and disease prevention. These are outlined in Chapter 10. No matter which of eight key roles CNLs are utilizing, Chapter 11 describes the importance of using the latest evidence in practice by learning about and implementing evidence-based practice (EBP). The key components of advanced clinical assessment that CNLs need to be able to implement in practice are included in Chapter 12.

Care environment management is the last major section of the exam outline for CNLs. This section opens with Chapter 13, which focuses on team coordination. CNLs are supposed to have a key role in facilitating and acting as members of a variety of interdisciplinary teams. CNLs have a significant role in outcomes, including decreasing costs. Thus, Chapter 14 describes health finance and economics, while Chapter 15 identifies health systems versus the specific microsystems in which CNLs work. In addition to being involved in outcomes, it is expected that CNLs be involved in health care policy (Chapter 16). The CNL role was developed specifically to help with quality and safety issues related to patient care. Thus, Chapter 17 focuses on quality management, which is as important as health care informatics (Chapter 18). Finally, Chapter 19 discusses ethics and ethical principles.

Clinical Nurse Leader Certification Review also includes four appendices. The first appendix contains the overall exam content, while the second appendix contains reflection questions to help nurses prepare for this examination. The third appendix includes multiple-choice questions and unfolding case studies. The final appendix contains the correct answer for these questions and the rationale for why the answer is correct.

Acknowlegments

Cyndy King would like to thank her parents, Dr. and Mrs. John A. King, for encouraging a career in nursing and for their love and support. She would also like to thank all her mentors, colleagues, students, and patients/families who have added to her love of nursing and lifelong learning. Lastly, Cyndy thanks her late husband, Michael A. Knaus, who believed in this book and who always provided love and support.

Sally Gerard would like to acknowledge the generosity of her colleagues who have mentored her in the wonderful journey of interprofessional improvement work. She would especially like to thank her CNL graduates, who are wonderful ambassadors of what this education was envisioned to create: creative, intelligent, collaborative leaders. In addition, the support of husband Bill and children Jack, Christian, and Holly is the key to all good things.

Cynthia R. King
Sally O'Toole Gerard

1

Information for Taking the Certification Exam

Cynthia R. King

Who Provides the Certification Exam?

The clinical nurse leader (CNL) certification program is managed by the Commission on Nurse Certification (CNC), an autonomous arm of the American Association of Colleges of Nursing (AACN). This exam is overseen by the CNC Board of Commissioners. CNC recognizes individuals who have demonstrated professional standards and knowledge through CNL certification. CNC promotes lifelong learning through CNL recertification requirements. The CNC Board of Commissioners and staff are the only ones who decide the policies and administration of the CNL certification program (www.aacn.nche.edu/cnl/cnc).

Information for Taking the Certification Exam

The CNL certification review prepares master's-prepared nurses to take the national CNL certification exam offered by the CNC, a division of the AACN. For some nurses completing a master's degree in a CNL program, it is required by their employer to complete and pass the CNL certification exam. However, by obtaining CNL certification, nurses gain power, credibility, and trust similar to other certified advanced practice nurses and board-certified physicians. It also demonstrates commitment and credibility. It acknowledges that a CNL has a certain amount of knowledge and skills.

In some organizations, there is an incentive, bonus, or differential pay raise given to become certified in one's area of expertise. Many hospitals that have achieved and maintain Magnet status further support and recognize certification as a part of professional development. It is up to employers as to whether they will reimburse candidates for the fee required to take the CNL certification exam. It is important to inquire before taking the exam whether you will be compensated.

The purpose of this chapter is to explain:
- Who provides certification
- Information about taking the exam
- The new exam format
- The exam content outline
- Total time
- Exam results
- Who is eligible
- The application process
- What to bring to the exam
- Resources

Certification Exam Format

As of April 2012, the CNC exam is one inclusive exam, with multiple-choice questions and unfolding case studies. However, for each section of the unfolding case study, there is only one multiple-choice question with one correct answer. More information in this regard is located in the Certification Guide at www.aacn.nche. edu/cnl/publications-resources.

The multiple-choice format allows examinees to test in one sitting and to receive automatic score results immediately following completion of the exam. In addition, the exam reflects the CNL job analysis that has recently been conducted. The format and content of the exam are robust, along with the unfolding case study items. The content outline is now part of the Certification Guide and is also listed separately as an Exam Content Outline. Both of these are available at www. aacn.nche.edu/cnl/publications-resources under Exam Resources, and a part of this content outline appears at the back of this review book (Appendix A).

The exam is only offered as a computer-based exam. The multiple-choice questions have an option of choosing one of four possible answers. Only one of the four answers is correct (even under the unfolding case studies), so examinees do not have to worry about choosing multiple correct answers out of the four choices. The exam has 150 questions (between regular multiple-choice questions and unfolding case studies).

Of the 150 questions, 130 will count toward the examinee's score. The remaining 20 questions are "trial" or "pretest" questions that are interspersed throughout the examination. Pretesting questions allows the Examination Committee and CNC to collect meaningful statistics about new questions that may appear as scored questions on future examinations.

The examination is based on three major content areas composed of four to twenty-three subcontent areas. These are listed in the Examination Content Outline in the Certification Guide. In addition, the percentage of examination questions devoted to each major content area is indicated. This can help the examinee decide what areas to emphasize when studying. Additionally, each question of the multiple-choice and unfolding case study sections is also categorized by a cognitive level that a candidate would likely use to respond. These categories are:

- Recall—the ability to recall or recognize specific information
- Application—the ability to comprehend, relate, or apply knowledge to new or changing situations
- Analysis—the ability to analyze and synthesize information, determine solutions, and/or evaluate the usefulness of a solution

The questions are developed by item writers and based on the AACN White Paper and a list of resources and bibliography. The purpose of the exam is to assess whether nurses are competent to work as CNLs in any health care setting. There is a CNL self-assessment exam that may be purchased at www.aacn.nche.edu/cnl/ publications-resources. There are also multiple-choice questions and unfolding case studies at the end of this review book that should be used to practice for the certification exam. Completing any practice question is strongly recommended. Additionally, it is helpful to review test-taking skills, as described in Chapter 2.

Detailed Test-Content Outline

This book is organized chapter by chapter according to the AACN/CNC Exam Content Outline (www.aacn.nche.edu/cnl/publications-resources). The Certification Guide (used to be Exam Handbook) with content outline, along with many other resources, may be found at www.aacn.nche.edu/cnl/publications-resources. This is the main resource section for the certification exam.

Total Time for the Test

The format of the certification exam is now scheduled as a 3-hour exam without any breaks. It is anticipated that most individuals will not need a full 3 hours for the exam, but all individuals may take the full 3 hours. You may go back and change your answers at any time. It is recommended that you arrive 20 minutes before the test begins. Any individual who arrives 15 or more minutes late will not be allowed to take the exam.

Exam Results

Candidates who take the CNL certification exam will receive automatic information as to whether they have passed immediately after the exam. Currently, individuals who pass the exam will only receive an e-mail that they have passed. Individuals who were unsuccessful will receive their exam scores and a diagnostic report.

In order to see the results, the successful examinee must click on the link that reads "View Results." In addition, exam results will be sent to the examinee's e-mail address that was provided on the certification application. The results will include scores in different content areas of the exam (the content areas outlined in the Certification Guide, at www.aacn.nche.edu/cnl/publications-resources). The final report of results will also show the examinee's scores in comparison with the highest possible score in each content area. The faculty contact for the institution/school will receive aggregate pass/fail reports within approximately 10 business days, following completion of the testing period (not exam date).

Who Is Eligible to Take the Exam?

An individual who meets the AACN eligibility requirements and passes the CNL certification examination will be awarded the CNL designation. In order to register for the certification exam, each individual must meet the requirements that follow (www.aacn.nche.edu/cnl/certification).

RN Licensure

The individual must hold a current and active RN license in the United States. Any individual will be ineligible if currently being disciplined by a state nursing board.

CNL Education

Graduation from a CNL master's or post-master's program, accredited by a nursing accrediting agency recognized by the U.S. Secretary of Education, which prepares individuals with the competencies delineated in the AACN *White Paper on Education and Role of the Clinical Nurse Leader* (2007) is required. All individuals scheduled to graduate from a CNL education program are encouraged to sit for the CNL certification exam. Students may apply to take the certification exam, but they must be in their last academic term. Students enrolled in a Model C program may sit for the exam before earning RN licensure. Students must then submit documentation of RN licensure to the CNC after successful completion of the CNL certification exam and meet all requirements to be awarded CNL certification.

Process for Enrolling for the Exam

All CNL certification application materials and resources provided by the CNC and AACN are located at www.aacn.nche.edu/cnl/certification. There are a number of steps that the student/candidate and faculty contact must take. The following list of steps includes:

1. Candidates must meet eligibility requirements established by the CNC and that are previously listed in this chapter.
2. The institution or school is required to schedule the testing date(s) within the testing period offered by the CNC. Then the institution must notify the CNC of the scheduled testing date, time, and proctor and contact information. Additionally,

the school or institution must submit (a) the Site Registration Form (www.aacn. nche.edu/cnl/exam-site-registration) and (b) School of Nursing CNL Education Program Verification Form (which needs to be signed by the dean/chief academic officer). This form is submitted only once for each school but must be approved and on file in the CNC office for candidates to be eligible to sit for the exam. A list of schools with forms on file is posted on the website.

3. The CNC will confirm proctor via e-mail and send a proctor manual to the faculty serving as proctor. If an online student or graduate is not near a CNL education program, he or she may take the exam at a testing center affiliated with Schroeder Measurement Technologies, Inc. (SMT). In this case, the proctor will be provided.

4. Another alternative is to take the test at one of several testing centers provided by SMT. These are sites that are available for CNL graduates and online students.

5. The candidate must also submit documents and a fee to CNC to register for the exam, whether they will be taking the examination at a School of Nursing or a site sponsored by SMT. Documents are located at www.aacn.nche.edu/cnl/ certification/app-documents and include:

   a. CNL Certification Examination Application

   b. Application Attestation

   c. Standards of Conduct Attestation

   d. CNL Education Documentation Form (signed by CNL program director)

   e. Request for Special Examination Accommodations and Documentation

   f. Disability-Related Needs Forms (if applicable)

6. Once the application is received, CNC sends electronic notification confirming receipt to the applicant; CNC also notifies candidates of outstanding documents.

7. CNC reviews the application.

8. The candidate confirms testing date, time, and location with the faculty contact/ proctor or testing site.

9. Once the candidates are confirmed, CNC sends a list of scheduled examinees to the faculty contact of the exam site or the site sponsored by SMT.

10. At least 2 days prior to the exam date, CNC sends an electronic notification to the faculty contact or testing site with names of eligible candidates and pass codes for each candidate to access the exam.

11. On the testing date, the examination is administered at the institution/school or testing site as scheduled.

12. Exam results and detailed scoring are electronically available to the candidate immediately after the exam.

13. Once the exam is over, the faculty contact may receive aggregate pass/fail results. This will occur approximately 10 business days following completion of the testing period.

14. After the exam, CNC also mails official notification and a certificate to each successful candidate. It is important to know that an individual is not officially certified until they receive a formal letter and certificate. Certification will be withheld from candidates who have outstanding documentation or payment.

15. The current examination fees are listed in the Certification Guide.

The Day of the Exam: What to Bring and What Not to Bring

On the day of the certification exam, the candidate must bring ONLY a current government-issued photo ID with them to the test site. The candidate will be required to sign in for verification of identity. **Any candidate without proper identification is not permitted to take the certification exam. Proper identification may include a valid driver's license with a color photograph and signature and a valid passport or military-issued identification card with a color photograph and signature.**

It is recommended that all examinees report to the scheduled designated testing site no later than 20 minutes before the scheduled testing time. **You will not be allowed to take the examination if you arrive more than 15 minutes after the scheduled testing time, and your examination fees will be forfeited.**

- EXCEPT your photo ID, no personal materials including purses, briefcases, hats, food/drink, paper, pen, books, or reference materials may be taken into the testing center. Car keys are permitted.
- No electronic devices are allowed in the testing room, including cameras, cell phones, pagers, PDAs, Blackberrys, laptop computers, or calculators.

Conclusion

Taking the certification examination is an important step for graduates of CNL programs. Tests and examinations always provide some anxiety and fear. However, when provided with concrete objective information about the exam and places to find resources, it can make taking the examination much easier and less anxiety provoking. It is hoped that this chapter and the entire review book will be helpful for CNL students now and in the future.

Resources

American Association of Colleges. (2012). *Clinical nurse leader publications and resources*. Retrieved April 15, 2012, from http://www.aacn.nche.edu/cnl/publications-resources

American Association of Colleges. (2012). *CNL certification guide*. Retrieved April 15, 2012, from http://www.aacn.nche.edu/cnl/publications-resources

American Association of Colleges. (2012). *CNL job analysis study*. Retrieved April 15, 2012, from http://www.aacn.nche.edu/cnl/publications-resources/job-analysis-study

American Association of Colleges. (2012). *Certification process overview*. Retrieved April 15, 2012, from http://www.aacn.nche.edu/cnl/certification

American Association of Colleges. (2012). *Commission on nurse certification*. Retrieved April 15, 2012, from http://www.aacn.nche.edu/cnl/cnc

American Association of Colleges. (2012). *Exam content outline*. Retrieved April 15, 2012, from http://www.aacn.nche.edu/cnl/publications-resources

American Association of Colleges. (2012). *Exam resources: Self-assessment exam*. Retrieved April 15, 2012, from http://www.aacn.nche.edu/cnl/publications-resources

American Association of Colleges of Nursing. (2007). *White paper on education and role of the clinical nurse leader*. Retrieved April 15, 2012, from http://www.aacn.nche.edu/publications/white-papers/ClinicalNurseLeader.pdf

Commission on Nurse Certification and Schroeder Measurement Technologies, Inc. (2011). *Exam content outline*. Washington, DC: Author.

2

Test-Taking Skills

Cynthia R. King

Taking any type of test or examination may provoke significant anxiety. This is also true for many individuals taking the clinical nurse leader (CNL) certification exam. There are a number of strategies that can be used to help prepare for a test or examination. These strategies may help an individual decrease his or her anxiety and ultimately increase his or her score. Unfortunately, test-taking strategies are not always taught in nursing school. Consequently, it is important for CNL students to learn these skills by reading or attending workshops.

Preparation Strategies for the CNL Certification Exam

When preparing for the exam, it is important for CNL students to remember they are experienced nurses and have completed all of the required courses for the certification exam. Thus, you are already prepared for the exam in many ways. However, this may not be enough to decrease anxiety and fear about taking the certification examination. What is most important to learn before the exam is how to analyze and dissect the examination questions.

Preparation Before the Examination

Before taking the CNL certification examination, there are specific resources to access and ways to prepare. Many of the resources are found in the Publications and Resources section of the American Association of Colleges of Nurses (AACN) website at www.aacn.nche.edu/cnl/publications-resources. Other ways to prepare include the following:

- Go to review sessions and pay attention to hints that the instructor may give about the test. Take notes and ask questions about items you may be confused about.
- Ask the instructor to specify the areas that will be emphasized on the test.

- Go over any material from practice tests, sample problems, and review materials.
- Increase your self-confidence (use guided imagery/visualization to decrease anxiety). Worry about how much you know and not how much others know.
- Manage your anxiety—different things work for different people—do NOT cram the day or night before, get enough rest, and arrive early for the exam.
- Minimize discomfort—dress comfortably, take a sweater (in case the air conditioning is too cold), sit near the front or wherever there are fewer distractions, sit away from windows if distracting.
- Get to the test site early to relax (do muscle relaxation or visualization); at least 20 to 30 minutes before the test starts.
- Be careful about taking too much sleeping medication the night before or drinking too much coffee before the exam.
- If given a piece of paper, write down quick notes of things you are afraid you might forget.
- Eat before the test. Having food in your stomach will give you energy and help you focus, but avoid heavy foods, which can make you groggy.
- Do not try to pull an "all-nighter." Get at least 6 to 8 hours of sleep before the test (normally 8 hours of sleep a night is recommended, but if you are short on time, get at least 6 hours, so that you will be well-rested enough to focus during the test).
- Put the main ideas/information/formulas onto a sheet that can be quickly reviewed many times; this makes it easier to retain the key concepts that will be on the test.
- Set your alarm and have a backup alarm set as well.
- Go to the bathroom before walking into the exam room. You do not want to waste any time worrying about your bodily needs during the test.

The Day of the Examination

There are also key ways to help decrease your anxiety and fear and be successful on the day of the certification test. Among these are the following:

- Bring a watch to the test, so that you can better pace yourself.
- Keep a positive attitude throughout the whole test and try to stay relaxed. If you start to feel nervous, take a few deep breaths to relax. Repeat throughout the test. This process will help you to stay relaxed and to make more energy available for remembering, thinking, and writing.
- Read directions carefully—do not over analyze questions or instructions.
- Do a quick "mind dump" of information you do not want to forget. Write it down on the paper or in the margin provided for the CNL examination.
- Look for tricky or key words (e.g., the best answer, the first step).

- At the end, go over the questions and answers to make sure you have read the question accurately.
- Do not change answers erratically.
- Look for CLUES in the question.
- Look for CLUES in the answer choices.
- If you have a tough question—answer it and keep it in the back of your mind, and as you go along you may return to it, as something else may trigger a different response.
- If all else fails, eliminate as many choices as you can and then make an educated guess.
- Generally, questions proceed from easy to difficult, so if you think you have a difficult question at the beginning, you are probably reading too much into it.
- If two answers look correct, give the most obvious answer.
- If no answer seems correct, choose the one that is most nearly correct.
- Look for clues within the questions. For example, if the question is in the past tense, but three of four of the multiple-choice answers are in the present tense, the one answer in the past tense is likely to be the correct answer.
- Do not stay on a problem that you are stuck on, especially when time is a factor.
- Pace yourself, so you do not rush.
- Read the entire question and pay attention to the details.
- Always read the whole question carefully. Do not make assumptions about what the question might be.
- Use good strategies for answering objective questions versus essay questions.
  - Look for the central idea of each question. What is the main point?
  - Statements that begin with *always, never, none, except, most,* or *least* are probably NOT the correct answer.
  - Try to supply your own answer before choosing an alternative listed on the test.
  - Mark an answer for every question.
- When problem solving, ask yourself:
  - What am I being asked to find?
  - What do I need to know in order to find the answer?
  - What information has been provided that will help me to find the answer?
  - How can I break the problem down into parts? What steps should I follow to solve the problem?
  - Does the answer make sense? Does it cover the whole problem?
- Keep an eye on the clock.
- If you do not know an answer, skip it. Go on with the rest of the test and come back to it later. Other parts of the test may have some information that will help you out with that question.

- Do not worry if others finish before you. Focus on the test in front of you.
- If you have time left when you are finished, look over your test. Make sure that you have answered all the questions.
- Change an answer only if you misread or misinterpreted the question, because the first answer that you put is usually the correct one. Watch out for careless mistakes.

Strategies for Analyzing Multiple-Choice Questions

It is essential for all students or nurses taking tests to understand the different parts of a question. In the CNL certification examination, all of the questions are essentially multiple choice. There are multiple-choice questions with four possible answers, only one of which is the correct answer. The unfolding case studies provide information on a case study and then generally have five multiple-choice questions that occur after new information is added to the case study. Each of these questions also has only four possible answers, only one of which is the correct answer. Consequently, it is helpful to understand strategies for analyzing multiple-choice questions. These include the following:

1. If the question asks for the **most correct answer,** remember it is not what you believe is the most correct that counts, but what the CNC/test writers believe is the most correct.
2. Read every word that counts. If the "stem" or the "given" section of the question includes several complicated statements, isolate each of them. Then when you have picked an answer, check it against each complicated segment. Your answer has to satisfy every part of the question.
3. In a multiple-choice question, in addition to the stem there are ALWAYS distractors (usually three or five) and a single correct answer. There may also be descriptive items, labels, an introductory sentence to be completed, or case studies.
4. Try reading the stem with each response.
5. Often all of the choices will seem somewhat plausible. In this case, there will probably be at least one clue word in the stem that makes one answer obviously better than the rest. Go back and read the stem looking for the clue word.
6. Discard as many ridiculous choices for answers as you can. Some answers are obviously wrong, so move quickly on to the next choice. Many answers are partly wrong. If they are wrong in ANY way, then they are not the right choice.
7. Many answers are correct statements by themselves, but they have nothing to do with the stem part of the questions.
8. A positive choice is more likely to be true than with a negative one.
9. A correct answer is often (not always) the choice with the longest and most precise information.
10. Answers that include *always*, *never*, *all*, and *none* are often incorrect.

11. Choose answers that include qualifying terms such as *often* and *most*.

12. If you have time to go over the questions and answers, check the one you were concerned about first and then go over the rest of the answers if you have enough time.

13. There is NO guessing penalty, so always take an educated guess.

Conclusion

For some individuals, test taking comes easily. Other individuals learn these skills early on but, for the majority, proper coaching and practice can increase their test-taking abilities. This chapter provides tips to help all individuals taking the CNL certification exam, so they can be successful. The tips for preparing for the examination, what to do the day of the examination, and tips for dissecting multiple-choice questions will hopefully decrease anxiety and fear for all CNL students.

Resources

Kesselman-Turkel, J., & Peterson, F. (2004). *Test-taking strategies*. Madison, WI: University of Wisconsin Press.

Nugent, P., & Vitale, B. (2008). *Test success: Test-taking techniques for beginners*. Philadelphia, PA: F. A. Davis Company.

Rozakis, L. (2003). *Test taking strategies & study skills for the utterly confused*. New York, NY: McGraw-Hill.

3

Horizontal Leadership

Teri Moser Woo

Clinical nurse leader (CNL) education provides the graduate with the ability to assume horizontal leadership within the health care team (American Association of Colleges of Nursing [AACN], 2007). A horizontal organization is one of decentralization of power and/or control, at least within specific departments. The emphasis is placed on horizontal collaboration. Horizontal leadership is where there may be multiple individuals who assume leadership of a team or teams in order to achieve a common goal. In contrast, vertical leadership is when there is always one team leader. Horizontal leadership is a philosophy of organizational leadership whereby the structure promotes equality and an "open-door policy." This allows team members to voice their opinions and to provide feedback freely. This is different from vertical leadership, which is a top-down style of leadership whereby team members are not encouraged to question or provide feedback. In order to provide horizontal leadership, the CNL must understand and apply leadership theories, work within the patient care team to plan and guide care, and promote an environment where nurses feel supported and empowered.

Theories of Leadership and Change

To provide horizontal leadership, the CNL is required to understand and apply theories of nursing, leadership, and change to practice.

- Nursing theories such as Orem's Self-Care or Leininger's Culture Care Diversity and Universality enable the planning of nursing care to be systematic, predictable, and purposeful.
- Leadership theories assist the CNL student to function within a microsystem by understanding leadership styles and grow as a leader.
- Complexity theory is used to understand a rapidly changing, unpredictable health care environment. It has its origins in the chaos model (e.g., changes are rapid, random, and frequent; Cannon & Boswell, 2010).
- Systems theory is used "in the design, delivery, and evaluation of effective health care" (AACN, 2007, p. 24).

- Change theory is critical to guiding clinical practice improvement. Using a theory such as Kotter's 8-Step Change Model provides and explains that there is a predictable process to practice improvement change. Another common change theory was developed by Kurt Lewin. Lewin's model described three stages of change: unfreezing, moving, and refreezing (Cannon & Boswell, 2010).

The Practice of Horizontal Leadership

In order to practice horizontal leadership, the CNL needs a "tool kit" of skills. These critical skills include guiding evidence-based practice, health care outcomes, lateral integration, use of feedback, coaching, and leading teams. The horizontal leadership may be formal or informal.

Evidence-Based Practice

The CNL uses evidence-based practice (EBP) to guide decisions regarding care and leadership decisions and to improve the quality of patient care in the micro-system. In order for EBP to be integrated into care, the CNL may need to educate the staff on the definition of EPB and how it can be applied to practice. The CNL may personally use or assist nursing staff in using evidence-based practice principles to design care for individuals or populations. Likewise, the steps of the EBP process can be used in making clinical decisions and assessing outcomes, such as preventing pressure ulcers or falls in the population (Thomas, 2010).

Health Care Outcomes

As leaders in the health care system, CNLs have a vital role in health care outcomes. For example, the Veterans Administration (Ott et al., 2009) has discovered numerous outcomes where CNLs have a positive effect. The outcomes may be financial (nursing hours per patient day), quality processes (e.g., pressure ulcers, discharge teaching, ventilator-associated pneumonia), patient and staff satisfaction, or changing practice to be based on evidence. As the role of the CNL has spread to other small and large health care organizations, executives are continuing to see positive effects by implementing the role and having CNLs as horizontal leaders.

Lateral Integrator

In describing the evolution of the CNL role, Tornabeni defines lateral integration as "the integration of care provided by multiple interdependent, and independent disciplines across a continuum of patient admission or experience" (2006, p. 6). The CNL lateral integrator role can be compared to that of the air traffic controller who has a balcony view of what is happening with the patient and health care team and system. By providing lateral integration of care for the patient, the CNL breaks down barriers and proactively manages care across the care continuum. This role is further discussed in Chapter 7.

Use of Feedback

Effective communication is an important skill for all CNLs. As Antai-Otong (2010) discusses, communication involves numerous aspects. A few of these include verbal and nonverbal communication, active listening, assertiveness, conveying clear and simple messages, and being specific. Giving and receiving feedback are part of horizontal leadership. Feedback should include some of the following skills: (a) clearly state what you plan to say, (b) emphasize the positive, (c) focus on the behavior or problem rather than the person, (d) use "I" statements rather than "you" statements, (e) avoid giving advice, and (f) avoid generalizations (Antai-Otong, 2010).

Coaching and Mentoring

The CNL has been identified as a crucial link in creating an environment of improved quality of care, safety, and performance. The CNL acts as a coach and mentor to all members of the health care team. Coaching and mentoring are ways the CNL can help new graduate nurses as well as experienced nurses. Mentoring involves a long-term relationship oriented toward nurses who are focused on advancing clinically. Instead, coaching is an ongoing two-way process in which the CNL can share knowledge and experience to help other nurses achieve desired professional goals. It focuses on learning, more complex ways of thinking and problem solving, rather than focusing on tasks (Clark, 2009). The CNL is perfectly positioned to coach new graduate nurses as they transition from education into practice. As the nurse gains skill and confidence, the CNL continues to act as a mentor in the design of care, as well as the professional development of the individual nurse. When coaching, the CNL is evaluating team members and constructively criticizing team members' performance. Other team members can also be coached; for example, in the use of EBP to improve care.

Leading Teams

The CNL is the logical choice to lead teams to improve the quality of care in the microsystem. The process of designing quality improvement requires the CNL to develop and lead a team of like-minded individuals toward a common goal. Likewise, the care of patients in a complex health care system demands an integrated team approach to care in order to have optimal outcomes. With education in leadership, change, and EBP principles, the CNL has or develops the skills to lead teams to reach the desired goal (Clark, 2009; Dye, 2010; Thomas, 2010). Thomas (2010) describes team leader tools for success and team charters. Furthermore, she provides team agendas, meeting-minutes templates, as well as team ground rules for CNLs to use. Dye (2010) actually describes team structure, team effectiveness, team activities and objectives, and rules and norms. These are all helpful for CNLs, especially when they first begin to lead teams.

Promoting a Safe and Ethical Environment

The CNL collaborates with the administration or nurse manager to promote an environment of safety and ethical care. To promote a culture of safety, the CNL learns how to evaluate and assess risks to patient safety and then works within the team to design and implement systems that support safe patient care (AACN, 2007, p. 36). An example of promoting safety is when the CNL is involved in the rate of falls for complex patients and determining methods to decrease the number of patient falls. Falls, especially among older adults, are a large national problem. CNLs need access to in-depth information related to safety both within their organization and regionally and nationally. When developing a plan of care for the individual or the microsystem, ethical principles are used in the design and delivery of the care. This is based on the fact that CNLs are well-informed of the traditional ethical principles of nonmalfeasance, beneficence, autonomy, and distributive justice. Additionally, the CNL must act in an ethical manner in providing safe, humanistic care (AACN, 2007, p. 15). Awareness of the many ethical dilemmas that are present for patients and families as well as for nursing staff is also an important part of the role of horizontal leadership for CNLs.

Horizontal Leadership Content on CNL Exam

According to the *Clinical Nurse Leader Job Analysis Summary and Certification Exam Blue Print* (2011), horizontal leadership questions represent 7% of the exam content. The content related to horizontal leadership covered on the exam is found in Table 3.1.

TABLE 3.1 Horizontal Leadership Content Outline for the CNL Exam

CATEGORY	WEIGHT
A. Horizontal Leadership	**7%**

  1. Applies theories and models (e.g., nursing, leadership, complexity, change) to practice

  2. Applies evidence-based practice to make clinical decisions and assess outcomes

  3. Understands microsystem functions and assumes accountability for health care outcomes

  4. Designs, coordinates, and evaluates plans of care at an advanced level in conjunction with interdisciplinary team

  5. Utilizes peer feedback for evaluation of self and others

  6. Serves as a lateral integrator of the interdisciplinary health team

  7. Leads group processes to meet care objectives

  8. Coaches and mentors health care team serving as a role model

  9. Utilizes an evidence-based approach to meet specific needs of individuals, clinical populations, or communities within the microsystem

  10. Assumes responsibility for creating a culture of safe and ethical care

  11. Provides leadership for changing practice based on quality improvement methods and research findings

Used with permission from the Commission on Nurse Certification.

Conclusion

Leadership is essential in the current health care climate in order to have optimal patient outcomes, yet the traditional model of top-down vertical leadership may not be an effective strategy for the CNL working with interdisciplinary teams. CNL education provides the CNL with the skills not only to assume leadership in patient care, but also to mentor others in sharing horizontal leadership to improve patient outcomes.

Resources

American Association of Colleges of Nursing. (2007). *White paper on education and role of the clinical nurse leader.* Retrieved February 15, 2012, http://www.aacn.nche.edu/publications/white-papers/ClinicalNurseLeader.pdf

Antai-Otong, D. (2010). Effective communication and team coordination. In J. L. Harris & L. Roussel (Eds.), *Initiating and sustaining the clinical nurse leader role: A practical guide.* Sudbury, MA: Jones and Bartlett Publishers.

Cannon, S., & Boswell, C. (2010). The clinical nurse leader as a transformed leader. In J. L. Harris & L. Roussel (Eds.), *Initiating and sustaining the clinical nurse leader role: A practical guide.* Sudbury, MA: Jones & Bartlett Publishers.

Clark, C. C. (2009). *Coaching and mentoring. Creative nursing leadership & management.* Boston, MA: Jones & Bartlett Publishers.

Dye, C. F. (2010). *Leadership in healthcare: Essential values and skills* (2nd ed.). Chicago, IL: Healthcare Administration Press.

Ott, K. M., Haddock, K. S., Fox, S. E., Shinn, J. K., Walters, S. E., Hardin, J. W., ..., Harris, J. L. (2009). The clinical nurse leader: Impact on practice outcomes in the Veterans Health Administration. *Nursing Economics, 27*(6), 363–371.

Sherman, R. O., Edwards, B., Giovengo, K., & Hilton, N. (2009). The role of the Clinical Nurse Leader in promoting a healthy work environment at the unit level. *Critical Care Nursing Quarterly, 32*(4), 264–271.

Thomas, P. (2010). Quality care and risk management. In J. L. Harris & L. Roussel (Eds.), *Initiating and sustaining the clinical nurse leader role: A practical guide.* Sudbury, MA: Jones and Bartlett Publishers.

Tornabeni, J. (2006). Evolution of a revolution. *Journal of Nursing Administration, 36*(1), 3–6.

4

Interdisciplinary Communication and Collaboration Skills

Denise M. Bourassa

Communication is an activity of conveying information and can be visualized in the form of a cycle. There is a sender of information, a receiver of information, and a method of sending information. In order for the communication cycle to be complete, the information must be received as it was intended by the sender to the receiver. Communication can be nonverbal, mainly through the use of body language; oral, as information that is shared face to face; and, finally, it can be written. Good communication skills are the cornerstone of interpersonal relationships, and as a result, are necessary for collaboration and interdisciplinary relationships among health care providers.

Communication and Collaboration as a Cultural Foundation of Health Care

Communication skills are acquired and learned through social interaction as we develop and mature. However, not everyone's experience with communication is the same, and therefore we all come to adulthood with different levels and types of communication skills. As health care providers, we are taught the essentials for communicating with patients, families, staff members, and other disciplines that are involved with the care of our patients. But do we understand the crucial importance of being able to communicate clearly and effectively? Do we know the inherent risk in poor communication? And how will we, as clinical nurse leaders (CNLs), lead the way to better interdisciplinary communication and collaboration skills?

The CNL role has been developed by the American Association of Colleges of Nursing (AACN) in an effort to answer a call to action by ground-breaking reports that have singled out communication and collaboration between health care workers and patients as leading causes of patient harm. *To Err Is Human: Building a Safer Health System* reports that an estimated 98,000 people die in hospitals every year as a result of medical errors. The specific types of errors outlined in this report include diagnostic errors, treatment errors, prevention, and failure of communication (Institute of Medicine [IOM], 1999). These errors often occur in a triangle of miscommunication between patients, providers, and other team members. Adding to the complexity of communication, health care providers are providing care among diverse individuals. As we become a more global society, our obligation as health care providers is to become aware of the diverse cultures for whom we are providing care. There is a complex myriad of social customs, religious practices, language barriers, belief systems, and cultural barriers that are faced every day. These factors can enhance or complicate communication and collaboration depending on the approach. As a CNL working within a microsystem, there is a unique opportunity to bridge that communication gap. Box 4.1 describes such a scenario.

BOX 4.1
Scenario

In a large tertiary hospital that delivers over 4,000 babies yearly, staff are accustomed to several different languages and cultures in their practices related to childbirth. At one point, however, a pattern emerged of patients coming from one particular clinic who had emigrated from a very small area of Burma, speaking a language called Karen. The nurses and other members of the health care team have been finding it difficult to find interpreters who speak anything close to Karen through the hospital language line, leaving a significant communication gap and posing a safety risk. This situation was brought to the CNL, who then researched the culture and spoke to key people at the clinic who were providing prenatal care for these patients. As it turns out, there are a large number of refugees who were brought to the area by a religious organization protecting them from war in their country. Based on these facts, in-services were offered to educate staff about this culture, why they are here, how many people have recently immigrated, and approximately how many were receiving prenatal care. This information went a long way to help bridge the gap that seemed impossibly large. The hospital language line became aware of this need, provided translations closer to the Karen language, and health care providers felt that their care and communication to these patients were enhanced.

Decentralization, fragmentation of the health care system, changing and nonintegrated technology systems, the increase in patient acuity, and the explosion of medical research have created a work environment that is difficult to keep up with. In 2001, the publication of *Crossing the Quality Chasm: A New Health System for the 21st Century* addressed these issues and more. The report stated that medical science and technology have advanced at an unprecedented rate and health care is increasingly more complex, while public health care needs are changing. People are living longer and, as a result, health care providers are seeing a higher prevalence of chronic conditions. The quality chasm is also due to a health care delivery system that is poorly organized, often overly complex, and uncoordinated, and does not lend itself to easy communication between health care providers. In this report, "10 rules for redesign" are suggested in order to redesign a fragmented system and provide better quality and safety for our patients. Of particular importance is rule number 10—"Cooperation among clinicians is a priority. Clinicians and institutions should actively collaborate and communicate to ensure an appropriate exchange of information and coordination of care" (IOM, 2001).

Communication Essentials

As outlined in the AACN *White Paper on the Education and Role of the Clinical Nurse Leader*, communication is complex, interactive, and ongoing, and forms the basis for building interpersonal relationships. These interpersonal relationships will include patients, health care providers, and other key stakeholders. Essential in good communication is critical listening, critical reading, and quantitative literacy, as well as oral, nonverbal, and written communication skills (American Association of College of Nursing [AACN], 2007). The White Paper challenges CNLs "to establish and maintain effective working relationships within an interdisciplinary team, communicate confidently and effectively with health care workers both collegial and subordinate, produce clear, accurate and relevant writing and communicate with diverse groups and disciplines using a variety of strategies" (AACN, 2007).

Critical Listening

The essentials of critical listening concepts originated 2000 years ago in Aristotle's treatise, *The Rhetoric* (www.rhetoric.eserver.org/aristotle/oneindex.html). Three major components of critical listening are ethos, or speaker credibility; logos, or logical arguments; and pathos, or psychological appeal.

1. Ethos refers to the credibility of the speaker. Two critical factors of speaker credibility are expertness and trustworthiness. As a CNL, you will need to listen critically while weighing decisions for practice and the implications they may have on staff and patients. On the other hand, your credibility as a CNL is rooted in your expert knowledge of your microsystem and the level of trustworthiness that you have earned with the people you interact with on a daily basis.

2. Logos—does the speaker make errors in logic? By accident, carelessness, inattention to detail, or lack of analysis? Well-supported arguments from speakers are expected—arguments that contain both true propositions and valid inferences or conclusions. Ask the following: Are the statements true? Are the data supplied the best and most recent? Are the data known and respected by the listener? Are the data accurately presented? Is there evidence of logical thinking by the speaker? And, as a speaker, are you logical; do you support your arguments with well-founded, recent, evidence-based knowledge?

3. Pathos—this is the psychological or emotional element of communication that is often overlooked or misunderstood. Pathos is when the speaker appeals to one or several needs or values of the audience to which he or she is targeting. The critical listener asks himself or herself: Is the speaker attempting to manipulate rather than persuade? What is the speaker's intent? Does the speaker combine logos with pathos?

Effective critical listening depends on the listener keeping all three elements of the message in the analysis and in perspective (Kline, 1996).

Critical Reading

Critical reading is the ability to discover information and ideas within text; this is the act of figuring out what is being said in text. It refers to careful, active, reflective, analytical reading. The critical reader understands that the writer has a job to do, address a topic, define terms clearly, present evidence, acknowledge common knowledge, and explain exceptions. Causes must be shown to precede effects and to be capable of the effect. Conclusions must be shown to follow logically from earlier arguments and evidence. Once the reader has determined that the former has been accomplished, he or she can decide to accept or reject the conclusions drawn from the writer. A successful CNL will need to be not only a critical listener, but also a critical reader (Kurland, 2000).

Quantitative Literacy

Quantitative literacy refers to the knowledge of and confidence with basic mathematical/analytical concepts and operations required for problem solving. It may also involve the skills needed to understand charts and performance metrics that reflect microsystem quality. As it becomes more prevalent that health care is driven by data, that is, patient satisfaction scores, infection rates, length of stay and readmission rates, the ability to interpret quantitative and qualitative data into meaningful, easy-to-communicate information is a skill that becomes necessary. In addition to a data-driven environment, evidence-based practice is the expectation, and without solid understanding of quantitative research and its interpretation, the CNL would not be able to lead the microsystem in a way that promotes safe quality care. It is essential that the CNL completely understands that the foundation of good communication is rooted in understanding what role critical listening, critical reading, and quantitative literacy play in acquiring communication skills.

Collaborative Partners

The White Paper identifies *Ten Assumptions for Educating the Clinical Nurse Leader,* and it is no mistake that of those 10 assumptions, 3 of them directly relate to interdisciplinary communication of information related to patient care.

Assumption 4 states that the CNL has the most comprehensive knowledge of the client and will be responsible for coordinating the variety of disciplines that will be participating in the plan of care. It goes on to caution that ". . . lack of communication results in a discontinuous and frequently unsafe, uncoordinated, inappropriate care. Learning to advocate for clients by communicating effectively with other interdisciplinary team members, including nurses in other setting" (AACN, 2007). Accordingly, Assumption 5 states that information will maximize self-care and client decision making, and Assumption 9 states that communication technology will facilitate the continuity and comprehensiveness of care.

The CNL is expected to possess essential qualities that are the foundation of effective communication and interdisciplinary collaboration. These essential qualities are known as therapeutic use of self, genuineness, warmth, empathy, acceptance, maturity, and self-awareness. These essential qualities enable the CNL to quickly establish trust and foster cooperative behavior with patients, staff members, and other health care team members. In addition to the essential qualities, a strong professional value system is necessary to garner cooperation and effective communication with interdisciplinary teams and patients. These values include altruism, accountability and responsibility, human dignity, integrity, and ethical principles. Strong professional values will distinguish the CNL as a trusted leader and facilitator of communication and collaboration that is for the sole benefit of patient care (Harris & Roussel, 2010). Thus, the CNL is at the center of many different communication systems (see Figure 4.1). The CNL communicates with patients, families, staff members at all levels, and providers of medical care.

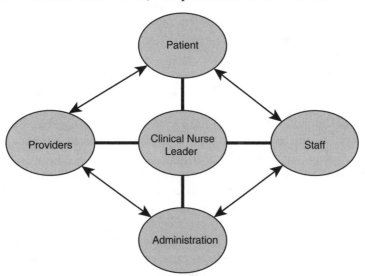

FIGURE 4.1 The CNL as a "center" of communication.

Bedside nurses and CNLs are at the frontline caring for patients, assessing interventions, and listening to patient concerns, and are therefore required to act accordingly. The CNL has the distinct advantage of basing clinical decisions on a perspective that encompasses family/patient preferences while adhering to clinical specific protocols and institutional constraints. If there is a family concern because a patient is unable to communicate, it is up to the RN (who is an advocate for that patient) to develop a therapeutic alliance to bridge the gap between patient and provider. A CNL may be instrumental in this process. This may be done in various ways, such as coaching by the CNL and supporting the nurse and the entire health care team to provide a plan of care for the patient that is respectful and safe. In November 2011, the U.S. Department of Health and Human Services' Agency for Healthcare Research and Quality (AHRQ) began a new initiative "Questions Are the Answer." This initiative encourages health care providers and patients to engage in effective two-way communication to ensure safer care and better health outcomes (AHRQ, 2011). In a series of patient testimonies videographed for this initiative, it was revealed that good communication between patient and provider resulted in more accurate diagnosis, a reduction in medications, and increased education to patients regarding when to seek medical help. As an end result, this led to better quality care for the patient and potential cost savings. It is very possible that The Joint Commission will be evaluating institutions to determine what work is being done to improve patient/provider communications (Case Management Advisor, 2012). As an advocate for the patient, bedside nurse, and lateral integrator, the CNL will be beneficial in facilitating communication and collaboration between patient and provider that will address this issue. If patient teaching is proving to be ineffective, it is important to investigate why. Is there a language or cultural barrier that has been overlooked by staff? Is staff communicating with patients in a way that will retain their attention? Are there more innovative ways to educate patients by computer? Has staff become stagnant and not grown with the technological changes that are facing us every day and our patients we serve? These questions can be asked by the CNL, and the discovery of the answers can be a joint effort between staff working with patients and CNLs.

Collaboration Among the Team of Care Providers

The consistent use of interdisciplinary communication and collaboration has been identified as not only important but also crucial to the safety of patient care. Although the word *interdisciplinary* conveys many assumptions, for the purposes of this chapter, it refers to registered nurses, physicians, midlevel providers, and all others associated with the medical care of a patient. Without free-flowing, timely, and accurate communication of test/lab results and changes in patient status between disciplines, care is compromised. When disciplines disagree with the plan of care and do not discuss it, care is compromised. When there is a lack of respect and trust between disciplines, care can be compromised. The goal is interdisciplinary communication and collaboration. However, in order to achieve that goal, the CNL must be able to communicate in a way that is understood and respected by the intended audience, most of them health care providers working within the multidisciplinary network of people engaged in the patient's care.

Documented studies show the extent to which poor communication and lack of respect between physicians and nurses lead to harmful outcomes for patients, while good working relationships between physicians and nurses have been cited as a factor in improving the retention of nurses in hospitals. A study conducted in 2005, regarding the behavior outcomes of nurses and physicians, sought to assess perceptions of the impact of disruptive behavior on nurse–physician relationships (Rosenstein & O'Daniel, 2005). The study specifically addressed the relationship between stress, concentration, frustration, team collaboration, information transfer, communication, and clinical outcomes, such as adverse events, errors, patient safety, quality of care mortality, and patient satisfaction. In the category of reduced communication, 94% of the nurses responded that disruptive behavior affected communication and 89% reported that information transfer was reduced (Rosenstein & O'Daniel, 2005). As delivery of care has become more complex, the need to coordinate care among multiple providers is necessary, putting the bedside nurse at the center of communication and the common denominator (IOM, 2011).

In the 2004 the IOM publication, *Keeping Patients Safe: Transforming the Work Environment of Nurses,* several recommendations are made to promote patient safety, in particular, fostering interdisciplinary collaboration. Bedside nurses interact with multiple levels of patient caregivers. In addition to the multiple levels, there are multiple changes from day to day and even shift to shift. It is not inconceivable that one nurse will interact with four different groups of health care providers for each patient she is assigned. As part of a study conducted by the IOM committee, a review of published research on team functioning and collaboration supports the effectiveness of teams and interdisciplinary collaboration in improving patient outcomes (IOM, 2004).

As the AACN has developed the CNL role with visions of better communication between health care workers, it is important to keep in mind the hallmarks of effective interdisciplinary collaboration: clinical competence, mutual trust, and respect. Clinical competence is crucial in gaining mutual trust and respect, implying that nurses and other disciplines are more likely to collaborate with each other when it is perceived that clinical knowledge is strong. Collaborative behaviors include shared goal and roles, effective communication, shared decision making, and conflict management strategies (IOM, 2004). Education goals of the CNL are aimed at addressing these issues to increase collaboration and communication between disciplines.

As a CNL who understands the importance of collaborative and interdisciplinary communication as it relates to patient safety, it is imperative that the CNL model communication that is clear, concise, and effective. This may be in the form of instituting bedside reporting, multidisciplinary rounding, intentional hourly rounding, or the situation background assessment recommendation (SBAR) form of communicating with health care workers. SBAR is a prime example of bridging the way medical professionals communicate with each other. When there is a patient concern, communication that is clear, concise, and to the point when making a recommendation for action is valued and respected. Box 4.2 displays SBAR for CNLs.

As you can see in Box 4.2, this type of communication is direct, provides specifics about the current situation, and a bit of background information that may be essential. There was no hesitation on the nurse's part that she wanted further evaluation. Instead of hinting around the matter and suggesting an evaluation from

---

BOX 4.2
SBAR Reporting of Patient Data to a Physician

After assessing a 3-day-old neonate, you discover that the heart rate is irregular, from 60 to 90 beats per minute. The conversation to the attending pediatrician should sound like this:

- **Situation:** Hi, this is Mary. I am taking care of the baby Jones in room 620. She is a 3-day-old newborn and I am concerned about her assessment findings.

- **Background:** Mom is a 3-day post-c-section for a nonreassuring fetal heart rate during labor. APGAR scores were 8 to 8 at birth. The infant has not breastfed well, has lost over 10% of birth weight; mom is working with lactation, and just accomplished a good feeding using supplementation.

- **Assessment:** Infant's temperature is 97.7°C, respirations 33, and heart rate is irregular, difficult to determine, and bradycardic between 60s and 90s; O_2 saturation is 94% to 97%. Infant is sleepy, tone is good, and skin slightly pale.

- **Recommendation:** I would like you to call the NICU and have someone come to further evaluate the infant.

NICU (neonatal intensive care unit), she recommended it as the natural course of action. As a result, the infant was seen promptly by a neonatal cardiologist.

This is just one example of some of the most current trends in health care communication that are being trialed by inpatient settings. However, change is not easy, so it is not surprising that there has been significant resistance from bedside nurses and others who do not understand (1) the need for better communication and (2) the significant research behind the success of these methods in creating a safer environment to deliver health care. This is where the CNL can blend his or her expert knowledge of the microsystem with the larger body of evidence that is guiding current practice. Although the concepts may change over time as health care continues to evolve, the CNL is the change agent that not only sees the need for change, but also seeks out literature to support best practice, relate it to staff at the bedside, and eventually track the progress of changes and make any necessary adjustments.

The CNL has been described as the lateral integrator of care; this role facilitates, coordinates, and oversees care provided by the heath care team. The goal of these actions is to meet care objectives by promoting a sense of shared responsibility for the patient between health care providers. Thus far the discussion has been focused on patient/provider/bedside RN/CNL. Within that lateral integration of care, there is the relationship between the CNL, staff nurse, and nursing administration. There will be times when the CNL will need to address issues to administration on behalf of staff to indicate why a new protocol is problematic. On the other hand, staff may need to hear communication from the CNL that certain protocols are not up for debate; that it has been required by a governing body such as The Joint Commission. However, what the CNL can and should do is look for reasons why the staff does not think it will work, investigate the barriers that staff point out, and either advocate for staff or coach them on developing ways to make the new protocol fit into the present microsystem. The end result will be adherence to protocol and increased patient safety due to the implementation of best practice.

TABLE 4.1 Interdisciplinary Communication and Collaboration Skills

CATEGORY	WEIGHT
B. Interdisciplinary Communication and Collaboration Skills	**7%**
1. Establishes and maintains working relationships within an interdisciplinary tea	
2. Bases clinical decisions on multiple perspectives including the client and/or family preferences	
3. Negotiates in group interactions, particularly in task-oriented, convergent, and divergent group situations	
4. Develops a therapeutic alliance with the client as an advanced generalist	
5. Communicates with diverse groups and disciplines using a variety of strategies	
6. Facilitates group processes to meet care objectives	
7. Integrates concepts from behavioral, biological, and natural sciences in order to understand self and others	
8. Interprets quantitative and qualitative data for the interdisciplinary team	
9. Uses a scientific process as a basis for developing, implementing, and evaluating nursing interventions	
10. Synthesizes information and knowledge as a key component of critical thinking and decision making	
11. Bridges cultural and linguistic barriers	
12. Understands clients' values and beliefs	
13. Completes documentation as it relates to client care	
14. Understands the roles of interdisciplinary team members	
15. Participates in conflict resolution within the health care team	
16. Promotes a culture of accountability	

Used with permission from the Commission on Nurse Certification.

BOX 4.3
Web Resources for Interdisciplinary Collaboration

Quality and Safety Education for Nurses—www.qsen.edu
National League for Nursing—www.nln.org
Institute of Medicine—www.iom.edu
Institute for Healthcare Improvement—www.ihi.org

Conclusion

The effective CNL is respected, relied on as an advanced clinician, and serves as a mentor for strong interdisciplinary communication and collaboration skills. The CNL will translate advanced knowledge in communication principles and technologies to staff, patients, and interdisciplinary providers. The CNL certification exam explores many areas of interdisciplinary communication and collaboration (Table 4.1). There are also many resources available from reputable online sources (Box 4.3). The CNL will model and facilitate collaboration, which will serve as a reminder that only with cooperation, collaboration, and clear communication will the patient's best interest be served.

Resources

Agency for Healthcare Research and Quality. (2011). *AHRQ initiative encourages better two-way communication between clinicians and patients.* Retrieved on February 10, 2012, from http://ahrq.gov/research/nov11/1111RA19.htm

American Association of Colleges of Nursing. (2007). *White paper on the education and role of the clinical nurse leader.* Retrieved February 10, 2012, from http://aacn.nche. edu/publications/WhitePapers/ClinicalNurseLeader.htm

Case Management Advisor. (2012). Communication critical with patient, provider. *23*(2), 18–20.

Harris, J. L., & Roussel, L. (2010). *Initiating and sustaining the clinical nurse leader role: A practical guide.* Sudbury, MA: Jones and Bartlett Publishers.

Institute of Medicine. (1999). *To Err is human: Building a safer health system.* Retrieved January 30, 2012, from http://www.nap.edu/books/0309068371/html/

Institute of Medicine. (2001). *Crossing the quality chasm: A new health system for the 21st century.* Retrieved February 6, 2012, from http://www.nap.edu/books/0309068371/html

Institute of Medicine. (2004). *Keeping patients safe: transforming the work environment of nurses.* Retrieved September 25, 2011, from http://www.nap.edu/catalog/10851.html

Institute of Medicine. (2011). *The future of nursing: Leading change, advancing health.* Retrieved on February 1, 2012, from http://www.iom.edu/reports/2010/the-future-of-nursing-leading-change-advancing-health.aspx

Kline, J. A. (1996). *Listening effectively-types of listening.* Air University Press, Maxwell Air Force Base, Alabama. Retrieved February 25, 2012, from http://www.au.af.mil/au/awc/awcgate/kline-listen/b10ch4.htm

Kurland, D. (2000). *How the language really works: The fundamentals of critical reading and effective writing.* Retrieved on February 29, 2012, from http://criticalreading. com/critical_reading_thinking.htm

Rosenstein, A. H., & O'Daniel, M. (2005). Disruptive behaviors & clinical outcomes: perceptions of nurses and physicians. *American Journal of Nursing, 105*(1), 54–64.

5

Advocacy and the Clinical Nurse Leader

Jonathan P. Auld

Advocacy is the act of expressing or defending the rights or causes of another. Professional nursing standards and the Code of Ethics for Nurses represent advocacy as an important characteristic of professional nursing. Advocacy plays a central role in professional nursing values as well as a core competency for the clinical nurse leader (CNL). The modern health care environment—with rapid advances in technology, increasing complexity, and a more critically ill and aging population—is an important reason advocacy is a prominent competency in the CNL role. Central principles of advocacy include the protection of patients' autonomy, acting on behalf of patients, advancement and protection of the profession, and social justice.

Protection of Patient Autonomy

A core nursing value is that patients or clients are autonomous beings who have the right to make their own decisions. The role of the CNL is to protect patients' rights to self-determination by working with the interdisciplinary team and the analysis of organizational structures and processes to ensure patient autonomy is maintained. The following are examples in which the CNL can protect patient autonomy:

- Ensure patients and families have information and understanding to facilitate informed decision making about their plan of care
- Analyze systems in organization to ensure informed consent is accessible and consistent
- Participate in the analysis of benefits and burdens of the treatment plan with consideration of the patient's cultural background
- Facilitate nurses' and the interdisciplinary team's communication of the treatment options to the patients and families, including the right to accept, refuse, or terminate treatment
- Ensure patients have the opportunity to make decisions with their desired support network of family, caregivers, and health professionals

Acting on Behalf of Patients

When patients are unable to make their own decisions, a foundational role of the nurse is to act on behalf of the patient. The CNL has the responsibility to work with the direct care nurses and the interdisciplinary team to uphold the patient's wishes to the extent that they are known. The following are ways in which the CNL can influence this aspect of advocacy:

- Assessing and analyzing organizational structures and processes that ensure advance directives are accessible to health care providers
- Facilitating communication with patient surrogates
- Providing guidance and support for patient surrogates in order for them to make informed decisions
- Policy or guideline evaluation and development to guide decision making when acting on behalf of patients
- Ensuring quality care through the development of evidence-based guidelines for care
- Coordination of care through referrals to other resources or services

Community Advocacy and Social Justice

Social justice is a guiding principle for the nursing profession. Through the analysis of the social, economic, and cultural environment in which health care is consumed and delivered, the CNL addresses the antecedents to poor health outcomes in communities and populations. The following are some examples of how CNLs incorporate social justice into the practice:

- Engaging policy makers and elected officials to influence health policy at institutional and governmental levels
- Engaging institutional leaders around health disparities and improving outcomes for populations and communities by
  - Talking with local, state, and federal lawmakers
  - Writing opinion articles for local or national newspapers
  - Lobbying elected officials to support programs that improve health outcomes for populations
- Building partnerships with community organizations to identify and address health disparities
- Applying knowledge of historical, social, and cultural contexts to address needs of patient or community populations
- Analyzing and developing evidence-based programs to ensure improved health outcomes for populations or communities

Advocacy for the Professional

The CNL is a leader in the nursing profession. An important aspect of this leadership is protecting and advancing nursing as a profession. Advocacy for the nursing profession can take a number of forms.

- Assessing and developing nurse competency and the development of the nursing professional role
- Establishing role clarity for nurses and the CNL in the interdisciplinary team and in an organization
- Developing and adhering to standards of practice for self and others to enhance quality outcomes
- Participating with professional organizations
- Participating in nursing education
- Influencing organizational and government policy that protects the rights of nurses in the workplace
- Engaging organizational and government leaders in establishing legislation that supports nurses practicing to the full extent of their licensure

Exam Content Outline and Advocacy

Advocacy is an important part of the CNL role. Additionally, it is a key topic on the CNL certification exam. The CNL certification exam has changed slightly on the basis of recent job analysis. Thus, Table 5.1 displays the new detailed content

TABLE 5.1 Health Care Advocacy

CATEGORY	WEIGHT
C. Health Care Advocacy	**5%**
1. Interfaces between the client and the health care delivery system to protect the client's rights	
2. Ensures that clients, families, and communities are well informed and engaged in their plan of care	
3. Ensures that systems meet the needs of the populations served and is culturally relevant	
4. Articulates health care issues and concerns to officials and consumers	
5. Assists consumers in informed decision making by interpreting health care research	
6. Serves as a client advocate on health issues	
7. Utilizes chain of command to influence care	
8. Promotes fairness and nondiscrimination in the delivery of care	
9. Advocates for improvement in the health care system and the nursing profession	

Used with permission from the Commission on Nurse Certification.

outline for the advocacy portion of the certification exam. This section of the exam is worth 5% of the total points.

Conclusion

As can be seen in the Examination Content Outline, advocacy is a clear part of the CNL role. CNLs are leaders, and through this role, they are responsible for advocacy in a variety of ways. For example, CNLs are involved in advocacy in the following ways: (a) health goals for patients/families, (b) determining plan of care with patients/families rather than for them, (c) by conducting evidence-based practice (EBP) and research, (d) promoting fairness, (e) using the chain of command, when needed, to advocate for clients, and (f) improving care for all patients and families. Advocacy has always been a part of the role of professional nurses, but it is also a critical role for CNLs as advanced generalists, role models, and leaders.

Resources

American Association of Colleges of Nursing. (2007). *White paper on the education and role of the clinical nurse leader.* Retrieved from http://www.aacn.nche.edu/publications/white-papers/ClinicalNurseLeader.pdf

American Nurses Association. (2001). *Code of ethics for nurses with interpretive statement.* Silver Springs, MD: Author.

Bu, X., & Jezewski, M. A. (2006). Developing a mid-range theory of patient advocacy through concept analysis. *Journal of Advanced Nursing, 57*(1), 101–110.

Commission on Nurse Certification. (2012). *Clinical nurse leader job analysis summary and certification exam blue print.* Retrieved from http://www.aacn.nche.edu/cnl/cnl-certification/pdf/ExamHndbk.pdf

Koiser, B. J., Erb, G., Berman, A. J., & Snyder, S. (2004). Values, ethics, and advocacy. In *Fundamentals of nursing: Concepts, process, and practice* (7th ed.). New Jersey: Pearson/Prentice Hall.

Paquin, S. O. (2011). Social justice advocacy in nursing: What is it? How do we get there? *Creative Nursing, 17*(2), 63–67.

Smith, A. P. (2004). Patient advocacy: Roles for nurses and leaders. *Nursing Economics, 22*(2), 89–90.

6

Integration of the Clinical Nurse Leader Role

Cynthia R. King

It is difficult for any nurse to integrate a new role into practice (e.g., nurse manager, nurse practitioner, clinical nurse leader [CNL]). The CNL role is the first new role in nursing in 35 to 40 years. Thus, transitioning into this role may be especially difficult for nurses. There are numerous nursing schools that now have CNL programs. The curriculum covers many of the key aspects that are the basis of the CNL role. However, not all programs help students learn to integrate their new role into practice. The CNL role, specifically, is aimed at managing a distinct population group through day-by-day management of clinical issues and decisions and focusing on patient outcomes. Moreover, the primary focus is on evaluating and supporting evidence-based decisions to ensure best possible clinical outcomes (Thompson & Lulham, 2007). Educated at the master's degree level, the nurse leader possesses a higher level of clinical knowledge and leadership that creates positive patient outcomes (Hartranft, Garcia, & Adams, 2007). Because the CNL role is new and is different from other nursing roles, it is not always easy to implement the role in health care settings. There are expectations from nursing administration and many other disciplines, as well as each CNL's individual expectations. It is preferable that all of these expectations align; however, they may be in competition, which can create tension and anxiety. Additionally, not all employers know how to help new CNLs integrate their role in their specific setting.

Essential Aspects of CNL's Role

The most critical period in your CNL career will be the transition from staff nurse to CNL. Your initial efforts as a CNL will set precedents and establish your basic style, and you may even have to change some of your attitudes. Before integrating the CNL role into a particular setting, it is crucial that the CNL understand his or her broad areas of responsibility. These are outlined by the American Association of College of Nurses and the broad areas are summarized as follows:

- *Clinician*: The CNL is designer/coordinator/integrator/evaluator of care to individuals, families, groups, communities, and populations. He or she is able to understand the rationale for care and competently deliver this care to complex and diverse populations. The CNL provides care at the point of care with particular emphasis on health promotion and risk reduction services.

- *Outcomes manager*: The CNL regularly synthesizes data, information, and knowledge to evaluate and achieve optimal client outcomes.

- *Client advocate*: The CNL becomes competent at ensuring that clients, families, and communities are well informed and included in care planning. The CNL also serves as an informed leader for improving care and as an advocate for the profession and the interdisciplinary health care team.

- *Educator*: The CNL uses appropriate teaching principles and strategies as well as current information, materials, and technologies to teach clients, health care professionals, and communities.

- *Information manager*: The CNL is proficient in using information systems and technology to improve health care outcomes.

- *Systems analyst/risk anticipator*: The CNL participates in systems review to improve quality of nursing care delivered and at the individual level to critically evaluate and anticipate risks to client safety with the aim of preventing medical error.

- *Team manager*: The CNL properly delegates and manages the nursing team resources and serves as a leader in the interdisciplinary health care team.

- *Member of a profession*: The CNL remains accountable for the ongoing acquisition of knowledge and skills related to his or her profession and to effect change in health care practice and outcomes and in the profession.

- *Lifelong learner*: Recognizes the need for and actively pursues new knowledge and skills as one's role and needs of the health care system evolves.

All CNLs need to be able to integrate these areas of responsibility. They may also have their role as a professional staff nurse focused on self-performance (e.g., self-direction) to a leader helping oversee the work of staff nurses (e.g., selfless service). Moreover, they need to be able to articulate the significant aspects of the CNL role to other nurses and other disciplines.

Articulating the Significance of the CNL Role

Once a CNL moves into his or her role or position, it is crucial to be able to state the essential aspects of that role. One method to learn how to articulate the key aspects of the CNL role is to practice a "2- to 5-minute elevator speech" during their residency. This simply means the CNL learns how to explain his or her role succinctly in 2 to 5 minutes. However, whatever the method, transitioning into a new role involves articulating newly acquired knowledge, skills, and abilities that differ from the ones used in the past role(s).

In order to articulate the significance of this new CNL role, individuals need to define the role for themselves, form expectations about the new role, describe to others, and encourage them to help make this role a success. However, there can be barriers to integrating and articulating the new CNL role. For example, there may be role conflict (when the role is different from what the new CNL expected) or isolation (e.g., if the CNL is the only one in the organization), or staff nurses or nurse managers do not perceive or embrace the new CNL role as being important.

In addition to being able to articulate what is involved in the CNL role to other disciplines, the CNL should be able to describe his or her role to patients and families. It is important to explain to patients/families that the CNL does not provide direct care for a particular group of patients, but instead is responsible for being a leader and guiding and influencing staff nurses with complex patient situations. Furthermore, CNLs should show a strong service orientation with a firm commitment to each patient/family.

Assuming Responsibility of One's Own Professional Identity and Practice

When CNLs begin their new role, and throughout their professional years in nursing, it is essential that they take responsibility for identifying their own professional practice and how that differs from other professional nurses. For example, CNLs must accept responsibility to demonstrate competence in their role and continually update their competencies, knowledge, and skills through professional education. Additionally, CNLs need to demonstrate they are competent leaders by (a) developing relationships with patients/families and many disciplines, (b) participating in and leading interdisciplinary teams, (c) being approachable and supportive, (d) appropriately delegating, (e) creating trust within relationships, (f) basing practice on evidence, and (g) effectively resolving conflict.

Networking is a vital strategy for CNLs, especially when beginning to integrate role into practice. Some individuals appear to have an easy time networking (e.g., extroverts), while others might need a mentor. Networking can be learned. However, it is not just simply meeting other individuals in your organization. It involves the cultivation of productive relationships for employment or business. The relationships developed become a supportive system of sharing information and services among individuals and groups having a common interest. For CNLs, networking is crucial both with staff on their unit (or setting) and with other disciplines. Developing a strong network early on will help CNLs with problems or issues they may face later.

Maintaining and Enhancing Professional Competencies and Lifelong Learning

As new CNLs learn to be responsible for professional development, it is important for these individuals to understand what it means to maintain professional competencies. This specifically encompasses a wide range of learning activities through which professionals (e.g., CNLs) maintain and develop through their career to ensure they continue to practice safely, effectively, and legally within their scope of practice. In order to maintain and enhance these initial competencies and lifelong learning, the CNLs will need to participate in a required number of hours of learning activities each year, maintain a personal professional profile of learning activities, and comply with any requests to audit how they have met the requirements.

As new CNLs, it is important to keep your supervisor informed of your career goals, as well as training and education needs. Express interest to your supervisor in succeeding in your new role and develop a plan for your professional development. Also remember to learn from your colleagues (other CNLs) in your health care organization, at conferences, and through nursing organizations.

Understanding the Scope of Practice and Adhering to Licensure Law and Regulations

All professional nurses, including CNLs, are required to understand and abide by their scope of practice and follow all requirements and regulations needed to maintain their license. In order to accomplish this, CNLs should provide a high standard of practice and care at all times and model this for staff nurses. Moreover, CNLs need to:

• Use the best evidence possible to help oversee care provided

• Keep skills and knowledge up to date

• Follow regulations on delegation of care and tasks to other nurses

• Maintain skills related to the eight roles outlined by the American Association of Colleges of Nursing

Advocating for Professional Standards of Practice Using Organizational and Political Processes

As a CNL transitioning into the new position, it is important to advocate for professional standards, policies, and procedures within your organization and politically. This is an even more urgent issue if the new graduate is the first CNL in the organization. He or she must blaze the trail for the other CNLs who will join the institution and the political arena. Some of the types of policies and standards to consider as a priority include (a) long-range goals, (b) immediate needs, (c) daily requirements, (d) organizational mandates, (e) quality issues, (f) safety issues, and (g) cost savings.

Politics is a process of finding solutions to universal concerns of humanity. This includes concern for public health. All nurses, including CNLs, advocate for the health of people and policies aimed at health promotion. Thus, it is imperative that CNLs become involved in making changes in public policy at the local, state, and national levels. Nurses are effective in the political process when they understand the sources of power and are willing to be involved and make a difference. Because the CNL role is the first new role in nursing in 40 years, it will be even more vital that CNLs become involved in the political process, as they will be able to speak most effectively to topics such as quality and safety issues related to patient care.

CNLs, and nurses in general, play a role in the development and implementation of policy. Ways in which nurses are involved in health policy are:

- Providing expertise
- Understanding consumer needs
- Experience with assisting consumers in making health care decisions
- A link to health care professionals and organizations
- Understanding the health care system
- Understanding interdisciplinary care

Articulating to the Public the Values of the Profession as They Relate to Client Welfare

When learning to integrate into their new role, CNLs need to be able to discuss both personal and professional values, which are individual and organizational expectations and ideas that help direct responsibilities, accountability, and proficiency. These values can influence decision making and communication, as well as judgment and daily routines. Professional values can include accountability, responsibility, and ethical principles.

As master's-prepared generalists, CNLs play a vital role in supporting and mentoring staff nurses at the bedside. Unfortunately, in some settings, staff have had little support from nursing.

Understanding and Supporting High-Quality, Cost-Effective, Safe Health Care

The CNL role is the first new role in nursing in 40 years. Improving patient outcomes was one of the main reasons the role was developed. The Institute of Medicine (IOM) found in several studies that the health care system was fragmented and in need of improvement. Development of the CNL was a step in the right direction. Specifically, the CNL role can help improve the quality of care provided to patients in terms of structure, process, and outcomes. Other areas in which the CNL role helps issues raised by the Institute of Medicine (IOM) are cost-effectiveness and safe care. The IOM suggests six goals for improvement in patient care: (1) safe, (2) effective, (3) patient-centered, (4) timely, (5) efficient, and (6) equitable. Keeping these goals in mind, using the best evidence, and collecting data, CNLs can have an impact on quality, safety, and cost-effectiveness of care.

Publishing and Presenting CNL Impact and Outcomes

As evidence-based research or quality improvement (QI) projects come to an end, enthusiasm may tend to wane; however, dissemination is crucial to further nursing knowledge. Dissemination is actually part of the EBP/research/QI process and should not be an afterthought. Several motivations for CNLs to disseminate findings include the following:

- Improve health
- Do better research
- Change policy
- Develop career
- Help someone
- Use resources wisely
- Increase funding

There are a variety of options for dissemination both for CNLs and for staff nurses. A number of these may include the following:

- Journal publication
  - full paper
  - short report/letter
  - news item
  - editorial
- Conference
  - local/national/ international
  - poster
  - oral presentation
- Report to funder
  - publish as a report
- Set up conference or seminar
  - within department
  - area or regional meeting
  - national
- TV/Lay press
  - hospital newsletter
  - newspapers, radio
- Internet
  - podcast
  - CD ROM
- Teaching

Dissemination can be scary if an individual has not been a part of this process previously. That is why CNLs should be educated during their curriculum and encouraged to disseminate the results of their master's program. They may be mentored by their faculty advisor to submit an article for publication and give presentations. Once CNLs have participated in dissemination of a project, they can serve as excellent role models for staff nurses who have completed projects and do not know where or how to disseminate.

Evidence-Based Practice and Nursing Research

Evidence-based practice (EBP) and nursing research are core competencies for the CNL and are connected to providing patient-centered care and to interdisciplinary teams. Increasing use of evidence helps the quality of care, safety of care, and avoidance of underuse, misuse, and overuse of care. CNLs understand the difference between nursing research (when there is a gap in knowledge) and EBP (when there are best outcomes that can be implemented in practice). In school, CNLs usually conduct an EBP or research project. This allows them to be role models for staff nurses when they transition into their CNL role. Equally important to the CNL role is the fact that each CNL learns in school how to search the literature for current evidence and research and apply it to clinical practice and potential patient outcomes.

It is also expected that CNLs will continue to be involved in EBP and nursing research once they have settled into their role. They may conduct nursing projects, serve on EBP/research shared governance councils, or work with other disciplines to conduct studies. The CNLs may also develop educational materials to help staff nurses better understand EBP and nursing research. They may also help staff nurses to plan, develop, and implement projects for clinical ladders.

Conclusion

Currently, the CNL role is being integrated in many different settings. There is potential for this role to be integrated in all areas of practice in all care settings (see Table 6.1). With the implementation of this new role comes the promise of streamlining coordination of care for all patients. For this role to be successful, it must be championed by executive leadership (e.g., the chief nursing officer) and understood by other nurses and disciplines as being a pivotal role at the point of care. The organizations that hire CNLs want to see them succeed just as much as the CNLs want to be successful. Furthermore, it is vital that CNLs implement the following roles: coordinate care for a specific microsystem (group of patients/families), oversee care across the continuum (lateral integration), and provide leadership to, and serve as a role model for, other professional nurses (Ott et al., 2009).

TABLE 6.1 Integration of the CNL Role

CATEGORY	WEIGHT
D. Integration of CNL Role	**8%**

1. Articulates the significance of the CNL role

2. Advocates for the CNL role

3. Assumes responsibility of own professional identity and practice

4. Maintains and enhances professional competencies

5. Assumes responsibility for lifelong learning and accountability for current practice and health care information and skills

6. Advocates for professional standards of practice using organizational and political processes

7. Understands the history, philosophy, and responsibilities of the nursing profession as it relates to the CNL

8. Understands scope of practice and adheres to licensure law and regulations

9. Articulates to the public the values of the profession as they relate to client welfare

10. Negotiates and advocates for the role of the professional nurse as a member of the interdisciplinary health care team

11. Develops personal goals for professional development and continuing education

12. Understands and supports agendas that enhance both high-quality, cost-effective health care and the advancement of the profession

13. Supports and mentors individuals entering into and training for professional nursing practice

14. Publishes and presents CNL impact and outcomes

15. Generates nursing research

Used with permission from the Commission on Nurse Certification.

Resources

American Association of Colleges of Nursing. (2007). *White paper on the education and role of the clinical nurse leader*. Retrieved from http://www.aacn.nche.edu/publications/white-papers/ClinicalNurseLeader.pdf

Burton, R., & Ormrod, G. (2011). *Nursing: Transition to professional practice*. Oxford, UK: Oxford University Press.

Clark, C. C. (2009). *Creative nursing leadership & management*. Boston, MA: Jones & Bartlett Publishers.

Dye, C. F. (2010). *Leadership in healthcare: Essential values and skills* (2nd ed.). Chicago, IL: Healthcare Administration Press.

Finkelman, A., & Kenner, C. (2010). *Professional nursing concepts: Competencies for quality leadership*. Boston, MA: Jones & Bartlett Publishers.

Hartranft, S. R., Garica, T., & Adams, N. (2007). Realizing the anticipated effects of the clinical nurse leader. *Journal of Nursing Administration, 37*(6), 261–263.

Kearney-Nunnery, R. (2008). *Advancing your career: Concepts of professional nursing.* Philadelphia, PA: F. A. Davis Company.

Ott, K. M., Haddock, K. S., Fox, S. E., Shinn, J. K., Walters, S. E., Hardin, J. W., ..., Harris, J. L. (2009). The Clinical Nurse Leader: Impact on practice outcomes in the Veterans Health Administration. *Nursing Economics, 27*(6), 363–383.

Thompson, P., & Lulham, K. (2007). Clinical nurse leader and clinical nurse specialist role delineation in the acute care setting. *Journal of Nursing Administration, 37*(10), 429–431.

7

Lateral Integration

September T. Nelson and Teri Moser Woo

The *White Paper on the Education and Role of the Clinical Nurse Leader* states, "the CNL provides lateral integration of care services within a microsystem of care to effect quality, client care outcomes" (American Association of Colleges of Nursing [AACN], 2007, p. 6). Tornabeni defines lateral integration as "the integration of care provided by multiple interdependent, and independent disciplines across a continuum of patient admission or experience" (2006, p. 6). This means not just in the acute care setting, but even in areas such as home care and hospice. It also means involving potential key stakeholders in addition to health care providers (health care administrators, financial individuals, and ombudsmen). This integration is necessary to remove the walls created by individual silos of fragmented care that impede communication and collaboration, thus contributing to errors and poor outcomes (Begun, Tornabeni, & White, 2006). A fundamental function of the clinical nurse leader (CNL) is to intentionally and proactively manage patient care services across professional boundaries (Begun et al., 2006). Additionally, the role involves communication with all the team members who are a crucial part of providing high quality and safe care (Hartranft, Garda, & Adams, 2007). According to Begun and associates (2006), the role of lateral integration of care is what has been missing in the care of patients with complex needs. There has been no nursing role that oversees care laterally and over time and that can then intervene and coordinate care.

Components of Lateral Integration

Understanding the interdependency of all disciplines in providing care is an essential part of the CNL role and lateral integration. Once the CNL understands the roles and expertise of the members of the interdisciplinary members, he or she can laterally integrate the team to deliver patient-centered care. Stanley (2010) described lateral integration as one of the defining aspects of CNL practice. Effective lateral integration requires multiple ongoing components:

- Communication
- Collaboration
- Coordination
- Evaluation

These components are not effective on their own, but require a coordinated flow between them. The CNL is integral to this process.

Communication

The CNL serves as a liaison between the members of the health care team, fostering the flow of information and serving as a translator (Stanley et al., 2008). As a lateral integrator, effective communication skills are essential. The quality of all relationships stems from effective communication and the rights and respect for others. Communication occurs in situations. It involves the transmission of feelings, attitudes, and ideas between people. This is an essential tool for the CNL, regardless of the setting. To foster this effective communication, Akper et al. (2006) suggest that the professional nurse should:

- Actively solicit input from all players
- Foster open rapport across professional boundaries
- Share clear goals, messages, and plans with all players
- Keep team members informed

Additionally, the CNL needs to be aware of both verbal and nonverbal communication. A crucial skill for CNLs to be successful communicators is active listening (Antai-Otong, 2010).

Collaboration

Collaboration is defined by McKay and Crippen as an "interdisciplinary process of problem solving that involves shared responsibility for decision making as well as the execution of specific plans of care while working toward a common goal" (2008, p. 110). In the context of health care, the role of the CNL is to develop an effective plan of care across settings in collaboration with all disciplines, professions, and stakeholders—including the patient (Begun et al., 2006).

To promote collaboration, the CNL:

- Seeks collaboration and consultation with all contributors to the health care delivery process, including the patient and family
- Synthesizes gathered input and information to find common goals
- Translates discipline-specific language to a common message, so that everyone has a clear understanding of the goals
- Evaluates information for relevance and appropriateness

- Not only communicates with members of the team, but also facilitates communication between members of the team
- Engages in and fosters shared decision making within the health care team

The CNL understands that the knowledge and perspective of just one discipline are limited and biased. Therefore, collaboration is essential to optimal outcomes and to provide a more complete, richer picture by incorporating multiple viewpoints into patient care.

Coordination

Coordination requires intentional planning and direction. The CNL is responsible for coordinating the flow of communication, activities of the team members, and the services provided to the patients.

The CNL coordinates care by:

- Organizing team members toward a common goal
- Creating and fostering systems that encourage communication, teamwork, and collaboration
- Coordinating care of patients and groups of patients using appropriate technology and information systems
- Managing the care of clients across settings and episodes of care
- Clearly delegating tasks and responsibilities
- Ensuring each member of the team has a clear understanding of each member's role

Within large health systems such as the Veterans Administration, the CNL role is implemented in all practice areas to provide streamlined, coordinated care across the spectrum, from acute care to ambulatory and long-term care (Ott et al., 2009). In other health care organizations, the CNL is implemented in the most critical areas first (e.g., medical–surgical units and units with the most acute patients). Then as more nurses graduate from CNL programs, the role is added to other units. Additionally, the CNL role is used in unique settings (e.g., home care, hospice, urgent care, and many others).

Ongoing Evaluation

Ongoing evaluation of care delivery systems and processes is an important component of lateral integration. The CNL monitors not only the final outcomes of care, but also the implementation and progression of care delivery strategies along the way. Evaluation of health care delivery teams and processes must be concurrent and ongoing. By seeing what is working as well as what is not, adjustments can be made to improve the overall outcomes.

Specific areas the CNL should monitor and evaluate include:

- The plan of care for specific patients and populations of patients
- Analysis of risk to promote client safety

- Perspectives of all team members
- Communication strategies and processes used by the team members
- Efficacy of coordination of services
- Use of technology and information systems
- Appropriateness and relevancy of current and newly emerging health care information
- Environment and system to optimize health care quality and outcomes
- Design and delivery of interventions and team processes

Through intentional, ongoing assessment of processes and systems, the CNL is able to implement changes and improve the efficiency, efficacy, safety, and quality of care as well as improve the satisfaction of those involved in the process (Baernholdt & Cottingham, 2010; Hix, McKeon, & Walters, 2009).

Lateral Integration Content on the CNL Exam

According to the *Clinical Nurse Leader Job Analysis Summary and Certification Exam Blue Print* (2011), lateral integration of care questions represent 6% of the exam content. The content related to lateral integration covered on the exam is found in Table 7.1 and Appendix A.

TABLE 7.1 Lateral Integration

CATEGORY	WEIGHT
D. Lateral Integration of Care Services	**6%**
1. Delivers and coordinates care using current technology	
2. Coordinates the health care of clients across settings	
3. Develops and monitors holistic plans of care	
4. Fosters a multidisciplinary approach to attain health and maintain wellness	
5. Performs risk analysis for client safety	
6. Collaborates and consults with other health professionals in the design, coordination, and evaluation of client care outcomes	
7. Disseminates health care information with health care providers to other disciplines	

Used with permission from the Commission on Nurse Certification.

For example, the CNL will generally need to involve multiple disciplines in the plan for discharge. Other disciplines may be needed for assistance in financial, social, and transportation issues if the patient has no family. Lateral integration may appear to be similar to client advocacy. However, client and family advocacy involves the CNL participating with other disciplines as well as the patient and family to decide current health care issues. One of the original four articles by *The Joint Commission Journal on Quality and Patient Safety* (Watson et al., 2008) describes the importance of team care with the CNL in an integral role and the difficulty of implementing change through lateral integration.

Conclusion

Health care delivery is an extremely complex process involving numerous disciplines, practitioners, and services. Each member of this health care team is at risk for practicing within the silo of one specific perspective. Through lateral integration, the CNL intentionally and proactively brings this team together to improve not only the health care delivery process but also patient outcomes. An important role of the CNL is to support and facilitate ongoing and evolving communication, collaboration, coordination, and evaluation among the multidisciplinary team, patient, and family.

Resources

American Association of Colleges of Nursing. (2007). *White paper on education and role of the clinical nurse leader.* Retrieved February 15, 2012, from http://www.aacn.nche. edu/publications/white-papers/ClinicalNurseLeader.pdf

Antai-Otong, D. (2010). Introducing the clinical nurse leader: A catalyst for quality care. In J. L. Harris & L. Roussel (Eds.), *Initiating and sustaining the clinical nurse leader role: A practical guide.* Boston, MA: Jones & Bartlett Publishers.

Apker, J., Propp, K., Ford, W., & Hofmeister, N. (2006). Collaboration, credibility, compassion, and coordination: Professional nurse communication skill sets in health care team interactions. *Journal of Professional Nursing, 22*(3), 180–189.

Baernholdt, M., & Cottingham, S. (2011). The clinical nurse leader—New nursing role with global implications. *International Nursing Review, 58,* 74–78.

Begun, J.W., Tornabeni, J., & White, K. R. (2006). Opportunities for improving patient care through lateral integration: The clinical nurse leader. *Journal of Healthcare Management, 51*(1), 19–25.

Commission on Nurse Certification and Schroeder Measurement Technologies, Inc. (2011). *Exam content outline.* Washington, DC: Author.

Hartranft, S. R., Garcia, T., & Adams, N. (2007). Realizing the anticipated effects of the clinical nurse leader. *Journal of Nursing Administration, 37*(6), 261–263.

Hix, C., McKeon, L., & Walters, S. (2009). Clinical nurse leader impact on clinical microsystems outcomes. *The Journal of Nursing Administration, 39*(2),71–76.

McKay, C. A., & Crippen, L. (2008). Collaboration through clinical integration. *Nursing Administration Quarterly, 32*(2), 109–116.

Ott, K. M., Haddock, K. S., Fox, S. E., Shinn, J. K., Walters, S. E., Hardin, J. W., ..., Harris, J. L. (2009). The clinical nurse leader: Impact on practice outcomes in the Veterans Health Administration. *Nursing Economics, 27*(6), 363–370, 383.

Stanley, J. M. (2010). Introducing the clinical nurse leader: A catalyst for quality care. In J. L. Harris & L. Roussel (Eds.), *Initiating and sustaining the clinical nurse leader role: A practical guide.* Boston, MA: Jones & Bartlett Publishers.

Stanley, J. M., Gannon, J., Gabaut, J. Hartranft, S., Adams, N., Mayes, C., Shouse, G. M., . . ., Burch, D. (2008). The clinical nurse leader: A catalyst for improving quality and patient safety. *Journal of Nursing Management, 16,* 614–622.

Tornabeni, J. (2006). Evolution of a revolution. *Journal of Nursing Administration, 36*(1), 3–6.

Tournabeni, J., & Miller, J. F. (2008). The power of partnership to shape the future of nursing: The evolution of the clinical nurse leader. *Journal of Nursing Management, 16,* 608–613.

Watson, J. H., Anders, S. G., Moore, L. G., Ho, L., Nelson, E. C., Godfrey, M. M., & Batalden, P. B. (2008). Clinical microsystems, part 2. Learning from micro practices about providing patients the care they want and need. *The Joint Commission Journal on Quality and Patient Safety, 34*(8), 443–452.

8

Illness and Disease Management

Audrey Marie Beauvais

The number of chronic diseases, such as cancer, diabetes, heart disease, stroke, asthma, arthritis, Alzheimer's disease, and depression, has been on the rise (Delaware Health Care Commission [DHCC], 2004). In fact, heart disease, cancer, and stroke comprise more than half of all deaths annually (Kung, Hoyert, Xu, & Murphy, 2008). Approximately one out of every two adults (133 of those Americans) has, at a minimum, one chronic illness (Wu & Green, 2000). This increase is related to the large population entering old age, and increased longevity in that category, and advances in health care that have enabled people to live a prolonged life with chronic illnesses (DHCC, 2004).

Chronic Illness

Unfortunately, chronic conditions are quite costly. In fact, care for individuals with chronic illness is estimated to account for over 75% of all health care spending (Hyman, Ornish, & Roisen, 2009; Matthews & Sewell, 2002; The Council of State Governments, n.d.). The good news is that these conditions are often preventable, as they are attributed to lifestyle and environmental factors such as lack of physical activity, poor nutrition, tobacco use, chronic stress, excessive alcohol use, and environmental toxins (Chambers & Grolman, 2011; DHCC, 2004; Hyman et al., 2009).

Individuals with chronic conditions are complicated and need someone to screen and address any physical, psychological, or social issues (Chambers & Grolman, 2011). Clinical nurse leaders (CNLs) can take an active role in illness and disease management, as they are knowledgeable about chronic diseases, able to assess and manage physical and psychological symptoms related to disease and treatment, able to recommend preventive measures, and able to engage in patient and family teaching (Chambers & Grolman, 2011).

When assessing and screening patients, CNLs need to be cognizant of both the nonmodifiable and modifiable risk factors for chronic diseases. Table 8.1 identifies some nonmodifiable risk factors using the example of diabetes. CNLs should assist in the development of individual interventions based on modifiable risk factors. Table 8.2 identifies some modifiable risk factors and potential interventions using the example of diabetes.

TABLE 8.1 Nonmodifiable Risk Factors for Diabetes

Age	As age increases, so does the risk for developing diabetes
Race/ethnicity	The risk of diabetes is greater in certain ethnic groups such as African Americans and Mexican Americans
Family history/genetics	An individual's chances of developing diabetes are greater if someone in their family has the disease

TABLE 8.2 Modifiable Risk Factor for Diabetes

	POTENTIAL INTERVENTIONS
Obesity	Provide nutritional education (such as portion control and food choices), increase physical activity, decrease calorie intake, modify lifestyle, behavior modification
High blood glucose	Follow dietary guidelines, regular home glucose testing, treat blood glucose as ordered by APRN or physician, medication education
Sedentary lifestyle	Help patients discover a way to put physical activity into their daily life. For example, the CNL may suggest that the patient take the stairs rather than the elevator, park farther away from his or her destination to encourage walking, wear a pedometer, join a walking group, join a gym, etc.
Smoking	Offer education regarding smoking cessation
Excessive alcohol intake	Offer alcohol counseling

CNLs will be most effective when part of a collaborative team of nurses, physicians, dietitians, social workers, and behavior health specialists (Chambers & Grolman, 2011). In addition, CNLs will want to develop community partnerships, which will enable them to connect their patients to programs that provide exercise, nutrition, and disease management education. CNLs should advocate for their patients to help them navigate the health care system as well as identify resources that will assist with health care and social needs (Chambers & Grolman, 2011).

CNLs, with their skills and abilities, are an asset for individuals with chronic illness, as they can assist with the creation of treatment plans and self-management approaches while anticipating and managing complications of disease progression. While creating treatment plans, CNLs should make certain that patients are partners in health care decisions. CNLs can help individuals with chronic illness by providing support, guidance, and education about the benefits of implementing a healthy lifestyle (Chambers & Grolman, 2011). Not only do CNLs play a vital role with developing plans and goals in partnership with patients as well as following up with ongoing health care needs, but they also play an essential role in evaluating and modifying the care that is received.

CNLs will need to be aware that focusing solely on the individual and his or her lifestyle will not be addressing the entire issue. Society as a whole has contributed largely to this problem by promoting such behavior as increasing portion sizes, consuming soft drinks, eating processed foods, and sitting for extended periods of time playing video games and watching television. CNLs can play an active role by advocating for social change that addresses these unhealthy lifestyle choices (Chambers & Grolman, 2011).

Disease Management

Disease management typically has three goals: to prevent chronic disease, improve quality of life, and reduce costs (DHCC, 2004). There are two types of disease management strategies that can help CNLs to reach these goals (DHCC, 2004). The two strategies, primary prevention strategies and secondary prevention strategies, are described in Table 8.3.

TABLE 8.3 Disease Management Strategies

Primary prevention strategies	Purpose	Prevent the onset of chronic illness
	Focus	On a healthy lifestyle Healthy habits and behaviors
	Intention	To result in long-term positive outcomes (Note: it is difficult to determine actual long-term cost savings)
	Examples	Healthy eating habits, maintaining a healthy weight, increased physical activity, smoking cessation
Secondary prevention strategies	Purpose	Lessen the effect of chronic disease once it has occurred Evade needless complications Avoid serious illness or disease advancement
	Focus	Assure that individuals with chronic illness receive the needed medical treatment and tests to manage their disease
	Intention	To produce faster outcomes Easier to measure improvement in health and cost saving outcomes
	Examples	Blood sugar testing and altering the diet of an individual diagnosed with diabetes

Source: DHCC (2004).

CNLs should incorporate primary and secondary prevention techniques into their practice (DHCC, 2004). Concentrating on secondary prevention will not yield favorable long-term outcomes with regard to better health condition or decreased cost (DHCC).

CNLs need to be aware of some key factors impacting chronic disease management. Table 8.4 highlights some of the important concepts in disease management. Additional information can be found at the Centers for Disease Control and Prevention website under "Chronic Disease Prevention and Health" or at the web

TABLE 8.4 Important Concepts in Disease Management

Patient-centered care/partnering	Patient-centered care is care that is grounded **in a mutually beneficial partnership** between the patient, family, and health care team. It involves the following: dignity, respect, information sharing, participation, and collaboration. CNLs should develop their partnering skills in order to enhance **shared decision making** with patients and the health care team (Saxe et al., 2007).
	CNLs should focus on individual assessment and needs of the patients in part with **effective interviewing and communication skills** (Saxe et al., 2007)
	CNLs should focus on self-care behaviors (e.g., taking medications correctly), emphasize patient choice, encourage shared decision making (Forbes & While, 2009), as well as assist individuals to make informed choices, develop a joint crisis plan, and a wellness recovery action plan (Kemp, 2011)
Education	CNLs should ensure that education is provided for patients, families, caregivers, employers, insurers, and legislators
	Outside agencies such as state health departments and national organizations may be able to provide educational materials on managing chronic diseases
	Accurate information about chronic illness and disease management is **necessary for effective plans, policies, and programs** to be developed and implemented (DHCC, 2004)
Data collection and analysis	CNLs will need to evaluate interventions by gathering and analyzing data to ensure they are obtaining positive outcomes. Accurate and current data regarding effective and efficient treatment guidelines will be needed as evidence to support and improve practice (Saxe et al., 2007).
	Data collection and analysis can be utilized to: • identify and monitor the most common chronic illnesses • identify effective strategies to manage chronic illnesses • identify effective treatment protocols (Saxe et al., 2007)
Information and communication technology	CNLs should utilize technology to help monitor care and outcomes of individuals with chronic diseases. This technology can be used to share information with patients and health care professionals (Saxe et al., 2007).
Motivation	Changing behavior and habits is difficult. As a result, it may be necessary to offer some incentives for individuals to make positive changes to their lifestyle and to embrace healthy behaviors. Incentives will need to be individualized to the person's interest. For example, incentives can be such things as saving money on medication and health care bills, improving the quality of life, and the ability to enjoy time with children or grandchildren.
Health literacy	According to the Institute of Medicine Report on Health Literacy, almost half of all Americans have trouble comprehending the health information that is provided to them. CNLs can play a valuable role in help ensuring that patients are educated as well as engaged and included in their health care decisions (DHCC, 2004).

(continued)

TABLE 8.4 *(continued)*

Identifying key population	CNLs need to remain cognizant of the public health perspective. Some groups are at increased risk for chronic illness than are other groups. In addition, certain strategies are more effective with particular diseases and populations. As a result, CNLs will need to identify target populations. Also, they will need to complete a needs assessment and develop strategies that work for that population, as there is no single set of strategies that will work for the needs of all individuals (DHCC, 2004; Saxe et al., 2007).
Determining resources	Operating a disease/illness management program will require financial and physical resources. As such, CNLs will need to identify approaches that are feasible, given the cost and availability of resources.
Identifying responsible parties	Operating a disease/illness management program will require that roles and responsibilities are assigned. In addition, it is essential to determine who will lead this effort and will be accountable for its success.
Key stakeholders	Key stakeholders are individuals or groups of people who have a vested interest in the disease/illness management program. They can prevent a project from reaching its goals as well as help a project be successful. Key stakeholders that may be involved with disease/illness management include employers, government agencies, health care providers, insurers, patients themselves, and family caregivers (DHCC, 2004; Jamison, 1998).
Clinical practice guidelines	CNLs should play an active role in developing and revising clinical practice guidelines for specific diseases/illnesses (Jamison, 1998). This involves monitoring the effectiveness of the guidelines as well as making modifications to the guideline based on the analysis of the data with the team. As mentioned above, information technology will help with the evaluation process (Jamison, 1998).

Source: DHCC (2004).

address www.cdc.gov/chronicdisease/index.htm. The website offers information on chronic diseases and health promotion, statistics and tracking, tools and resources, state profiles, and health equity.

Transitions Between Levels of Care and Readiness for Discharge

CNLs will need to remain aware that transitions between levels of care are a critical time for patients (Weiss, Yakusheva, & Bobay, 2010). A patient who returns to the emergency department or is readmitted to an acute care facility within a month after hospital discharge may not have been ready to leave, may not have been adequately prepared, may not have had a well-coordinated aftercare plan, or not have been able to deal with the demands of self-management at the next level of care (Weiss et al., 2010). A return to the hospital may result in outcomes that are adverse, potentially avoidable, and costly (Weiss et al.).

CNLs can assess readiness for discharge on the basis of the following information:

- **Physical readiness:** Is the patient stable? What is the patient's functional ability? How strong is the patient? How are the patient's vital signs, elimination, and intake and output? Is the patient able to ambulate and climb stairs? How is the pain control? Is the patient nauseous or vomiting (Bernstein et al., 2002; Clark, Steinberg, & Bischoff, 1997; Fenwick, 1979, Kortial, 1991; Stephenson, 1990; Titler & Pettit, 1995; Weiss & Piacentine, 2006; Wong & Wong, 1999)?

- **Personal status:** What is the patient's and family's perception regarding readiness for discharge? How does the patient feel on the day of discharge (Weiss et al., 2010)?

- **Knowledge/Education:** Does that patient understand the discharge information regarding self-management at home? For example, is the patient knowledgeable about their medications, medical treatments, restrictions, and access to care providers (Weiss et al., 2010)? Does the patient understand his or her illness/disease process, treatment, potential complications, and expected recovery (Lerret, 2009)? Is the patient prepared and competent to manage his or her self-care (Weiss & Piacentine, 2006)?

- **Identification of unique and individual needs:** What are the patient's and family's unique stressors (i.e., monetary, ambivalence about being discharged from the care of the hospital health care professionals, acclimation need to integrate the patient back into the family, family ability and competence, perceived weakness, and fear of death; Lerret, 2009)?

- **Communication and coordination:** Has there been coordination and communication between the patient, family, and health care team? Discharge planning should start on admission. Patients tend to experience less anxiety and are better able to cope when the discharge is planned ahead and involves the patient and family. In addition, improved communication helps to foster continuity of care and a collaborative relationship (Lerret, 2009).

- **Perceived coping ability:** How well does the patient think he or she is able to manage his or her care at home? What are the psychosocial factors?

- **Expected support:** How much financial, emotional, and social support will be available?

- **Access to care:** Does the patient have access to the health care system and community resources (Weiss & Piacentine, 2006)?

When a patient transitions to another level of care, the CNLs need to support patient safety. This can be accomplished by focusing on self-management of medication and medication reconciliation, follow-up with primary care provider and specialists, patient understanding regarding key clinical signs about his or her condition, as well as ensuring that support systems and sufficient services are arranged (Agency for Healthcare Research and Quality [AHRQ], 2010).

Pain Management, Palliative Care, and End-of-Life Issues

If CNLs are going to play a role in managing diseases, they will most certainly be involved with managing pain, palliative care, and end-of-life issues. The following sections will briefly cover pain management, palliative care, and end-of-life issues.

Pain

According to the Institute of Medicine (IOM; 2011), approximately 116 million adult Americans are affected by chronic pain. Medical treatment and lost productivity attributed to chronic pain are said to cost our nation approximately $635 billion annually (IOM). In light of this information, CNLs will need to find ways to improve pain assessment and management. CNLs will need to assess, design, and provide interventions for moderation of pain and suffering and try to maintain, restore, and optimize patients' level of functioning. CNLs need to complete pain assessments to help ascertain the cause, understand how it influences the individual, specify suitable pain strategies, and evaluate the helpfulness of these strategies (Briggs, 2010). Table 8.5 provides some key aspects regarding pain assessment.

Additional information on pain can be found at the following websites:

- American Pain Foundation: www.painfoundation.org
- American Pain Society: www.ampainsoc.org
- Institute of Medicine: www.iom.edu/Reports/2011/Relieving-Pain-in-America-A-Blueprint-for-Transforming-Prevention-Care-Education-Research.aspx

Palliative Care

Palliative care is health care that focuses on improving the quality of life for individuals who are suffering with a serious illness or disease (Matzo & Sherman, 2001). Palliative care concentrates on pain and symptom management, communication, and coordinated care. It can be provided from the time of diagnosis and can be provided along with curative treatment. Palliative care does not accelerate or delay death. Rather, it offers respite from pain and other symptoms, incorporates the psychological and spiritual components of care, and provides assistance for patients to actively participate in life until they die. In addition, it offers support to families through the patient's illness and death, as well as throughout the family's grieving process (Matzo & Sherman, 2001).

TABLE 8.5 Key Aspects of Pain Assessment

Site	Identify the **location** of the pain
	Where does it hurt?
Amount/severity	How **intense** is the pain? How bad is the pain?
	Pain is an individual experience, so the CNL will need to have the patient rate it. Ask patients to rate their pain during movement and at rest.
	There are a variety of pain assessment tools available
Characteristics/description of pain	What is the quality and type of pain?
	Describe the pain. Does the pain radiate/spread anywhere? Is the pain throbbing, burning, aching, tender, dull, sharp, crushing, gnawing, stabbing, cramping, sore, discomfort, etc.?
	There are several kinds of physical causes of pain
	Nociceptive pain: typically localized, constant, aching, throbbing. Typically time limited and responds well to treatment
	Neuropathic pain: often described as burning, shooting, and pins and needles. The pain can also result from light touch. Typically chronic
	Mixed category of pain: a combination of the above two
Onset and timespan	When did it begin? Was it sudden or gradual?
	How long did it continue?
	Is there a pattern to the pain? Does the pain vary during the day? Is it sporadic?
	Is it constant? What started the pain?
	What things make it hurt more (i.e., activity)?
Prior pain management techniques used and relief from pain	What medications and nonmedication approaches have been tried? Were they successful?
	What makes the pain better or worse?
Related symptoms and effect on level of functioning/activity	Do you have any other symptoms associated with the pain (nausea, photosensitivity, stiff neck, etc.)?
	What effects has the pain had on you and your family?
	Has the pain affected your mood, your dietary intake, your functioning, your sleep?

Source: Briggs (2010).

Hospice and End-of-Life Care

Palliative care differs from end-of-life care and hospice care. Hospice/end-of-life care provides quality care to people in the last months of their life who have decided to stop curative treatments. CNLs should help ensure that individuals in the last phase of life get the dignity and respect they deserve. Every person should be afforded the chance to discuss how they would like to be treated. They should be given an opportunity to formulate a "living will" and determine a health care proxy. CNLs can play an important role by making certain that physical and psychological suffering will be attended to and by taking measures to ensure comfort will be sought out. For additional information, CNLs can access the National Hospice and Palliative Care Organization (NHPCO) website (www.nhpco.org/templates/1/homepage.cfm).

Common Geriatric Problems

Given the aging population, CNLs will need to be knowledgeable about common geriatric problems. There are 13 principal clinical issues for geriatric care listed below:

- Cognitive impairment
- Depression
- Behavioral issues
- Gait/mobility
- Incontinence
- Nutrition
- Sleep
- Vision
- Hearing
- Caregiver issues (social support/isolation)
- Home safety
- Driving safety
- Health and financial planning (Bogardus, Richardson, Maciejewski, Gahbauer, & Inouye, 2002)

CNLs will need to bear in mind these common issues as they consider the plan of care most appropriate for the geriatric population. In addition, the CNL should recognize that there are certain patterns of problem occurrences in the population as a whole, such as:

- Several acute-care admissions
- Two or more visits to the emergency department during a 6-month period
- Discharge from a hospital or skilled nursing facility
- Inadequate nutrition
- Medication nonadherence
- Lack of psychosocial support necessary to sustain wellness
- Expected increased use of medical services following hospital discharge
- Asthma in children, which is chronic and severe (AHRQ, 2010)

Being aware of these patterns will help CNLs anticipate needed interventions.

Assessing Health Literacy

CNLs will need to be able to identify whether patients have issues with health literacy (Cornett, 2009). Patients will frequently hide their deficits due to feelings of embarrassment and shame. They develop coping skills that help them conceal their limited literacy, and that may lead health care providers to misjudge their ability to comprehend patient teaching. A recent article by Dr. Cornett provides some practical ways to identify behavioral clues for low health literacy. For example, patients who provide incomplete forms, make excuses such as they forgot their glasses, or state that they will complete the paperwork at home may be trying to hide low literacy. Low literacy skills can be uncovered when CNLs ask certain nonthreatening assessment questions (Cornett, 2009). Dr. Cornett provides some useful sample questions. For example, a CNL could say the following to a patient: Many people have trouble understanding the health care information given to them. Do you ever have (or would you like to have) someone help you with your forms, your insurance information, and your medication labels?

The information above can be supplemented with additional useful resources:

- U.S. Department of Health and Human Services (Office of Disease Prevention and Health Promotion) *Quick Guide to Health Literacy* can be accessed at the following website: www.health.gov/communication/literacy/quickguide/quickguide.pdf

- The Council of State Governments *Health Literacy Tool Kit* can be accessed at the following website: www.csg.org/knowledgecenter/docs/ToolKit03HealthLiteracy.pdf

Cultural Sensitivity

CNLs will be expected to offer illness and disease management while also providing culturally competent care. Culturally competent care requires that the CNL is sensitive to matters related to culture, race, gender, and sexual orientation. There is evidence to support a relationship between patient outcomes and nurses' cultural competence (Boyer, 2006). In order to become culturally competent, Boyer suggests that there are several stages through which CNLs will need to progress:

- Cultural awareness: CNLs need to recognize their own individual values, beliefs, and prejudices. CNLs should reflect on their own cultural practices.

- Cultural knowledge: CNLs should stay unbiased and find information concerning other cultures to establish educational underpinnings.

- Cultural skills: CNLs need to demonstrate the ability to communicate efficiently. Additionally, they should have the ability to identify, assess, and incorporate the values, beliefs, and cultural customs of the person under their care.

TABLE 8.6 Illness and Disease Management

CATEGORY	WEIGHT
A. Illness and Disease Management	**7%**

1. Assumes responsibility for the provision and management of care at the point of care in and across all environments

2. Coordinates care at the point of service to individuals across the lifespan, with particular emphasis on health promotion and risk reduction services

3. Identifies client problems that require intervention, with special focus on those problems amenable to nursing intervention

4. Designs and redesigns client care based on analysis of outcomes and evidence-based knowledge

5. Completes holistic assessments and directs care based on assessments

6. Applies theories of chronic illness care to clients and families

7. Integrates community resources, social networks, and decision support mechanisms into care management

8. Identifies patterns of illness symptoms and effects on clients' compliance and ongoing care

9. Educates clients, families, and care givers to monitor symptoms and take action

10. Utilizes advanced knowledge of pathophysiology and pharmacology to anticipate illness progression, and response to therapy, and to educate clients and families regarding care

11. Applies knowledge of reimbursement issues in planning care across the life span

12. Makes recommendations regarding readiness for discharge, having accurately assessed the client's level of health literacy and self-management

13. Applies research-based knowledge from nursing and the sciences as the foundation for evidence-based practice

14. Develops and facilitates evidence-based protocols and disseminates these among the multidisciplinary team

15. Understands the role of palliative care and hospice as a disease management tool

16. Understands cultural relevance as it relates to health care

17. Educates clients about health care technologies using client-centered strategies

18. Synthesizes literature and research findings to design interventions for select problems

19. Monitors client satisfaction with disease action plans

20. Evaluates factors contributing to disease, including genetics

21. Designs and implements education and community programs for clients and health professionals

22. Applies principles of infection control, assessment of rates, and inclusion of infection control in plan of care

23. Integrates advanced clinical assessment

- Cultural interaction: CNLs will need to work with individuals from various cultural backgrounds to expand their understanding and become more at ease and self-assured.
- Cultural sensitivity: CNLs will need to understand and accept the individual's values and beliefs. The CNL will need to show presence, support, empathy, flexibility, and tolerance (Boyer, 2006).

Cultural Considerations Near the End of Life

In addition to the general principles of cultural considerations noted above, there are some special considerations for those individuals who are nearing the end of their lives (Matzo et al., 2002). CNLs should begin by ensuring that a cultural assessment of the dying patient and family has been completed, as the understanding that should arise from this information has a potential influence on care. For example, the following dimensions of care can be of significance to those near the end of life (Matzo et al., 2002):

- Ethnic group
- Gender
- Age
- Differing abilities
- Sexual orientation
- Religion and spirituality
- Socioeconomic factors
- Place of residency

Additional information on many aspects of cultural competency can be accessed through the U.S. Department of Health and Human Services Office of Minority Health at the following web address: minorityhealth.hhs.gov/templates/browse.aspx?lvl=1&lv1ID=7.

Conclusion

CNLs can play a vital role in disease and illness management given their ability to assess and manage symptoms related to disease and treatment, ability to recommend interventions, and ability to provide education to patients, families, and communities (Chambers & Grolman, 2011). In order for CNLs to manage diseases and illnesses appropriately, they will need to consider certain key factors. For example, CNLs will need to be aware that transitions in level of care are a critical time for patients and will thus need to ensure that patients are assessed for their readiness for discharge. Given the nature of disease management, CNLs will also need to be involved in managing pain, palliative care, and end-of-life issues. In addition, as our population ages, CNLs will need to be well versed in issues that affect our geriatric population. Finally, CNLs will need to be cognizant of their patient's health literacy as well as cultural considerations. The concepts of illness and disease management included in the CNL exam are broad and challenging for CNL students (Table 8.6).

Resources

Agency for Healthcare Research and Quality. (2010). *Chronic care and disease management improves health, reduces cost for patients with multiple chronic conditions in an integrated health system.* Retrieved August 27, 2011, from http://www.innovations.ahrq.gov/content.aspx?id=1696

Bernstein, H. H., Spino, C., Baker, A., Slora, E. J., Touloukian, C. L., & McCormick, M. C. (2002). Postpartum discharges: Do varying perceptions of readiness impact health outcomes? *Ambulatory Pediatrics, 2*(5), 388–395.

Bogardus, S. T., Richardson, E., Maciejewski, P. K., Gahbauer, E., & Inouye, S. K. (2002). Evaluation of a guided protocol for quality improvement identifying common geriatric problems. *Journal of the American Geriatrics Society, 50*(2), 328–335.

Boyer, D. (2006). Cultural competence at the bedside. *Pennsylvania Nurse, 61*(4), 18–19.

Briggs, E. (2010). Assessment and expression of pain. *Nursing Standard, 25*(2), 35–38.

Chambers, P., & Grolman, C. (2011). The emerging role of disease management nurses for chronic disease care. *Viewpoint,* January/February, 4–6.

Clark, M., Steinberg, M., & Bischoff, N. (1997). Patient readiness for return to home: Discord between expectations and reality. *Australian Occupational Therapy Journal, 44,* 132–141.

Cornett, S. (2009). Assessing and addressing health literacy. *Online Journal of Issues in Nursing, 14*(3), 1.

Council of State Governments. (n.d.). *State officials guide chronic illness.* Retrieved August 26, 2011, from http://www.csg.org/knowledgecenter/docs/SOG03ChronicIllness.pdf

Delaware Health Care Commission. (2004). *Chronic illness and disease management: House joint resolution 10 task force key findings and recommendations.* Retrieved August 26, 2011, from http://dhss.delaware.gov/dhss/dhcc/files/chronicillnessreport-final0804.pdf

Fenwick, A. M. (1979). An interdisciplinary tool for assessing patients' readiness for discharge in the rehabilitation setting. *Journal of Advanced Nursing, 4,* 9–21.

Forbes, A., & While, A. (2009). The nursing contribution to chronic disease management: A discussion paper. *International Journal of Nursing Studies, 46,* 120–131.

Hyman, M., Ornish, D., & Roisen, M. (2009). Lifestyle medicine: Treating the causes of diseases. *Alternative Therapies, 15*(6), 12–14.

Institute of Medicine. (2011). *Relieving pain in America: A blueprint for transforming prevention, care, education, and research.* Washington, DC: The National Academies Press.

Jamison, M. (1998). Chronic illness management in the year 2005. *Nursing Economics, 16*(5), 246–253.

Kemp, V. (2011). Use of "chronic disease self-management strategies" mental healthcare. *Current Opinion in Psychiatry, 24,* 144–148.

Kortial, K. (1991). Anaesthesia for ambulatory surgery: Firm definitions of "home readiness" needed. *Annals of Medicine, 23*(6), 635–636.

Kung, H. C., Hoyert, D. L., Xu, J. Q., & Murphy, S. L. (2008). Deaths: Final data for 2005. *National Vital Statistics Reports Center for Disease Control, 56*(10), 1–121.

Lerret, S. M. (2009). Discharge readiness: An integrative review focusing on discharge following pediatric hospitalization. *Journal for Specialists in Pediatric Nursing, 14*(4), 245–255.

Matthews, T. L., & Sewell, J. C. (2002). *State official's guide to health literacy.* Lexington, KY: The Council of State Governments.

Matzo, M. L., & Sherman, D. W. (2001). Palliative care nursing: Ensuring competent care at the end of life. *Geriatric Nursing, 22*(6), 288–293.

Matzo, M. L., Sherman, D. W., Mazanec, P., Barber, M. A., Virani, R., & McLaughlin, M. M. (2002). Teaching cultural considerations at the end of life: End of life nursing education consortium program recommendations. *The Journal of Continuing Education in Nursing, 33*(6), 270–278.

Saxe, J., Janson, S. L., Dennehy, P. M., Stringari-Murray, S. S., Hirsch, J. E., & Waters, C. M. (2007). Meeting a primary care challenge in the United States: Chronic illness care. *Contemporary Nurse, 26*(1), 94–103.

Stephenson, M. E. (1990). Discharge criteria in day surgery. *Journal of Advanced Nursing, 15*, 601–613.

Titler, M. G., & Pettit, D. M. (1995). Discharge readiness assessment. *Journal of Cardiovascular Nursing, 9*(4), 64–74.

Weiss, M. E., & Piacentine, L. B. (2006). Psychometric properties of the readiness for hospital discharge scale. *Journal of Nursing Measurement, 14*(3), 163–180.

Weiss, M., Yakusheva, O., & Bobay, K. (2010). Nurse and patient perceptions of discharge readiness in relation to post discharge utilization. *Medical Care, 48*(5), 482–486.

Wong, J., & Wong, S. (1999). Criteria for determining optimal time of discharge after total hip replacement. *British Journal of Clinical Governance, 4*(4), 135–141.

Wu, S. Y., & Green, A. (2000). *Projection of chronic illness prevalence and cost inflation.* Santa Monica, CA: RAND Health.

9

Knowledge Management

Deborah C. Jackson

The clinical nurse leader (CNL) White Paper dictates that the CNL is an outcomes manager who synthesizes data, information, and knowledge to evaluate and achieve optimal client outcomes (American Association of Colleges of Nursing [AACN], 2007). The CNL has the ability to acquire a wealth of data from multiple sources within the microsystem and throughout the mesosystem. Beginning with listening to shift-to-shift reports at the start of her day, to multidisciplinary rounds, physical assessments of patients, lab reports, hourly rounding, and reviewing electronic medical record (EMR) documentation, there is no lack of topics upon which the CNL might focus to evaluate for potential outcome improvement.

Driving Forces and Outcomes

Starting in October 2012, hospitals are trying to adjust to the newest wrinkle in the world of health care: the impact of linking patient-satisfaction scores to Medicare payments. Formerly, in the fee-for-service payment system, the Centers for Medicare and Medicaid Services (CMS) paid all health care providers without discriminating on the basis of quality of care (Fenter & Lewis, 2008). Ascertaining that this method is no real incentive to improve outcomes, CMS is promoting a pay for performance (P4P) reimbursement strategy that links payment to the quality of care provided by clinicians, offering financial incentives for improvements in care, as well as disincentives for care that does not achieve adequate outcomes. The standardized tool being utilized that measures patient perception of the quality of care received is the HCAHPS (Hospital Consumer Assessment of Healthcare Providers and Systems). Since 2007, CMS has required most hospitals to submit HCAHPS; failure to do so has resulted in payment reductions (Dunn, 2011). However, beginning in 2013, CMS will switch from pay-for-reporting to one based on pay-for-performance. Although HCAHPS measures patients' perception of quality, the results are also directly connected to quality, such as medication information, preprocedural education, and discharge instructions (Dunn, 2011).

So now, the role of the CNL regarding knowledge management has been expanded. Figure 9.1 depicts the cycle of knowledge management. Data from nurse sensitive indicators, quality improvement initiatives, patient satisfaction, advancing technology, and competent clinical care are even more critical in the age of the P4P, owing to the transparency of data. The CNL will synthesize all microsystem data, including information obtained from HCAHPS scores, and strive to achieve improvement outcomes, which will favor improving patient outcomes. The P4P indicators are another defining, justifying feature of the CNL role—to promote cost-effectiveness.

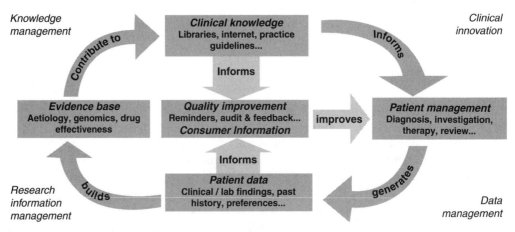

Source: World Health Organization (2012).

FIGURE 9.1   The clinical knowledge cycle.

AACN (2007) has challenged nursing educators and professionals to accept the "unparalleled opportunity and capability to address the critical issues that face the nation's current health care system." The nursing profession can have an impact on changing our current health care system by reshaping nursing practice. Nursing has been and continues to be described as an art and a science. Science is based on facts and evidence. Going forward, nursing practice must be established by the same method, which is the most recent evidence. The CNL, practicing within a microsystem, has the ability to, and is obligated to, obtain this evidence by a variety of methods: literature search using electronic search engines such as Cumulative Index of Nursing and Allied Health Literature (CINAHL) or Cochrane Database of Systematic Reviews and online software programs such as Mosby's Nursing Consult. In addition, the CNL utilizes access to EMR documentation of patient care and medication administration, multidisciplinary rounds on the microsystem, nursing grand rounds, and first-hand observation of the problems and challenges presented at the bedside with the ability to obtain quantitative and qualitative data. The transformation of nursing practice should have evidence-based research as the prototype for changing all aspects of practice such as policies, procedures, guidelines, and standards of care. "The credibility of health professions will be judged by practices based on the latest and the best evidence from sound scientific studies in combination with clinical expertise, astute assessment, and respect for patient values and preferences" (Melnyk & Fineout-Overholt, 2005).

The value of a clinical nurse leader will be measured by the high-quality outcomes in individuals and groups of clients, as well as ability to manage waste and control costs within a microsystem. The CNL compares desired effect outcomes with national benchmarks against like institutions. Going along with the goals of the CMS, the CNL strives to identify quality measures that need improvement, incorporates new evidence into practice, implements new guidelines for patient care, tracks data on these projects, and is able to show improved clinical outcomes that are cost effective within the microsystem. The CNL needs to understand economies of scale, how to read a balance sheet, the difference between fixed and incremental costs, how to establish per unit costs, and some basic marketing strategies (Boxes 9.1 and 9.2). Basic business skills and organizational theory must become accepted components of CNL education (AACN, 2007).

BOX 9.1
Examples of Outcomes Tracked in Acute Care

- Falls
- Falls with injuries
- Pressure ulcers
- Central line catheter infections
- Catheter-related urinary tract infections
- Ventilator-acquired pneumonias (VAPs)
- Use of restraints
- Hospital readmission rates

BOX 9.2
HCAHPS Categories of Data

- Care from nurses
- Care from doctors
- Experience in the hospital
- Preparation for discharge
- Overall rating of hospital

The CNL's Role in Epidemiology

As the CNL is accountable for designing and implementing measures that modify risk factors within the microsystem, it is also an expectation that data will be collected in an effort to predict expected health problems and health care–associated infections (HAIs). Knowledge of the epidemiological triad is essential as the starting point, prior to the collection of data, for the identification and prevention of present and future diseases and infections within the microsystem.

The epidemiological triad, a model explaining the spread of disease, consists of an agent, a host, and an environment; the agent being the organism, such as a virus or bacterium, that infects the host (person or animal) in an environment or place with the appropriate conditions that allow for the host to be infected. Epidemiology provides the CNL with a method or direct approach to uncovering the cause of a sudden increase in infections within the microsystem, such as multiple methicillin-resistant *Staphylococcus aureus* (MRSA). Of course, this applies to a variety of hospital-acquired infections that are a significant challenge in today's health care. Epidemiology allows for the development of and testing for hypotheses pertaining to occurrence and prevention of serious infections that increase morbidity and mortality. By collecting specific data related to each patient affected, discovery of either the agent or the environment will allow for future prevention of the disease.

Epidemiology has been described as the sum of factors that influence the incidence and distribution of disease (Morath & Turnbull, 2005). The evolution surrounding current thinking related to poor outcomes and errors has shifted around this "sum of factors." Medical errors and poor outcomes are now ascribed to faulty systems, not to an individual. "The focus on error in the research was a reflection of the medical culture's flawed, entrenched belief that the actions of individuals, 'bad apples,' were responsible for harm to patients" (Leape, 2001). By working closely with the professional disease professionals in nursing and medicine, the CNL can support this more productive approach to improvement by using knowledge of epidemiologic data in the microsystem to enact change.

The CNL on any microsystem would do well to focus on the two guiding principles that have emerged: (a) error is best viewed as a broken health care system and (b) errors will always exist and should be viewed as a data source, which can help to avoid harm (Leape, 2001). Research demonstrates that accidents and near misses are a result of faulty systems, culture- and system-based failures in teamwork, communications, and transitions (Morath & Turnbull, 2005). Data and errors of the microsystem must be made transparent, allowing the CNL to understand the epidemiology of the error, to learn from it, to alleviate it, and to prevent future mistakes in the care delivery system. Also, not to be dismissed is the public's outcry related to being held financially accountable for the cost of these medical errors. Consumers of health care are demanding that action be taken to reduce harm to patients. What better incentive to reduce and prevent these adverse events than to have the consumers demand that health care providers account for their erroneous actions?

In accordance with the information regarding epidemiology of the microsystem, the CNL will develop a disease surveillance plan, if one has not already been created. Knowing which resources within the microsystem are available and can be targeted for use, the CNL will begin by collecting evidence-based research (EBR) and best practice guidelines on the specific disease identified. EBR can help identify probable causes within the specific microsystem (acute care facility, extended care facility, community clinic, physician's office, etc.) as well as recommended treatments and prevention of future outbreaks. The Agency for Healthcare

Research and Quality states that HAIs are one of the top 10 leading causes of death in the United States (AHRQ, 2010). Knowing this, the CNL incorporates infection control as a fundamental aspect of preventing disease on the microsystem, where the patient population already has a compromised immune system.

In addition, the CNL must be aware of surveillance compliance with state and local infection control agencies. Some diseases must be reported. Most hospitals are enrolled in the national health care safety network (NHSN), an Internet-based surveillance system that integrates and expands a facility's own surveillance program to a national level. One purpose of NHSN is to conduct collaborative research studies with NHSN member facilities to describe the epidemiology of emerging HAIs, assess the importance of potential risk factors, further characterize HAI pathogens and their mechanisms of resistance, and evaluate alternative surveillance and prevention strategies (NHSN, 2011). The CNL should have a working knowledge of the data collected within the organization, who is responsible for what data, and to what data registries the organization is reporting.

Risk Anticipation and Evaluation ✳

Individuals seeking health care can be at risk in a variety of settings. Since October 2008, when CMS refused to reimburse hospitals for conditions acquired after admission, such as falls, pressure ulcers, central line infections, and deep vein thrombosis, it has become fiscally prudent for each hospital to identify which patients may be at risk for such conditions during the admission process. Assessments initiated in the emergency department (ED), on admission to the microsystem, and then again, on a daily basis (sometimes each shift), are utilized in an attempt to prevent such occurrences. Millions of dollars are spent annually on items used to prevent falls (bed alarms, safety slippers, etc.), pressure ulcers (skin creams, specialty beds, constant repositioning of the patient), and central line infections. Resources have been utilized in many environments for the Institute for Healthcare Improvement (IHI)'s use of bundles—order sets specific to prevent different HAIs and safety hazards. Hourly rounding by staff on units is meant specifically to prevent such conditions. Each hour, the nurse or another member of the health care team must enter the patient's room and address patient needs such as pain assessment, elimination, and physical positioning. This level of risk identification and risk reduction is a significant shift in health care. Often it is the CNL who is leading the development or implementation of these changes.

For adequate treatment to be provided, all of the patient's conditions and health needs must be addressed upon admission to the hospital. Previous medical records and treatments for conditions such as diabetes, hypertension, congestive heart failure, chronic kidney disease, and chronic obstructive pulmonary disease must be carefully considered when treating the present condition. Failure to do so might result in a lengthier hospital stay or readmission. It is essential to review current hospital medications and treatments and how they interact with the list of comorbid conditions, developing an integrated, evidence-based treatment plan that considers primary diagnosis and comorbidities (Institute for Healthcare Improvement, 2012; Box 9.3).

BOX 9.3
Medication Management

Medication management is a significant challenge in health care and that challenge must be addressed by all members caring for individuals across systems. Issues for the CNL:

• What tool is currently being used to address medication management/ reconciliation?

• What are the most common high-risk medications patients are prescribed at discharge?

• How is the process of medication review, education, and intervention incorporated into the routine practices of the microsystem?

• What resources are available to support this issue?

Example: The STOPP and START criteria were developed in 2007 to serve as a screening tool for comprehensive assessment of safety and quality of prescription in patients 65 years and older (Topinková, Mádlová, Fialová, & Klán, 2009). Using STOPP criteria, potentially inappropriate drugs are identified in drug regimens, which could be stopped altogether or replaced by a safer drug alternative. Both screening tools represent a new method for improving quality of geriatric prescribing in clinical practice (Topinková et al., 2009).

Risk anticipation, the ability to critically evaluate and anticipate risks to client safety, is a critical component of the CNL role. The CNL also uses risk analysis tools and quality improvement methodologies at the systems level to anticipate risk to any client and intervenes to decrease the risk (Commission on Nurse Certification, 2007). Root cause analysis (RCA) is a structured method used to analyze serious adverse events. It is now widely deployed as an error analysis tool in health care (AHRQ, 2012)

The major concept of RCA involves identifying underlying problems related to the system, rather than concentrating on the mistakes made by an individual. If one should occur on the microsystem, the CNL would follow a "prescribed protocol that begins with data collection and reconstruction of the event through record review and participant interviews" (AHRQ, 2012). A multidisciplinary team should then analyze the sequence of events leading to the error, with the goals of identifying how and why the event occurred. The ultimate goal of RCA, of course, is to prevent future harm by eliminating the latent errors (the hidden problems within the systems that contribute to adverse events) that so often underlie adverse events (AHRQ).

Another tool for risk analysis in health care is "failure mode effect and analysis" (FMEA). "A healthcare failure mode and effect analysis process is conducted in an effort to help identify weak points in a process, to prevent failures of a process/ system and to reduce or prevent medical errors, before these processes have the chance to occur" (Wilcox, 2012). Reporting of "near misses" in many organizations is a key opportunity to conduct a FMEA and analyze the components of the system that could allow for errors. Reports by nurses of medication "near misses" are a wonderful opportunity for this process. Suppose a CNL observes a nurse draw up a dose of insulin that seems much greater than the dose the patient normally requires. The staff nurse reports that the computerized medication administration record indicates the patient is due for the large dose when, in fact, the CNL realizes that the nurse has misread the insulin coverage. This near miss with a high-risk medication is an opportunity to analyze the factors involved, because if one nurse made the mistake, it can certainly happen again.

Electronic Medical Record

Modern technology has created an explosion in the world of health care related to new equipment designed to prevent medical errors and keep the patients' medical records safe. The electronic medical record (EMR) was implemented to prevent medical errors and plays a significant role in reducing the cost of health care, reducing complications, and achieving better outcomes (Harris & Roussel, 2010). With the implementation of the EMR, health care workers have the ability to access patient records nationwide. This process, now supported (and being made mandatory by 2015) by the federal government, is in the form of a health information exchange (HIE). It refers to the sharing of clinical and administrative data across the boundaries of health care institutions and other health data repositories (Harris & Roussel, 2010).

The CNL performs a critical part in developing, training, and auditing all documentation into the EMR. Order sets may be created at the request of physicians or staff in order to provide consistency in disease management and prevent variations in care when able. Clinical support systems can be put into place to share information with nurses at critical times to avoid or reduce the risk of error. The EMR affords greater access to data collection, facilitates communication across microsystems, and addresses some areas of safety. Physicians and CNLs may have the potential to communicate electronically with their patients after discharge, checking that patients are doing well, taking medications as instructed, and knowing when to call if not feeling well, all in an attempt to prevent readmissions. The complexity, functionality, and compatibility of EMRs vary greatly by institution and health care system. The CNL will be instrumental in supporting the development and integration of an EMR system that will continue to be developed in the coming decades.

Lastly, an important aspect for electronic communication is patient privacy. The CNL must do everything possible to ensure that patient records are not viewed inappropriately by anyone who is not directly caring for the patient. Enforcement of safety measures, for the CNL as well as the staff on the microsystem, such as closing EMRs when completed, not leaving any paperwork for others to view, or giving passwords to fellow employees, is mandatory to protect privacy. Issues related to ethics and privacy in the EMR are discussed further in this book.

Benchmarking Data

On any given microsystem, the CNL continually strives to improve the quality of care for the patient population. Since good performance reflects good quality practice, it is essential that performance be measured both against other microsystems within the institution and against like microsystems on a national level. Competition can be healthy among these like microsystems, the goal being to strive for continually better outcomes and practices. The progress of quality improvement initiatives can be tracked by using measures of quality and safety. There is always a need to improve the quality of care or the safety of practice for a microsystem. The use of external benchmarks allows the CNL to determine whether or not improvement has truly been made. Benchmarking in health care has been defined as the continual and collaborative discipline of measuring and comparing the results of key work processes with those of the best performers in evaluating organizational performance (Hughes, 2008).

Benchmarking in health care allows the organization to improve the efficiency, cost-effectiveness, and quality of services performed in a meaningful manner. On the microsystem level, data collected by the CNL on each of the quality indicators can be compared to like microsystems nationwide and gauged on the effectiveness of protocols used. If falling below the national benchmark, the CNL reflects on practice used, researches on best practices, and seeks out knowledge on what is used by like systems whose achievement levels are excellent. Likewise, if the microsystem is well above the benchmark (considering this the expectation), the CNL reflects on the methodology in place for this indicator and analyzes whether or not the same can be used elsewhere.

Designing Care to Optimize Outcomes

On a weekly, monthly, and quarterly basis, nursing administration, nursing management, and CNLs seriously evaluate the results of quality indicators for the individual microsystems, as well as the mesosystem as a whole. Comparisons are made against national benchmarks with like microsystems. As previously stated, in the near future, CMS will reduce reimbursement for health care facilities that do not perform up to par. For those indicators whose rates lie below (or above, as the case may be) the benchmarks, it is necessary to determine where the variations lie. In addition to the most commonly thought attribution to variation in the work of the practitioners, the CNL must consider variability in the methodology of the

---

BOX 9.4
Methods to Support Knowledge Sharing to Optimize Outcomes

- Electronic medical record
- Informational hurdles at the microsystem and mesosystem levels
- Shared governance council
- Unit practice councils
- Journal clubs
- Unit practice councils
- Data boards with benchmarks
- Staff involvement in RCA

system, which can produce variations in access and outcomes, as well as other significant results (Box 9.4). Specific variations must be dissected separately for true determination of causes. Each variation should have the following addressed: Is there a need to identify it? How will it be measured? Does it necessitate improvement? *Can improvement occur?*

Optimal client outcomes best occur when the health care team has the patient's *total* history: physical, social, and psychological. Without this being complete, the CNL begins with a handicap when trying to establish goals for this patient. Collaboration with the nursing staff, especially the primary nurse, and the entire interdisciplinary team is advantageous to the CNL in developing a specific, individualized plan of care that allows for optimal outcomes. Each of these health care workers is an expert in his or her field, and their suggestions are taken seriously. The AACN's Synergy Model stresses that responsibility and accountability for outcomes is a shared responsibility between the patient and the health care provider (Curley, 1998).

Keeping in mind that the patient's perception of what is an "optimal patient outcome" is most important in today's world of patient satisfaction scores, HCAHPS, and future reimbursement from CMS, it is imperative that the CNL educate the staff on the importance of developing a comprehensive plan, assessing risk, and individualizing care on admission to the microsystem. A proactive, evidence-based approach by the entire team will best support outcomes related to the patient's disease state.

Accountability for Knowledge Management

The American Nurses Association (ANA) Code of Ethics for Nurses (4.2) states, "Accountability means to be answerable to oneself and others for one's actions. In order to be accountable, nurses act under a code of ethical conduct that is grounded in moral principles of fidelity and respect for the dignity, worth, and self-determination of patients. Nurses are accountable for judgments made and actions taken in the course of nursing practice, irrespective of healthcare organizations' policies or providers' directives" (ANA, 2011).

Harris and Roussel (2010) further address accountability for the CNL by emphasizing that responsible people account for what they do and how well they perform, work effectively with others, complete tasks, and achieve outcomes. Accountability includes developing trust, being known to follow through on problems, keeping promises, and being persistent on problem resolution even when anticipated outcomes are not obtained.

These statements relate to the CNL even more than to the staff nurse, as the CNL plans, evaluates, and revises plans of care; develops and provides staff and patient education; and has input on many of the decisions made for the microsystem. The CNL on the microsystem assumes responsibility for the total care of the patients and families on a fair and equitable basis, advocating that all patients receive continuity of care without bias or unfair judgment. Being accountable, this leader asks for and offers feedback in an attempt to create desired improvements. Skills needed for accountability include remaining engaged when a situation continues to be problematic, persistence in seeking new and creative solutions, asking for advice of the experts and superiors when needed, and thinking outside the box to accomplish new pathways for accomplishment of goals. Continually striving to achieve the best results, the CNL does not give up when outcomes are under par; revision of strategies and further evidence-based research demonstrate a determination that outcomes will be of the best quality possible!

Also taken into consideration here is the cultural diversity of the patient population within the microsystem. Sensitivity and cultural competency must be displayed for each and every individual plan of care. It is the judgment of the CNL, usually through evidence-based research, that formulates many of these decisions. If the patient's plan of care is less than adequate, or contains misinformation, harm may come to the patient. Utilizing input from patients and families, the CNL can support optimal care for diverse populations on the microsystem. The CNL assumes accountability for outcomes through the collection and application of research-based information to design, implement, and evaluate client plans of care (AACN, 2007). If there are errors in judgment made, the CNL is ethically accountable, and must correct, reevaluate decisions made, and develop new strategies. As stated earlier, the value of the CNL position is judged by the patient outcomes and cost efficiency that result from decisions made for the microsystem. The business case for the CNL role is intricately involved in the outcomes of a microsystem and the associated cost savings for the organization.

Knowledge of Complementary Therapy

Along with the standardized and common medical treatments, complementary and alternative medicine (CAM) has again made a place for itself in medicine in the 21st century. Long before doctors and hospitals were commonplace, there were individuals who practiced medicine utilizing what was on hand: plants, herbs, spices, and prayers. The shaman in China, the medicine man in America, and those who practiced witchcraft and voodoo were all familiar in towns and villages when one was sick or hurt. Yoga has been practiced for more than 5,000 years and improves flexibility, increases strength, develops better concentration, improves posture, and promotes breathing. Reiki healing promotes overall balance to feel and function well, is safe, and supports any medical treatment plan. Acupuncture and chiropractic medicine are other examples of CAM.

Over the past 20 years, many patients are turning to and adding CAM to the treatment plans prescribed by their doctors. Some avoid prescribed medicines at any cost, hoping that CAM will be sufficient. The CNL on any microsystem would be wise to impress upon the staff that it is prudent to consistently ask the patients upon admission if they take any vitamins, minerals, herbs, or supplements. Many of these CAMs potentiate, decrease, or negate the medicinal effects of traditional medications being taken. The CNL must educate the staff to be aware of such interactions. For example, garlic and ginko can increase the effect of some anticoagulants, while goldenseal can decrease the effectiveness; women who are on oral contraceptives may be surprised if also taking St. John's Wort to fight depression, as it may also render the contraceptives ineffective (Ehrlich, 2011).

Herbs are unregulated and there are no standard doses, so it becomes imperative for the admission nurse to deliberately ask if the patient takes any vitamins or herbs, since many people do not think of them as medicine. On the other hand, when traditional treatment plans are not working or are not fully effective, the CNL might suggest CAM to the staff as well as the interdisciplinary team. This can be especially true for patients with refractory pain, such as cancer patients or those with migraine headaches. Together the staff nurse and the CNL might evaluate the success or failure of combined treatment care plans. If it proves that the CAM is unsuccessful, exploration of other CAMs is deemed necessary.

In addition to the traditional route of using evidence-based research, today's nurse needs to also inquire about the possibility of CAM for patients. The CNL might be wise to include educational programs on this topic, so that staff will be prepared for this additional inclusion in medicine in today's world.

TABLE 9.1 Knowledge Management

CATEGORY	WEIGHT
B. Knowledge Management	**5%**
1. Applies research-based information	
2. Improves clinical and cost outcomes	
3. Utilizes epidemiological methodology to collect data	
4. Participates in disease surveillance	
5. Evaluates and anticipates risks to client safety (e.g., new technology, medications, treatment regimens)	
6. Applies tools for risk analysis	
7. Uses institutional and unit data to compare against national benchmarks	
8. Designs and implements measures to modify risks	
9. Addresses variations in clinical outcomes	
10. Synthesizes data, information, and knowledge to evaluate and achieve optimal client outcomes	
11. Demonstrates accountability for processes for improvement of client outcomes	
12. Evaluates effect of complementary therapies on health outcomes	

Used with permission from the Commission on Nurse Certification.

Conclusion

The CNL certification exam covers a broad range of content related to knowledge management (Table 9.1). Clinical instructors and nurse educators continually educate and impart knowledge to students, nurses, and administration. The dilemma lies in having them retain and store this knowledge. Knowledge management promotes learning, the acquisition of new knowledge, and a systematic way of retaining this resource for future use. Acknowledging that explicit knowledge is easily retained and documented, we give credence to tacit knowledge within the minds of the most experienced nurses and seek ways to keep their knowledge and experience if they leave the institution. If we do not retain what we have discovered and learned, we will forever be reinventing the wheel.

Having discussed the various methodologies for obtaining data, the CNL synthesizes this data and applies it to developing improvement on the microsystem. Knowledge management permits quality improvement throughout the unit, strengthening practice and protocols, utilizing the latest in technology, and creating and strengthening a professional staff capable of continuing to acquire assets of knowledge. The CNL is continuously accountable for patient safety, HCAHPS results, and the discretionary use of CAMs on the microsystem. The future success of all of the above depends on how the acquisition of knowledge is stored and retained. Well-managed knowledge will serve to strengthen both the microsystem and the organization, enable both to avoid repetition of problems, and store valuable evidence from research, readily accessible for practice when needed.

Resources

Agency for Healthcare Research and Quality. (2010, November 4). AHRQ awards $34 million to expand fight against healthcare-associated infections. *U. S. department of health and human services. Press Release.* Retrieved January 21, 2012, from http://www.ahrq.gov/news/press/pr2010/haify10pr.htm

Agency for Healthcare Research and Quality. (2012). *Patient safety primers—Root cause analysis.* Retrieved January 23, 2012, http://psnet.ahrq.gov/primer.aspx?primerID=10

American Association of Colleges of Nursing. (2007). *White paper on the role of the clinical nurse leader.* Washington, DC. http://www.aacn.nche.edu/publications/white-papers/cnl

American Nurses Association. (2011). *Code of ethics for nurses with interpretative statement.* http://ana.nursingworld.org/MainMenuCategories/EthicsStandards/CodeofEthicsforNurses/Code-of-Ethics.aspx

Commission on nurse certification. (2007). *Clinical nurse leader. Standards of conduct.* Retrieved January 22, 2012, from http://www.aacn.nche.edu/cnl/certification/SOC.pdf

Curley, M. (1998). Patient-nurse synergy: optimizing patient outcomes. *American Journal of Critical Care, 7*(1), 64–72.

Dunn, L. (2011). Studer group: Raising HCAHPS is about more than better service. *Becker's hospital review.* Retrieved from http://www.studergroup.com/dotCMS/knowledgeAssetDetail?inode=713350

Ehrlich, J. (2011). *Herbal medicine. University of Maryland medical center.* Retrieved February 26, 2012, from http://www.umm.edu/altmed/articles/herbal-medicine-000351.htm

Fenter, T., & Lewis, S. (2008). Pay-for-performance initiatives. *Supplement to Journal of Managed Care Pharmacy. 14*(6, Suppl. C), S12–S15.

Harris, J. L., & Roussel, L. (2010). *Initiating and sustaining the clinical nurse leader role. A practical guide.* Sudbury, MA: Jones & Bartlett Publishers.

Hughes, R. (2008, April). *Patient safety and quality: An evidence-based handbook for nurses: vol 3.* AHRQ publication no. 08-0043.

Institute for Healthcare Improvement. (2012, January 20). *Disease specific care for common comorbidities.* Retrieved January 22, 2012, from http://www.ihi.org/search/pages/results.aspx?sq=1&k=Risk%20Assessment%20Tool%20For%20CHF

Melnyk, B., & Fineout-Overholt, E. (2005). *Evidence-based practice in nursing & health-care. A guide to best practice.* Philadelphia, PA: Lippincott Williams & Wilkins.

Morath, J., & Turnbull, J. (2005). *To do no harm. Ensuring patient safety in health care organization.* Foreward by Lucian L. Leape. San Francisco, CA: John Wiley & Sons.

National health care safety network. (2011). About NHSN. Home page. *Centers for disease control and prevention.*

Topinková, E., Mádlová, P., Fialová, D., & Klán, J. (2009). New evidence-based criteria for evaluating the appropriateness for drug regimen in seniors. Criteria STOPP (screening tool of older person's prescriptions) and START (screening tool to alert doctors to right treatment). *Vnitřnie lékařství, 54*(12), 1161–1169.

Wilcox, J. (2012). Failure mode effect and analysis—Nursing. *Phillips Learning Center.* Retrieved January 23, 2012, from http://www.theonlinelearningcenter.com/Catalog/product.aspx?mid=6357

World Health Organization. (2012). The clinical knowledge cycle. *Image source page.* Retrieved February 1, 2012, from http://www.who.int/management/general/knowledge/en/index.html

10

Health Promotion, Disease Prevention, and Injury Reduction

Sally O'Toole Gerard

The stage is set for an unprecedented chapter in the history of nursing, as factors impacting health promotion and disease prevention come together in a time of great need. Health care has begun a new era of reform with an emphasis on prevention of illness, rather than treating existing diseases as they occur. The need for this change in ideology is apparent in the explosion of preventable conditions and associated illnesses. Obesity, for example, illustrates the impact of a preventable condition with a ripple effect that will greatly impact the health care resources of the future. The clinical nurse leader (CNL) stands poised to encompass health promotion and risk reduction in diverse settings to support individuals, families, and the American health care system.

Health promotion and risk reduction take on a variety of diverse scenarios for the master's-prepared generalist. Today's CNLs have expanded beyond the original vision of acute care and include community/public health, home health, outpatient settings, long-term care, hospice, and more (Stanley, 2010). Considering the variety of settings, CNLs can be involved in primary, secondary, and tertiary disease prevention in an array of clinical situations. The needs of the population being served in the CNL's particular microsystem will drive the specific approach to ensure positive patient outcomes. The CNL assumes the responsibility for those patient-centered outcomes through the assimilation and application of evidence-based information to design, implement, and evaluate appropriate health promotion interventions for individuals (American Association of Colleges of Nursing [AACN], 2007).

The complexity and fragmentation of the current health care system supports the role of the CNL as an advocate in the arena of health promotion and risk reduction. Integrating research, technology, best practice models, and individualized family care within a fast-moving, outcome-driven health care environment requires the CNL to practice to the fullest extent of the role. This chapter will review significant themes of health promotion and provide examples of CNL activities related to health promotion, risk reduction, resource management, and the common challenges of maintaining optimal health.

Health Promotion and Healthy People 2020

The impact of health promotion efforts by health care members is supported by the identification of national health issues. Key resources for health care providers include the U. S. Department of Health and Human Services (USDHHS) publications of Healthy People: National Health Promotion and Disease Prevention Objectives for health promotion programs. The Healthy People initiative provides science-based, 10-year national objectives for improving the health of all Americans. The program has established benchmarks for three decades and monitored progress over time to encourage collaboration across sectors, guide individuals in health decisions, and measure the impact of prevention activities (Healthy People, 2011). The vision of this work is to establish a society in which people live long and healthy lives (see Table 10.1 for additional details of the latest report, Healthy People 2020 [HP 2020]).

TABLE 10.1 Healthy People 2010 Summary

HEALTHY PEOPLE 2020	RELEASED IN DECEMBER 2010
Mission: Healthy People strives to	• Identify nationwide health improvement priorities • Increase public awareness and understanding of determinants of health, disease, and disability and opportunities for progress • Provide measurable objectives and goals that are applicable at the national, state, and local levels • Engage multiple sectors to take action to strengthen policies and improve practices that are driven by the best available evidence and knowledge • Identify critical research, evaluation, and data collection needs
Overarching goals	• Attain high-quality, longer lives free of preventable disease, disability, injury, and premature death • Achieve health equality, eliminate disparities, and improve the health of all groups • Create social and physical environments that promote good health for all • Promote quality of life, healthy development, and healthy behaviors across all life stages
Health measures: 4 categories will serve as indicators of progress toward the HP 2020 goals	• General health status • Health-related quality of life and well-being • Determinants of health • Disparities

Source: Healthy People (2011).

The HP 2020 initiative empowers CNLs, in all settings, to be aligned with the nation's health care priorities, focus areas, and goals. This most recent report continues to support all aspects of health promotion and gives specific guidance to the nurse's role. Undoubtedly, the CNL's academic preparation has introduced the Healthy People data as a valuable resource. These professionals can incorporate the mission, vision, and goals of HP 2020 into their own approach to health promotion as appropriate to their population. The CNL is strategically positioned to partner with individuals to initiate and maintain healthier lifestyles focusing on the human response to symptoms and diagnoses (Carranti, 2010). This collaboration of a national vision with a CNL who can individualize care, utilize resources, and support the uniqueness of the human response to health is invaluable to the challenge of attaining the HP 2020 goals.

The CNL Role in Health Promotion, Risk Reduction, and Disease Prevention

Regardless of the microsystem for which the CNL is responsible, the work of health promotion requires a multitude of skills. The CNL must have a strong theoretical foundation in health promotion. Not only does the master's curriculum introduce course content in health promotion, but the CNL also integrates the curriculum of epidemiology, health policy, research, health assessment, pathology, and pharmacology to be a clinical expert in designing care. The goal of this care is to allow for an optimal level of wellness. The application of this knowledge is supported through practicum experience, which specifically involves health promotion activities and patient/family education. Effective health promotion, risk reduction, and disease prevention also require effective teaching and evaluation skills and knowledge, including knowledge of available resources, teaching, and communication methods and learning principles (AACN, 2007). A patient scenario is introduced and

---

BOX 10.1
Patient Scenario

Mrs. Louis, a 56-year-old Haitian woman, is admitted to the emergency room with a chief complaint of severe headache.
Clinical data of note:

Blood pressure: 220/118 mmHg

Pulse: 90 bpm

Respirations: 22/minute

Temperature : 97.9°F

ECG: normal

Routine lab work unremarkable with the exception of a random glucose of 245 mg/dl

Body mass index: 32

Other client information: Patient is non–English speaking, works full time as a maintenance worker for a large hotel, and lives with multiple family members, including a spouse and children of varied ages. Her father died of a heart attack, age unknown, and her mother died of unspecified causes at the age of 79. She has medical insurance through her employer. She has no private physician in the community.

(continued)

> *(continued)*
>
> **Treatment** The patient is monitored for a number of hours. She is started on an antihypertensive and given a prescription to continue the medication after discharge. Prior to discharge, the patient is informed that she had high blood sugar and was prescribed a medication to treat this as well. She is told to follow up with a physician in the community in 1 week. Her teenage son acts as the interpreter for the patient. She is given written instructions for discharge from the emergency room regarding her medications and follow-up treatment. No appointment was made with a primary care provider (PCP) for her follow-up.
>
> **Patient Follow-Up** The patient filled the two prescriptions believing both were to treat the cause of her headache, which she vaguely understood to be high blood pressure. She took the medications daily until the bottle was finished, at which time her headaches had ceased. She had no understanding of her new diagnosis of diabetes.
>
> Keep this patient scenario in mind as more commentary follows, including her readmission to the emergency department (ED) 2 years later.

discussed through the chapter to help illustrate how relatively common patient situations can benefit from a CNL's approach to health promotion (Box 10.1).

Levels of Prevention

Primary prevention involves measures to prevent illness or disease from occurring. For a CNL in the public health or occupational health arena, this could include exercise programs, nutrition programs, weight loss initiatives, smoking cessation, stress reduction activities, and increased awareness of the body's well-being. The HP 2020 data continue to cite exercise as a top goal for our country. In examining Mrs. Louis, we see that the adoption of regular exercise could have supported decreased weight, decreased blood pressure, stress reduction, and improved insulin utilization. This type of primary prevention can occur at the workplace, through churches, or other community organizations or health care–sponsored outreach programs. As CNLs continue to establish roles outside of acute care, the careful planning of culturally appropriate community programming and resource utilization is critical.

Secondary prevention refers to methods and procedures to detect the presence of disease in the early stages, so that the effective treatment can be initiated and complications decreased (Greiner & Edelman, 2010). Screenings of all types play a key role in secondary prevention. Cancer, cardiovascular, and diabetes screens are some of the most common. Heart disease is the leading cause of death in the United States, resulting in the death of 2,200 Americans daily, many of whom were unaware of their condition (American Heart Association, 2011). A screening program for Mrs. Louis could have alerted her to the presence of hypertension, hyperglycemia, or possibly both. A referral to a health care provider for management of her health could have prevented the emergency room visit and facilitated more appropriate use of resources.

The insidious nature of these often asymptomatic diseases allows for microvascular and macrovascular damage, leading to poorer outcomes. Initiation of health-promoting behavior can have a great impact on the course of a disease. Categories of prehypertension and prediabetes offer evidence-based research on the impact of behavior modification. Studies on prediabetes indicate that lifestyle interventions can reduce the rate of conversion to type 2 diabetes from 30% to 43% (Ackerman & Marrero, 2007). As the incidence of these types of diseases increases, CNLs in all areas of health care can be instrumental in developing age-appropriate, culturally appropriate, and accessible programs that promote health, reduce disease burden, and improve outcomes.

Tertiary prevention refers to prevention strategies needed after a disease or condition has been diagnosed in an attempt to return the client to an optimum state of health (Kaser & Grossman, 2011). This type of prevention can also occur in a variety of CNL settings. Acute care of the patient with coronary artery bypass graft (CABG), stroke, asthma, and cancer treatment are just a few of many types of tertiary care. Often this type of care includes a team of professionals such as physical therapists, dietitians, occupational therapy, social workers, case managers, and more. The CNL has a vital role in the coordination of care within the interdisciplinary group.

Barriers to Health Promotion/Risk Reduction

The Healthy People documents have some overarching goals, one of which is to increase the quality and years of healthy life for an individual. Members of the health care team can support this goal in a variety of ways, but the ultimate determination for adopting positive health behaviors or lifestyle changes is ultimately up to the individual. The best possible scenario is that members of society are raised with healthy lifestyle choices such as a healthy diet, tobacco-free environment, adherence to personal safety standards, and high levels of exercise. Unfortunately, many individuals have lifestyle indicators that are inconsistent with health and risk reduction. For this reason, it is commonly necessary for health care professionals to educate and support individuals and families in the adoption of behavior changes. CNLs may have studied a variety of theoretical models of behavior change, such as the health belief model and Pender's health promotion model.

A classic model of examining how people intentionally change their behaviors is described in Prochaska's work on behavior change, which is based on the study of addictions. It may be referred to as the transtheoretical model of change. The concepts and phenomenon of intentional change within an individual were studied to uncover more depth to support professionals in their appreciation of successful change (Prochaska, DiClemente, & Norcross, 1992). This research produced a theory of stages in the process of change: precontemplation, contemplation, preparation, action, and maintenance (see Table 10.2). These stages are not linear, but spiral in nature, in which an individual may vacillate, moving forward and back with a varying degree of success toward change. The concepts of this model can be associated with other theoretical models of behavior change, all of which support an evolving and individualized approach to change.

TABLE 10.2 Stages of Change

STAGE OF CHANGE	DESCRIPTION
Precontemplation	Individuals are not considering change within the next 6 months. They may be resistant, have a lack of knowledge, or be overwhelmed by the problem.
Contemplation	Individuals are seriously thinking about changing within the next 6 months, but because of ambivalence, they may remain in this stage for years
Preparation	Individuals are seriously planning to change within the next month and have already taken some steps toward action
Action	This stage involves overt modification of the problem behavior; can last from 3 to 6 months
Maintenance	This period begins after 6 months of continuous successful behavior change. Individuals can remain in maintenance from 3 to 5 years and still experience temptations to relapse and often do revert to the behavior.

Source: Prochaska et al. (1992).

Let us take, for example, the CNL's role in adoption of healthy lifestyles regarding use of tobacco products. A CNL involved in public health or community health may assess the population/microsystem being served and provide educational interventions to deter individuals from trying tobacco products. Programming would be individualized to the target group, age appropriate, culturally appropriate, and may involve some type of incentive program. This primary prevention is the preferred situation, in which a person does not adopt a lifestyle that is inconsistent with health. For those in the community who do use tobacco, a series of cessation initiatives would also be individualized and deemed appropriate to the active smokers. In most cases, a CNL would have a diverse team of professionals to plan, implement, and evaluate program efforts. This team should analyze available data related to national, state, and local smoking trends, effectiveness of previous interventions, and available evidence for optimal outcomes related to tobacco use. For those smokers who are not ready to enter the action phase, the interventions can fuel the contemplative stage, as they understand the consequences of their actions, although they are not ready to change.

In the acute care setting, a tobacco user who had been in the precontemplative stage, in which there is no intention of changing behavior, may be catapulted into the action phase by an acute health issue. A heavy smoker who is admitted to the hospital with shortness of breath and diagnosed with pneumonia may be strongly motivated to take action, quit smoking, and commit to a smoke-free life. The concerns of serious health issues, cancer, and death that were present in the precontemplative phase may now be actualized into a readiness to take action. Although the person may truly be committed to quit, the maintenance phase often requires work to prevent relapse. Because many health-related behaviors truly stem from a physical and psychological addiction, relapse is the rule rather than the exception (Prochaska et al., 1992). The CNL can maximize success in the maintenance phase through patient education, preparing the client for the struggles of maintenance and offering strategies to promote success. Again, utilizing the resources of an interdisciplinary team in the acute care environment and in the community supports health promotion.

Health Care Literacy

The issue of health care literacy challenges all aspects of health promotion and risk reduction. On a national level, this issue is gaining traction through a variety of sources. The Healthy People initiative, the Institute of Medicine (IOM), and the Centers for Disease Control are some of the national leaders in highlighting the importance of this central health issue, which goes beyond the ability to read. Health care literacy is the capacity to obtain, process, and understand basic health information and services to make appropriate health decisions (Baur, 2011). The Office of Disease Prevention and Health Promotion (ODPHP), USDHHS launched a National Action Plan to Improve Health Literacy (the "Action Plan") to draw attention to limited health literacy as a major public health issue (Baur, 2011). This collaborative work from a multitude of public and private sector organizations provides a framework to identify the most important actions to take to improve the society-wide problem of limited health literacy. The Action Plan outlines strategies for all disciplines to address this widespread problem and work to support a more health-literate society.

Nurses in all settings have a vital role in improving health care literacy, and CNLs in particular can be leaders in this initiative. In the complex setting of our current health care system—namely polypharmacy, ambiguous health recommendations, unclear medication instructions, insurance forms, multiple medical specialists, and medical terminology—navigating the health care system is challenging in the best of situations. Add to that an individual's illness, comprehension of medical issues, varied cognitive abilities, fears, cultural conditioning, vision, and hearing loss, and you have a vastly difficult situation for most people. Now add the complexity of poor health care literacy and the outcomes can be quite problematic. Clearly communicated information to support health issues would seem to be a foundation for navigating this maze toward good health.

As the vision of the CNL is to have direct contact with individuals receiving care, the comprehensive assessment of knowledge, literacy issues, cultural circumstances, and spiritual and socioeconomic factors is essential to support health. Through discussions with patients, families, members of the health care team, and community services, the CNL can support individualized care of complex patients. Through increased awareness of literacy issues and utilization of the Action Plan's resources, CNLs and all team members can support the vision of this work. The vision has been summarized in three points: A health-literate society is one that (a) provides everyone with access to accurate and actionable health information, (b) delivers person-centered health information and services, and (c) supports lifelong learning and skills to promote good health (Baur, 2011). The specific goals of the Action Plan are broad and lend support to CNLs in all settings. You may access these goals at www.health.gov/communication/literacy.

Let Us Go Back to Mrs. Louis

Admission Scenario

Two years after her ED visit described previously, Mrs. Louis is admitted back to the ED. She had not been feeling well for a few days and began to have chest pain on a Friday night while working at her housekeeping job in the local hotel. A family member in attendance helps to communicate this information to the ED staff and shares the patient's medical history of being treated for headaches due to high blood pressure. She is admitted for a cardiac workup and to rule out a myocardial infarction. She is admitted to the cardiac telemetry unit at 3 a.m. on Saturday morning. The nursing report from the emergency room gives a medical history of hypertension but notes that the patient's blood sugar is 536 mg/dl, and a new diagnosis of type 2 diabetes is assumed to be present.

Arrival at Inpatient Unit

The patient arrives at the unit sleepy with no family members present. The English-speaking nurse orients the patient to the room and tries to elicit some basic information for the admission process in addition to the objective data about her patient such as vital signs, weight, and physical assessment data.

Day 1: On Saturday at 8 a.m., the hospitalist assigned to this patient obtains her medical records from her previous ED visit 2 years earlier and notes that the type 2 diabetes was diagnosed at that time. The communication regarding this patient now changes from "new onset diabetes" to "a 2-year history of diabetes in which the patient was noncompliant in follow-up as instructed by the ED staff."

Family members were updated on the status of the cardiac testing and also told that the patient had indeed done the right thing by being evaluated for chest pain, but that it was most likely caused by her high blood sugars. The family stated they did not know she had blood sugar problems. In response to this conversation, the nurse gave the family information on diabetes, which was written in English.

Day 2: On Sunday, Mrs. Louis has a new nurse. This nurse recieved the following information about Mrs. Louis:

- Testing for a myocardial infarctive (MI) was negative.
- She had a 2-year history of hypertension and diabetes
- The patient was being treated with an antihypertensive, and blood pressure was now within acceptable limits
- Blood glucose was still high, measuring in the high 300 range and was being treated with oral medicines and insulin
- The patient was scheduled for a stress test, and pending the results of that test she may be discharged
- This nurse was also told that the family had been given information on care for people with diabetes

Discharge Planning

Later in the day, when the charge nurse, who is in a CNL program, receives an overview of the patient, she questions the nurse caring for Mrs. Louis regarding discharge planning. The primary nurse responds by saying she had just met the patient but that the patient was negative for an MI and had a 2-year history of her medical issues but was noncompliant. In addition, the patient did not seem to speak English and the family was not present at this time, but that it was reported to her that patient education had been done the previous day. The nurse in charge of the unit then brought up the following questions to the more novice nurse:

- Have you spoken directly to the patient to assess what she may or may not know about her diabetes? (The patient did not know she had diabetes at all and did not know that the high blood pressure for which she was previously treated was a lifelong condition.)
- What language does the patient speak? (Creole)
- Have you checked the hospital's education database to provide the patient with information in her own language? (It was not available but was retrieved from the reputable government website.)
- Did you utilize the telephone interpreter system to communicate with the patient rather than using a family member to interpret? (No)
- Does the patient know how to check blood sugar and have the equipment to do so at home? (No, she did not know she had diabetes.)
- Have you discussed with the physician what medications the patient will go home on and how the team can best educate her about this plan? (No)
- Will she go home on insulin and does she know how to administer the medication? (Subsequent findings: the doctor would discharge her on insulin and no teaching had been started.)
- With what outpatient and community resources can we connect her with to develop a deeper understanding about caring for herself and managing her two chronic conditions? (The hospital has a comprehensive outpatient diabetes management program at a nearby location, which the staff nurse knew little about.)
- Did you know there are social workers and nursing care managers who are available by request on weekends to support our safe discharge of this patient? (The novice nurse did not know this.)
- Have you notified the dietary department to come and speak regarding the dietary implications of both diabetes and hypertension? (Requesting a dietary consultation for a patient is an independent nursing function.)
- What risk factors for heart disease can you identify in this patient and how can you address them? (Patient has many modifiable risk factors for heart disease.)

On the basis of collaboration with her nursing peers, the primary nurse provided the patient with appropriate educational materials regarding diabetes, hypertension, and risk factors for related cardiovascular disease. After providing this information in the patient's language and asking her to review it, the nurse utilized a telephone interpreter system to communicate more effectively regarding these complicated issues. It became clear to this nurse that the patient clearly did not understand the information provided by the ED about her conditions and follow-up care on her last admission. The nurse also assessed that the patient seemed to be illiterate even in her own language. In discussing discharge with the health care team, the physician shared that the patient would be discharged on insulin and a variety of oral medications; would need to check blood sugar regularly; and should be advised to follow a low-salt, calorie-restricted diet and exercise regularly to promote weight loss. The physician made no reference to the health care organization's comprehensive outpatient diabetes education center, but did make the referral for when it was requested by the primary nurse.

When the nurse had accurate knowledge of the discharge plan and a more accurate assessment of the patient's needs, she worked with the various members of the team to properly prepare the patient for discharge, including connecting the patient with the outpatient diabetes office, where the patient would be seen the following day. Prior to discharge, the nurse worked with the patient and family on the procedures needed to check blood sugar and safely administer insulin. Knowing that insulin is a high-risk medication, and in light of this individual's situation, the nurse advocated that social services provide visiting nurse services to support the transition of the patient to her home environment. The nurse had previously been told that the patient did not qualify for home services because she was not homebound. This patient was discharged Sunday evening with a plan that addressed her immediate safety needs, her limited comprehension of her complex conditions, basic technical skills on necessary procedures, and outpatient resources to bridge the continuum of care and support long-term behavior changes to decrease the risk of associated illnesses.

The situation described for Mrs. Louis is based on actual facts of a particular patient; these scenarios present themselves in varied settings every day. Without an assessment of individualized needs, including knowledge levels and health care literacy components, the system that works to treat and heal can go very much off course. The complexity of the health care system coupled with the complexity of a diverse population of consumers requires insightful and open-minded nurse leaders to improve care. In this scenario, Mrs. Louis could have been discharged with a longer list of instructions that she did not understand, leading to future admission for stroke, uncontrolled diabetes, or hypertension. The health care community could once again seek to blame Mrs. Louis for being noncompliant rather than examining their own system. The opportunities for health promotion and risk reduction with Mrs. Louis are vast, but they are not simple. Managing chronic illness, adopting health-promoting lifestyle changes, and eliminating risks such as smoking, sedentary lifestyle, and obesity are challenging in the best of situations. Often these situations are more complicated by low literacy, language barriers, cultural considerations, finances, family dynamics, and a lack of desire. These difficult situations are best optimized by nurses who welcome the challenges presented and collaborate with patients, families, and health care team members to provide care.

The CNL's Role in Risk Reduction and Patient Safety

Measures of health care quality and outcomes have become an integral part of the nursing profession from the bedside to the boardroom. Measures of patient outcomes, financial outcomes, and transparency of organizational quality measures have forever changed the health care playing field. Much of this change can be attributed to landmark reports from the IOM and the work of The Joint Commission regarding patient safety (IOM, 2009). The work of these organizations has been part of the impetus for the American Association of Colleges of Nursing (AACN) to bring the vision of the CNL to reality. For this reason, it is logical that patient safety is at the core of the CNL role. Concepts of health promotion and disease prevention are aligned with patient safety to maximize the most positive patient outcomes in any health care setting.

The Joint Commission is dedicated to a safe health care environment and is a valuable resource for practicing CNLs. Annual patient safety goals for acute care and ambulatory care help all health care leaders to prioritize initiatives to improve the environment, which seeks to care for, help, and heal people of infinite diversity. Some of the very public reports regarding health care mistakes that have resulted in injuries and death have spurred a new level of awareness from the public, regarding risks of seeking care. Media reports of wrong-site surgeries, fatal and near-fatal medication errors, and lethal hospital-acquired infections are plentiful, not to mention Internet access to credible or less credible information. Nonetheless, these factors all add up to a new era of public awareness of safety issues in health care settings. CNLs should be very knowledgeable of The Joint Commission's annual goals, which can be found at www.jointcommission.org.

The influence of patient safety metrics cannot be minimized in the role of today's health care settings, and the CNL must possess not only an understanding of these metrics but also an ability to share that understanding with direct care providers in all settings. Nurses have traditionally been a profession of caregivers who were not educated in data measures, run charts, control charts, and histograms. These types of data may be involved in the "dashboard" measures of their care area. These are the areas that have been chosen for a particular unit to measure the quality of care in that area. Patient satisfaction, fall rates, infection rates, and so on may be posted on a monthly or quarterly basis for staff to evaluate. For many, the direct link between the care they provide every day and those metrics of quality are not well connected. The CNL and others who are often accountable to those measures have a vested interest in a staff of professionals and ancillary caregivers who can provide safe, high-quality care and can understand the metrics surrounding that care in a measurable way. Dashboard indicators should also be aligned with the strategic mission of the organization, and so the direct link can be made from the bedside to the boardroom.

The running scenario of Mrs. Louis in this chapter is a very familiar and relatively uncomplicated situation considering the complex conditions encountered in all areas of health care. Our population of health care consumers is aging rapidly and living longer. Multiple chronic diseases, polypharmacy, complex social issues, lack of adequate health care coverage, and spiritual needs can complicate the care of persons in all settings. The relatively new role of the CNL originated in the current and future need to have someone directly involved in care who can see "the big picture."

TABLE 10.3 Health Promotion and Disease Prevention Management

CATEGORY	WEIGHT
C. Health Promotion and Disease Prevention Management	**5%**

1. Teaches direct care providers how to assist clients, families, and communities to be health literate and manage their own care

2. Applies research to resolve clinical problems and disseminate results

3. Engages clients in therapeutic partnerships with multidisciplinary team members

4. Applies evidence and data to identify and modify interventions to meet specific client needs

5. Counsels clients and families regarding behavior changes to achieve healthy lifestyles

6. Engages in culturally sensitive health promotion/disease prevention intervention to reduce health care risks in clients

7. Develops clinical and health promotion programs for individuals and groups

8. Designs and implements measures to modify risk factors and promote engagement in healthy lifestyles

9. Assesses protective and predictive (e.g., lifestyle, genetic) factors that influence the health of clients

10. Develops and monitors holistic plans of care that address the health promotion and disease prevention needs of client populations

11. Incorporates theories and research in generating teaching and support strategies to promote and preserve health and healthy lifestyles in client populations

12. Identifies strategies to optimize client's level of functioning

Used with permission from the Commission on Nurse Certification.

Conclusion

The conditions of society are ever changing as are the needs of that society. Nurses have always been at the forefront of health promotion and continue to be strengthened in that role with the CNL. The liberal education for the master's prepared generalist supports the vast array of settings for the CNL throughout the health care continuum. The CNL certification exam covers many of the concepts of health promotion that are applied in a variety of clinical situations (Table 10.3). The practicum experience of CNL students allows for practical application of the multiple and diverse roles described. As we stand on the edge of health care reform, all citizens have a vested interest in how health care can be safer, more cost effective, less fragmented, and focused on health promotion rather than on disease treatment. Our current resources are being burdened with many preventable illnesses, and primary prevention is critical to the health of our nation. Achievement of improved outcomes must take into account issues of health literacy.

As CNLs are establishing practice in a number of health care settings, national resources can help to recognize and focus care based on patient safety goals, health care indicators, and best-practice publications. From public health, school settings, acute care, outpatient facilities, and long-term care, the CNL has vast opportunities to make improvements. The skill set acquired through a liberal education at a graduate level prepares these expert clinicians for the challenge.

Resources

Ackerman, R., & Marvero, D. (2007). Adapting the Diabetes Prevention Program Lifestyle intervention for delivery in the community. *The Diabetes Educator, 33*(1), 68–78.

American Association of Colleges of Nursing. (2007). *White paper on the education and role of the clinical nurse leader*. Washington, DC. Retrieved from http://www.aacn. nche.edu/publicaitons/Whitepapers/ClinicalNurseLeader07.pdf

American Heart Association. (2011). *Heart disease and stroke statistics–2011 update: A report from the American Heart Association*. Retrieved from http://circ.ahajournals. org/content/123/4/e18.full.pdf

Baur, C. (2011). Calling the nation to act: Implementing the national action plan to improve health literacy. *Nursing Outlook, 59,* 63–69.

Carranti, B. (2010). CNL role in health promotion and disease prevention. In J. Harris, & L. Roussel (Eds.), *Initiating and sustaining the clinical nurse leader role: A practical guide* (pp. 197–218). Sudbury, MA: Jones & Bartlett Publishers.

Greiner, P., & Edelman, C. (2010). Health defined: Objectives for promotion and prevention. In C. Edelman & C. Mandle (Eds.), *Health promotion throughout the life span* (pp. 3–21). St. Louis, MO: Elsevier.

Healthy People. (2011). *About healthy people*. Retrieved from http://www.healthypeople. gov/2020/about/default.aspx

Institute of Medicine. (2009). *Informing the future–Critical issues in health*. Retrieved from http://www.iom.edu/~/media/Files/About%20the%20IOM/ITF2009.pdf

Kazer, M. K., & Grossman, S. C. (2011). *Gerontological nurse practitioner. Certification review*. New York, NY: Springer Publishing.

Prochaska, J., DiClemente, C., & Norcross, J. (1992). In search of how people change. Applications to addictive behaviors. *American Psychologist, 47*(9), 1102–1114.

Stanley, J. (2010). Introducing the clinical nurse leader: A catalyst for quality care. In J. Harris & L. Roussel (Eds.), *Initiation and sustaining the clinical nurse leader role. A practical guide*. Sudbury, MA: Jones & Bartlett Publishers.

11

Evidence-Based Practice

Cynthia R. King

Evidence-based practice (EBP) has been clearly defined in general and for nursing. However, there continues to be confusion about what EBP is and how nurses should utilize this important concept in clinical practice. It is important that clinical nurse leaders (CNLs) and other health care providers not confuse the term *research utilization* (RU) with EBP. RU refers to the review and critique of scientific research and then the application of the findings to clinical practice. EBP is a broader concept that includes using the best and current evidence, the patient's preferences, and the clinician's expertise or judgment. Thus, the three key components in EBP are:

- Use of evidence
- Patient preferences and values
- Clinical or professional judgment based on clinical expertise

It is also important to remember the difference between research and EBP. Research is conducted when there is a gap in knowledge, whereas EBP is conducted when there are one or more best practices that can be applied to clinical practice.

The American Association of Colleges of Nursing (2007) established a number of assumptions about the CNL role. EBP is threaded throughout a variety of assumptions, such as the following:

Assumption 2: Client care outcomes are the measure of quality practice

Assumption 3: Practice guidelines are based on evidence

Assumption 5: Information will maximize self-care and client decision making

Assumption 6: Nursing assessment is the basis for theory and knowledge development

Basing nursing care on the best evidence is characteristic of clinical leadership. This is the expectation of CNLs as leaders.

The Evidence-Based Process

Once a CNL clearly understands the definition of EBP, it is crucial to understand the steps in the process. Most professional nurses have learned the research process during nursing school, but it is only in recent years that faculty have spent much time describing the EBP process and the difference between that and the research process. Table 11.1 displays the steps in the EBP process and the research process.

TABLE 11.1 EBP Process Versus Research Process

EBP PROCESS	RESEARCH PROCESS
Identify clinical problem	Identify clinical problem
Review literature/search for evidence	Review literature/search for evidence
Critique evidence	Design study
Synthesize evidence and patient view	Write research proposal
Implement evidence-based change	Obtain IRB* approval
Evaluate outcomes	Collect and analyze data
Present or publish findings	Present or publish findings

* Institutional Review Board.

As is shown in Table 11.1, both the EBP and the research process start the same way. The key to both processes is identifying a clinical question or issue. From there, the CNL must review the literature and obtain evidence (e.g., data from admissions or Human Resources). Only after the literature is reviewed can an individual decide if they need to conduct an EBP project or conduct research. The decision is based on whether there is a gap in knowledge (then the CNL designs research) or whether there are one or more best practices in the literature (then the CNL can conduct an EBP project). Although some of the middle steps are different, the final step should be the same in each process—disseminate findings via presentations or publications.

The Clinical Question or Issue

As seen in Table 11.1, both EBP and research start with a clinical question or issue. Therefore, a well-designed clinical question is crucial. Once CNLs learn how to design thorough clinical questions, they can easily design the remainder of the EBP (or research) project. Although most research and EBP books briefly describe the importance of the clinical question, Melnyk and Fineout-Overholt's (2011) seminal book on EBP provides an excellent chapter on developing the clinical question or issue. Not only do the authors describe the most common method for developing a clinical question (called PICOT), but they also provide a variety of examples of well-designed questions.

The most common way to develop the clinical question is using the PICOT method. By carefully developing each of the five components of the question, it helps to clearly articulate the question, which then drives the remainder of the steps of the EBP process. Table 11.2 helps to describe the various components of the PICOT method.

TABLE 11.2 The PICOT Method for Developing Clinical Questions

LETTER AND DESCRIPTION	EXAMPLE(S)
P = patient population/disease	Elderly with congestive heart failure; obese adolescents
I = intervention or issue of interest	A specific therapy or educational intervention
C = comparison intervention	An alternative therapy, placebo, disease vs. no disease
O = outcome	Outcome expected from therapy, patient outcome
T = time	The time it takes for intervention

While Melnyk and Fineout-Overholt (2011) provide an excellent description of PICOT, they also give a template to use for practice and many excellent examples. The more CNLs and professional nurses practice writing clinical questions, the easier it will become.

Where and How to Locate Evidence

Once the clinical question has been refined, the next step is to locate appropriate evidence in the literature. In general, CNLs and other disciplines will find the most current evidence in academic journals and by utilizing databases such as CINAHL, PubMed, and Medline. Other ways to access journals are via (a) the journal website, (b) a search engine (e.g., Google Scholar), (c) an electronic library, (d) Cochrane Databases (e.g., they contain systematic reviews), or (e) *British Medical Journal of Clinical Evidence* (e.g., it provides summaries of evidence with recommendations). Sometimes evidence or data is also found in other departments (e.g., admissions, physical therapy, human resources). Searching for evidence can be overwhelming. In order to increase the chances that CNLs and other disciplines access the right information, some of the following strategies can be implemented:

- Be familiar with and practice different methods for searching for evidence and data
- Search for literature reviews and meta-analyses
- Set up e-mail alerts to receive content lists of the most relevant journals
- Attend EBP workshops and conferences
- Set up a journal club

Melnyk and Fineout-Overholt (2011) provide detailed descriptions regarding how to search for evidence. They also provide specific websites for specific EBP databases and screenshots of how the databases and websites will look. Furthermore, they provide descriptions on specialized search functions. Because nursing schools often do not provide thorough lectures on searching literature, the information contained in the EBP book by Melnyk and Fineout-Overholt (2011) is even more valuable to CNLs conducting EBP projects.

Critically Appraising the Literature and Determining the Strength of the Evidence

Once the literature is obtained, it has to be synthesized and critically appraised. The literature may be quantitative or qualitative or both (e.g., mixed methods). There are many sources that list questions to ask when critically appraising the literature. Many of these questions are used in EBP projects but also in journal clubs. When appraising the literature, CNLs must also evaluate the literature for the strength of evidence or credibility.

There are different methods for CNLs to use to select the most credible evidence. The competencies developed by AACN for CNLs include a role to make point-of-care decisions on the basis of best possible evidence (AACN, 2007; Herrin & Spears, 2007). There are a variety of hierarchies that can be used to determine how credible the collected evidence is. Each of these hierarchies has different levels. Some are designated by letters (A–D or A–F) and some are designated by numbers (e.g., Level 1–Level 4 or Level 1–Level 7). Melnyk and Fineout-Overholt (2011) recommend using a hierarchy with seven levels based on the design as follows:

- Level 1: Systematic review or meta-analysis of randomized controlled trials (RCTs) and evidence-based clinical practice guidelines
- Level 2: One well-designed RCT (randomized controlled trial)
- Level 3: Quasi-experimental studies documented without randomization
- Level 4: Well-designed case–control and cohort studies
- Level 5: Systematic reviews of descriptive and/or qualitative studies
- Level 6: Single descriptive and/or qualitative studies
- Level 7: Expert opinion and/or expert committee reports

As described, CNLs must have the skills to critically appraise the literature gathered for the EBP project. Critical appraisal involves the structured process of examining research in order to determine its strengths and limitations and therefore the relevance it should have in addressing the clinical question. Moreover, CNLs need to understand the difference between quantitative and qualitative articles and data. Quantitative studies investigate clinical questions that involve the collection of data in numeric form, whereas qualitative studies involve the collection of data in nonnumeric form (e.g., using words in forms such as personal interviews, observation). Although the terminology used to describe whether evidence is quantitative or qualitative is slightly different, it is still important that CNLs learn to critically appraise both quantitative and qualitative evidence.

CNLs are not only expected to develop and implement EBP projects, but they are also required to partner with patients/families and other disciplines to improve patient outcomes within their microsystem. There are many different ways to use evidence to improve patient outcomes. For example, CNLs may use evidence to (a) start journal clubs, (b) start nursing grand rounds, (c) develop or update policies and procedures, or (d) create care pathways or protocols.

Use of Measurement Tools During the Implementation of the EBP

As CNLs are accountable for health care outcomes in a particular microsystem, unit, or setting, it is crucial they accept responsibility for the assimilation and application of evidence to design, implement, and evaluate client plans of care with staff nurses. When working with staff nurses on plans of care for patients, it is important to teach staff nurses how to locate current practices and evidence as well as measurement tools to apply to plans of care. Frequently in practice settings, assessment tools are used for clinical decisions because they have been used in that microsystem or setting for many years. This does not mean the tool is the most appropriate for that patient population or acuity of patients. Thus, one key skill that CNLs may need to teach staff nurses is how to locate measurement tools for assessment that are reliable and valid and are based on solid evidence. It may be that while searching, reviewing, implementing, and evaluating a new assessment tool for a specific microsystem, the staff nurses and CNLs discover that the new measurement tool may actually be best applied in multiple microsystems, the mesosystem, or throughout the entire organization.

Putting Evidence Into Practice

Once the literature has been critically appraised and one or more of the best practices have been identified, it is time to put the evidence or best practice into the clinical practice. However, there continue to be barriers for staff nurses and CNLs in implementing EBP in the practice setting. Some of these barriers include:

- Lack of staff understanding about EBP and research
- Failure to understand importance of EBP and research in the clinical setting
- Difficulty in determining a clinical question or issue
- Lack of time and/or competing priorities
- Lack of knowledge and skills related to searching current literature
- Lack of access to library and/or computers
- Lack of support from administration (e.g., director of nursing, chief nursing officer)
- Lack of money for EBP and research projects

Despite potential barriers, there are many different types of interventions or best practices that can be implemented as part of EBP. It seems simple to say that CNLs should apply the "best evidence" in a clinical decision. However, it is crucial to remember that the EBP involves considering the patient's concerns and preferences. Thus, CNLs need to use their good clinical judgment as well as the current evidence and the way in which it is most relevant to a specific patient's concerns.

There are definite advantages to CNLs overcoming barriers and creating a culture where patient care is based on evidence. Some of the more global advantages include (a) increased professionalism, (b) increased collaboration, (c) decreases in length of stay and costs, and (d) increased patient safety and quality of care. Besides conducting a specific EBP or nursing research project, there are specific strategies that CNLs can use to create a culture where patient care is based on evidence. Some of these strategies include

- Ensure all policies and procedures are based on the latest research-based literature
- Start a journal club on the unit for staff nurses
- Post a summary of research studies on a topic of interest to staff
- Update staff on the latest evidence in short staff gatherings (e.g., 15 minutes)
- Link quality indicators to EBP
- Invite nursing faculty members to unit meetings or to help with a project
- Mentor staff nurses who have to complete EBP activities for school or clinical ladder

Results of Intervention and Evaluation

After implementing a change based on the critical appraisal of the literature for a specific period, the CNL needs to analyze the results and evaluate the implemented change. The CNL may be analyzing a wide array of important outcomes. Some of these may include patient health outcomes, provider and patient satisfaction, efficacy, and economic analysis. The question is, how does a CNL apply the results of the project to patient care? For instance, are there patient differences (e.g., biological, socioeconomic) that may diminish the response to the intervention? Based on the evaluation, the CNL may need to alter the intervention slightly, expand the intervention to other settings, or decide the intervention is not appropriate for this clinical setting.

Communication of Results in a Collaborative Manner

Although any nurse with the appropriate knowledge and skills can implement EBP in a clinical setting, most staff nurses are not taught these skills. However, if they do learn how to search for best practices and evidence (e.g., finding reliable and valid measurement tools for assessment), rarely are staff nurses taught how to disseminate and communicate their findings to other nurses and disciplines. CNLs, however, learn how to use leadership skills as well as interdisciplinary collaboration and communication skills to successfully help staff communicate important EBP and research results within the microsystem, clinical setting and, specifically, to other disciplines. There are a variety of options for dissemination both for CNLs and staff nurses. A number of these may include the following:

- Journal publication
  - full paper
  - short report/letter
  - news item
  - editorial

- Conference
  - local/national/international
  - poster
  - oral presentation
- Report to funder
  - publish as a report
- Set up conference or seminar
  - within department
  - area or regional meeting
  - national
- TV/Lay press
  - hospital newsletter
  - newspapers, radio
- Internet
  - podcast
- CD–ROM
- Teaching

TABLE 11.3 Evidence-Based Practice

CATEGORY	WEIGHT
D. Evidence-Based Practice	**8%**
1. Communicates results in a collaborative manner with client and health care team	
2. Uses measurement tools as foundation for assessments and clinical decisions	
3. Applies clinical judgment and decision-making skills in designing, coordinating, implementing, and evaluating client-focused care	
4. Selects sources of evidence to meet specific needs of individuals, clinical groups, or communities	
5. Applies epidemiological, social, and environmental data	
6. Reviews datasets to anticipate risk and evaluate care outcomes	
7. Evaluates and applies information from various sources to guide client through the health care system	
8. Interprets and applies quantitative and qualitative data	
9. Utilizes current health care research to improve client care	
10. Accesses, critiques, and analyzes information sources	
11. Provides leadership for changing practice based on quality improvement methods and research findings	
12. Identifies relevant outcomes and measurement strategies that will improve patient outcomes and promote cost-effective care	
13. Synthesizes data, information, and knowledge to evaluate and achieve optimal client outcomes	

Used with permission from the Commission on Nurse Certification.

What is most important is to disseminate findings in some manner. If nurses do not disseminate the results of EBP and research projects, nursing knowledge will not advance. Additionally, other staff and CNLs will not have access to best practices that have been developed at other institutions. Thus, the last step of the EBP project is not analysis of the results, but dissemination of the findings.

Conclusion

Understanding and using EBP is a part of the leadership role of CNLs (Table 11.3). It is imperative that CNLs understand the EBP and research processes and be able to describe them to staff nurses. It is part of the CNL's role to be sure that he or she creates a culture of evidence. The steps in the EBP process have been described here as well as other strategies that can be used to assist CNLs in creating a working environment based on evidence.

Resources

American Association of Colleges of Nursing. (AACN). (2007). *White paper on the education and role of the clinical nurse leader.* Washington, DC: Author.

Aveyard, H., & Sharp, S. (2011). *A beginner's guide to evidence based practice in health and social care professions.* New York, NY: Open University Press, McGraw Hill.

DiCenso, A., Guystt, G., & Ciliska, D. (2005). *Evidence-based nursing: A guide to clinical practice.* Philadelphia, PA: Elsevier.

Herrin, D., & Spears, P. (2007). Using nurse leader development to improve nurse retention and patient outcomes: A framework. *Nursing Administration Quarterly, 31*(3), 231–243.

Malloch, K., & Porter-O'Grady, T. (2006). *Introduction to evidence-based practice in nursing and health care.* Boston, MA: Jones & Bartlett Publishers.

Melnyk, B., & Fineout-Overholt, E. (2011). *Evidence-based practice in nursing & healthcare* (2nd ed.). Philadelphia, PA: Wolters Kluwer: Lippincott Wilkins and Williams.

Powers, B. A., & Knapp, T. R. (2010). *Dictionary of nursing theory and research* (4th ed.). New York, NY: Springer Publishing Company.

Schmidt, N. A., & Brown, J. M. (2012). *Evidence-based practice for nurses: Appraisal and application of research.* Boston, MA: Jones & Bartlett Publishers.

12

Advanced Clinical Assessment

Grace O. Buttriss

The skills of advanced clinical assessment are essential for the clinical nurse leader (CNL) to master, comprehend, and perform on clients within their individual microsystems. The information acquired from the clinical assessment will provide the CNL with the data needed to continuously monitor client care and enhance the quality of ongoing care. Client assessments require competent observation techniques, clinical reasoning skills, and individual consideration of all cultural aspects related to their care. Linguistically appropriate services must be provided, and religious beliefs and genetics should be considered in planning all client care. These specific components will provide the CNL with the foundation to collect and differentiate, verify and organize the collected data, and initiate the documentation of client data.

Advanced clinical assessment also includes the collection of data about an individual's past and current health status as well as their health promotion and disease prevention strategies. The state and concern of the whole person is considered to be the foundation of holistic health. Holistic health views the total mind, body, and spirit and interdependent and functioning as a unit. A client's health status depends on all areas working together to promote an individual's optimal health (Jarvis, 2012).

Designing, Coordinating, and Evaluating Plans of Care

The advanced clinical assessment commences with the collection of data related to an individual's current and past health care condition. This process involves the initial client survey and the collection and analysis of both subjective and objective data. The information obtained in conjunction with the client's health care record and diagnostic information will be utilized to formulate an individual client database. The database will provide a baseline for client care and an ongoing assessment of the client response to all medical and nursing interventions that are executed.

The database also provides the CNL with the foundation for formulating both clinical judgments and diagnoses through the process of diagnostic reasoning. These components are essential for client care planning with the advanced clinical physical assessment serving as the foundation for this process.

Additionally, the CNL will coordinate the process of risk reduction for assigned clients and will refer to the "Guide to Clinical Preventive Services," which is updated annually for the evidence-based, gold-standard recommendations used for populations. These recommendations are associated with specific, proven screening, counseling, and preventive strategies (Jarvis, 2012).

The CNL will also use the Healthy People 2020 Leading Health Indicators to coordinate client care. These indicators are identified every decade to communicate the high-priority health issues for individuals living within the United States. It is important to include them in providing care for clients within the CNL's microsystems. They can be utilized to guide clients and support the promotion of health and avoiding preventable illness by empowering individuals to make informed health choices (HealthyPeople.gov, 2012). These 12 leading health indicators have associated actions that can be taken by individuals and communities to address the importance of promoting health improvement to support the maintenance of a healthy lifestyle (Box 12.1).

The CNL is responsible for designing, coordinating, and evaluating the plan of care for all individuals within their assigned microsystems. This plan of care should be synchronized with the entire health care team in order to identify expected client outcomes and evaluate ongoing achievement of these outcomes.

BOX 12.1
Healthy People 2020 Leading Health Indicators

- Access to health services
- Clinical preventive services
- Environmental quality
- Injury and violence
- Maternal, infant, and child health
- Mental health
- Nutrition, physical activity, and obesity
- Oral health
- Reproductive and sexual health
- Substance abuse

(HealthPeople.gov, 2012)

Developing a Therapeutic Alliance With the Client

The CNL begins the clinical assessment by developing a therapeutic alliance with his or her assigned clients. This alliance begins with the first client encounter and continues throughout their affiliation. The client is always considered to be the principal source for personal information and this is identified as primary data. Additional information obtained about the client from family members, support persons, members of the health care team, diagnostics, or the utilization of current research are considered to be secondary or indirect sources of data. These secondary sources are important, but should always be validated for accuracy.

The exchange of health care information between the CNL and the client can be achieved by many techniques, including observation, one-on-one client interviews, past medical records, and through physical assessment techniques. The client interview is a structured form of communication that provides the basis for acquiring specific client information related to his or her current needs and symptoms. The procedure is conducted to obtain a confidential, comprehensive health history and should be held in a private and comfortable setting, if possible, for both the CNL and the client. The comprehensive health history should include those items found in Box 12.2.

BOX 12.2
Comprehensive Health History

- Biographic data
- Present health or history of present illness
- Medications/allergies
- Medical/surgical history
- Family history/genogram
- Review of systems
- Psychosocial history
- Diagnostic results

The present health or history of present illness is the reason the client is currently seeking care. This relates to the client's description of what he or she is experiencing and the signs and symptoms related to his or her decision to seek medical attention at this time. There are eight critical characteristics used to summarize the client's presenting symptoms (see Box 12.3):

BOX 12.3
Characteristics to Describe Symptoms

- Location
- Character or quality
- Quantity or severity
- Timing

- Setting
- Aggravating or relieving factors
- Associated factors
- Client's perception

The mnemonic PQRSTU can also be used to organize the client's symptoms (see Box 12.4).

BOX 12.4
Mnemonic for Symptoms

- P: Provocative or palliative
- Q: Quality or quantity
- R: Region or radiation
- S: Severity scale
- T: Timing
- U: Understand patient's perception of problem

(Jarvis, 2012)

Current medications, including over-the-counter medications and any supplements, dosages, and frequency should also be recorded for the client. Allergies to medications are also important and should be included. The specific type of allergic reaction is important to clarify and record during the data collection. An immunization history should also be determined and documented for any client seeking care.

The client's past medical and surgical history are significant because of the potential effect on his or her current health. This history includes childhood illnesses; accidents or injuries; serious or chronic conditions; any hospitalizations, surgeries, obstetric history; last physical exam; dental, vision, hearing, or applicable screenings. The client's family history is essential to obtain and relate to his or her ongoing care and risk factors. A genogram is an important tool for the CNL to create for organizing and tracking a client's family history for a minimum of three generations (Jarvis, 2012).

A review of systems is performed on each client to evaluate the health condition of systems and to assess the effectiveness of his or her individual health promotion practices. According to Jarvis (2012), the review of systems should include subjective and objective data areas (see Box 12.5).

BOX 12.5
Review of Symptoms

- General health status
- Skin
- Hair
- Head
- Eyes
- Ears
- Nose and sinus
- Mouth and throat
- Neck
- Breast
- Axilla
- Respiratory
- Cardiovascular
- Peripheral vascular
- Gastrointestinal
- Urinary
- Male and female genital
- Musculoskeletal
- Neurological
- Hematological
- Endocrine
- Pain
- Nutrition

A mental status examination that includes cognitive functioning data should be included with all advanced clinical assessments and should evaluate those areas listed in Box 12.6.

BOX 12.6
Mental Status Examination

- Consciousness
- Language

(continued)

(*continued*)
- Mood and affect
- Orientation
- Attention
- Memory
- Abstract reasoning
- Thought process
- Thought content
- Perceptions

Substance use and abuse should be a component of the assessment based on the negative effects on many body systems. The most commonly used questionnaires include the CAGE, which takes less than a minute to complete, but is less effective in women and minorities. The TWEAK questionnaire helps to identify at-risk women who drink, particularly pregnant women. This tool measures the client's tolerance to alcohol consumption (see Boxes 12.7 and 12.8).

BOX 12.7
CAGE Questionnaire

- Have you ever felt you should *cut down* on your drinking?
- Have people *annoyed* you by criticizing your drinking?
- Have you ever felt bad or *guilty* about your drinking?
- Have you ever had a drink first thing in the morning to steady your nerves or get rid of a hangover (*eye-opener*)?

BOX 12.8
TWEAK Questionnaire

- **Tolerance**—Number of drinks tolerated or how many drinks it takes to feel "high."
- **Worry**—Do you have close friends or relatives worried about your drinking in the past year?
- **Eye-opener**—Do you sometimes take a drink in the morning when you get up?
- **Amnesia**—Has a friend or family member ever told you things you said that you could not remember saying?

(*continued*)

- **Kut Down**—Do you sometimes feel the need to cut down on your drinking?

  Score 2 points for Tolerance and Worry
  Score 1 point for others.
  >2 points = a drinking problem, and further assessment is needed
  (Jarvis, 2012)

Intimate partner violence, child abuse, and elder abuse are health problems that the CNL must recognize and assess. These assessments include both physical and sexual violence and psychological and emotional abuse or neglect, or financial abuse. There are multiple tools and questionnaires available for use in all clinical settings. The key is recognition and documentation to include photography and the use of forensic terminology for legal purposes.

A sleep assessment should be conducted on every client due to the detrimental cumulative effects of sleep loss and disorders on the body systems. The assessment should consider factors associated with sleep loss to include insomnia caused by age, medications, psychological factors, gender, and lifestyle. An assessment of sleep apnea should also be included to help in determining the cause of the sleep loss (Wilson & Giddens, 2009).

A functional assessment is an additional important assessment tool and should be completed on each client to evaluate his or her activities of daily living. This information will provide the CNL with the information to evaluate the client's self-care abilities, current and past relationships, and his or her individual coping techniques. A functional assessment is performed during the interview phase and should include those areas listed in Box 12.9.

BOX 12.9
Functional Assessment

- Self-Esteem/Self-Concept
- Activity Level/Exercise
- Sleep/Rest
- Nutrition/Elimination
- Interpersonal relationships/Resources
- Spiritual resources
- Coping/Stress management
- Use of tobacco, alcohol, illegal substances
- Environment/Exposures
- Sexual history
- Abuse

(Jarvis, 2012)

Identifying Client Problems That Require Intervention

The advanced clinical assessment is a systematic data collection method that utilizes the techniques of:

- Inspection
- Auscultation
- Palpation
- Percussion

These techniques are organized according to the CNL's preference for head-to-toe (cephalocaudal) or the body system approach. These techniques are also prioritized on the basis of the client's current diagnosis and symptoms. The primary focus will be on the individual physiological system that correlates with the client's current symptoms and diagnosis (Smith, Duell, & Martin, 2012). The immediacy of the symptoms can also necessitate a change by performing a rapid and accurate focused review of systems to address the presenting urgent, potentially life-threatening client complaint.

The CNL will implement the nursing process to organize all nursing actions and interventions. This approach offers a systematic, problem-solving method for providing client care in all health care settings. The provision of client care will also be guided by the utilization of evidence-based practice concepts and practices. These concepts will promote quality client outcomes through the client interventions of the CNL.

Holistic Assessment

The advanced physical assessment is based on a holistic approach and a systematic method of problem solving and care planning identified as the nursing process. This method is goal directed and ensures that the client receives consistent, continuous, quality care. It also provides the foundation for professional nursing accountability while taking into account the input of the client's support persons and the entire health care team.

This process is put into practice to identify a client's health status and the actual or potential health care problems or needs of the client. It is used to diagnose and treat the human response to actual or potential health or illness problems (American Nurse Association [ANA], 1980).

The plan of care is developed for interdisciplinary and collaborative implementation with all members of the health care team.

A plan is developed to meet and deliver care based on identified areas utilizing the following components:

- Assessment
- Analysis/Diagnosing
- Planning
- Implementation
- Evaluation (Smith et al., 2012)

Client assessment is the first step in this process. This involves the establishment of a client database, skilled observation, and documentation of the findings. This is an essential step because subsequent components depend on the precision and consistency of the initial assessment process. The plan must also include the client's health values and beliefs, individual priorities, available resources, the urgency of the current health problem, and the proposed medical and nursing treatment plan.

Assessment is followed by the formulation of applicable diagnoses. This step involves critical thinking to develop all applicable diagnoses to guide ongoing client care.

The planning process involves priority setting and establishment of client goals and outcomes based on the client response. These include both short- and long-term goals that are written on the basis of the client and the health care team member's plans. This is based on the health care needs and is specific to each client.

The implementation or intervention stage provides for execution of the plan based on scientific principles to reach specific client goals. This is established from the clinical assessment of the client, data interpretation, client needs, goals, and outcomes.

The evaluation process assesses the client outcomes and goal attainment from the implementation phase. This is the final phase of holistic care and includes any changes to the plan based on the nursing evaluation. The treatment plan will be continuously reevaluated to determine whether it should be continued, modified, or terminated based on the client reassessment and general response. The CNL can significantly impact a client's overall health through implementation and follow-through of the individualized plan of care. This plan can influence a client's current lifestyle, promote healthy behaviors, and prevent the development of future disease processes.

The CNL can serve in the roles of client educator and care coordinator to promote an ongoing lifestyle of health promotion for clients. The role of patient educator is supported by professional standards and provides the client with consistency and individualized care. This plan of care should include mutually agreed upon client management of health, nutrition, exercise, medications, and lifestyle modifications to improve an individual's sense of well-being (Harris & Roussel, 2010).

Pathophysiology, Assessment, and Pharmacology

The pathophysiological alterations of the clients will be determined upon completion of an advanced clinical assessment of the client. Any health alterations will be diagnosed in conjunction with the members of the health care team and can be treated with a variety of therapies to include pharmacotherapy as required. The assessment should take into consideration the developmental stage of the client and his or her achievement of developmental milestones throughout the life span.

Clinical Judgment and Decision-Making Skills in Client-Focused Care

The CNL's use of clinical judgment is constant and must be dynamic while remaining goal-directed and client-centered. It involves collaborative care that can be universally applied through the implementation of a methodical approach to client care. It is essential that this approach involve gathering input from all members of the health care team to form a cohesive conclusion about future care.

CNLs are positioned, educated, and prepared to coordinate the total care of clients within their microsystems. This coordinated effort includes the use of clinical judgment and decision-making skills to develop, coordinate, implement, and evaluate comprehensive client care. The mastery of advanced clinical assessment techniques will enhance the decision-making process of client care and provide the information necessary to reinforce the decisions related to future care.

The CNL may use multiple methods to document the advanced clinical assessment based on the clinical agency's preference for documentation. A common method for organizing a client's clinical record is the use of SOAP notes.

- S—Subjective Data—the primary information provided by the client
- O—Objective Data—direct observations from sight, smell, touch, and hearing
- A—Assessment—interpretation, conclusions, potential diagnoses, actual, and potential problems
- P—Plan—diagnostic tests, therapeutic modalities, consults, and rationales (Seidel, Ball, Dains, Flynn, & Solomon, 2011)

Illustrations can provide a better explanation than a narrative description in conveying a client's pain location, radiation, or the size, shape, or location of lesions (Figure 12.1). They can also be used to document pulse amplitude and deep tendon reflexes (Seidel et al., 2011).

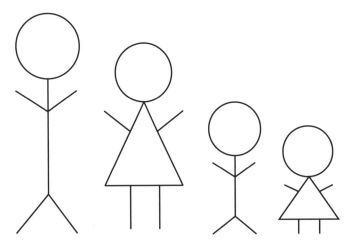

FIGURE 12.1 Put an "X" at each part of the body where you have pain.

Emergency or life-threatening conditions require the CNL to complete a rapid primary assessment to determine and manage life-threatening conditions. This rapid assessment should be completed within seconds, and the priorities should be established on the basis of pathophysiological processes and the ABCDEs as follows (see also Box 12.10).

- Airway—assessment and cervical spine stabilization
- Breathing—ventilation is assessed and assisted
- Circulation—assessed and bleeding is controlled
- Disability—assessment of neurological status
- Exposure—complete assessment unclothed

BOX 12.10
Level of Responsiveness: AVPU

- A—Alert
- V—Verbal stimuli: responsive to
- P—Painful stimuli: responsive to
- U—Unresponsive

The secondary assessment begins when stabilization of emergency conditions is under control. The assessment will include SAMPLE:

S—Symptoms

A—Allergies

M—Medications

P—Past illnesses

L—Last meal

E—Events preceding the precipitating event (Seidel et al., 2011)

Evaluating the Effectiveness of Pharmacological and Complementary Therapies

The CNL will use advanced skills assessment to evaluate the effectiveness of both the pharmacological and the complementary therapies ordered for his or her clients. These therapies will be monitored by use of clinical assessment techniques, diagnostics, and overall client responses to ordered therapies.

TABLE 12.1 Advanced Clinical Assessment

CATEGORY	WEIGHT
E. Advanced Clinical Assessment	**5%**

1. Designs, coordinates, and evaluates plans of care

2. Develops a therapeutic alliance with the client as an advanced generalist

3. Identifies client problems that require intervention, with special focus on those problems amenable to nursing intervention

4. Performs holistic assessments across the lifespan and directs care based on findings

5. Applies advanced knowledge of pathophysiology, assessment, and pharmacology

6. Applies clinical judgment and decision-making skills in designing, coordinating, implementing, and evaluating client-focused care

7. Evaluates effectiveness of pharmacological and complementary therapies

Used with permission from the Commission on Nurse Certification.

Conclusion

The role of the CNL is important for the provision of holistic care to clients. Advanced clinical assessment skills provide the CNL with valuable information to make ongoing decisions about client care. These skills correlate with the provision of quality practice and optimal client care outcomes to promote comprehensive care at all levels (Table 12.1).

Resources

American Nurse Association. (1980). *The nursing process*. New York, NY: Author.

Harris, J. L., & Roussel, L. (2010). *Clinical nurse leader role*. Sudbury, MA: Jones & Bartlett Publishers.

Healthy People 2020 Leading Indicators. (2012). Retrieved from www.healthypeople.gov/

Jarvis, C. (2012). *Physical examination & health assessment* (6th ed.). St. Louis, MO: Elsevier.

Seidel, H., Ball, J., Dains, J., Flynn, J. A., & Solomon, B. S. (2012). *Mosby's guide to physical examination* (7th ed.). St. Louis, MO: Elsevier.

Smith, S. F., Duell, D. J., & Martin, B. C. (2012). *Clinical nursing skills: Basic to advanced skills* (8th ed.). Boston, MA: Pearson.

U.S. Preventive Services Task Force. (2011–2012). *Guide to clinical preventive services 2011–2012*. Retrieved March 10, 2012, from www.ahrq.gov./clinic/prevenix.htm

Wilson, S. F., & Giddens, J. F. (2009). *Health assessment for nursing practice* (2nd ed.). St. Louis, MO: Elsevier.

13

Team Coordination

Bonnie Haupt

The *Future of Nursing: Leading Change, Advancing Health* report calls for interprofessional collaboration in health care: "As the delivery of care becomes increasingly complex across a wide range of settings, and the need to coordinate care among multiple providers becomes ever more important, developing well-functioning teams becomes a crucial objective throughout the health care system" (Institute of Medicine [IOM], 2010a). Historically, the health care delivery system has functioned in a practice of hierarchical order. The physician-driven orders have long been the model for the health care team in decision making. Little feedback or input was sought from other team members regarding the patient's plan of care. Health care team members are no longer operating in silos; they are working together for better patient care outcomes. Today's health care system involves active participation of all interprofessional team members when coordinating and delivering care. Physicians, nurses, lab technicians, health assistants, and physical therapists are a few of the direct care professionals coming together to improve patient stays, satisfaction, and outcomes. In the health care setting, patients are also interfacing with indirect care professionals who are members of the interprofessional team. Indirect team members may include dietary staff, medical clerks, pharmacists, clinical informatics, housekeepers, patient advocates, and leadership individuals, all of whom affect the patient's care.

Leading Teams

Strong leaders in nursing are needed to collaborate and build effective teams. It is essential for nursing leaders to act as full partners with direct and indirect health professionals, being accountable for establishing high-quality care outcomes, while working collaboratively with members of the interprofessional health care team. *Dorland's Medical Dictionary* (2007) identifies coordination as "[a] nursing intervention in the nursing minimum data set; action geared to the integration of multidisciplinary treatment plans with the goal of smooth, continuous patient or client care." Coordinating the required services will streamline the health care process, improve communication among providers, and improve patients interaction with the health care team.

The clinical nurse leader (CNL) is emerging as a strong leader and team coordinator in the health care system. Introduction of the CNL role into the health care setting has increased nursing membership's role in collaborating for patient care outcomes. The American Association of Colleges of Nursing (AACN) White Paper (2007) envisions the CNL role as designing, coordinating, and evaluating client care outcomes (p. 12). CNLs have taken a lead role in team collaboration and coordination, bringing all members of the interprofessional team together. For example, the following scenario highlights the CNL's role here.

A CNL on a 30-bed acute care unit has identified a patient who requires the coordination of his care. Mr. J, a 75-year-old male patient, was admitted yesterday to the unit with weight loss and failure to thrive. The medical team believes he has been aspirating. Mr. J has a medical history of hypertension, diabetes, alcohol use, is legally blind, and smokes one pack of cigarettes per day. Mr. J's visiting nurse has logged 10 out of the last 14 days with periods of hypotensive blood pressure. Mr. J complains that he has felt dizzy at times and unsteady on his feet this past week. It is noted that he has several cigarette burns on his clothes and lower extremities. His daughter is concerned about her father's living conditions, ability to care for himself, and overall health status. Mr. J lives alone in a two-story home and has been independent and active in the community up to 3 months before admission, when his wife of 50 years passed away. When coordinating care for Mr. J, what members of the interprofessional team should be included? The team might include a pharmacist, physician, registered nurse, care coordinator, dietician, psychiatrist, social worker, physical and occupational therapists, and let us not forget the patient and his family as active members of the health care team. Daily CNLs are charged with coordinating care teams for various patients in the health care system. These care teams focus on patient care, patient safety, and clinical outcomes. CNLs are involved with assessing and identifying needs, formulating plans, and implementing and objectively evaluating the outcomes.

CNL Curriculum Framework for Client-Centered Health Care

A master's-prepared education provides the CNL with the necessary skills and leadership abilities to form and lead effective teams. AACN (2007) identifies team coordination competencies necessary for success in the CNL curriculum framework for client-centered health care as delegation, supervision, interdisciplinary care, group process, handling difficult people, and conflict resolution.

Delegation

Health care professionals view delegation as a process of assigning a task or tasks to team members. The CNL must feel comfortable and confident in this role, whether assigning simple tasks to subordinates, or complex assignments to peers and executive leadership when working in teams. An important aspect of delegation is knowing your team member's skills, experiences, and competencies. The CNL should define interprofessional team member abilities and identify responsibilities that are appropriate to complete assigned tasks. If team members lack certain abilities, the CNL is responsible for educating individuals in proper processes and procedures.

Supervision

Supervision of team members is a vital component of the collaborative process, whether supervising the team member in a simple task or chairing a committee identifying flow issues affecting patient outcomes. The CNL, as team coordinator, is the individual who assumes accountability and responsibility for supervising and leading the team to a common goal. Acting as a coach and mentor, the CNL is responsible for not only team goals but also individual member goals. Seamless supervision leads to enhanced safety and well-being of patients and interprofessional team members in the health care environment.

Interdisciplinary Care

Interdisciplinary care is now referred to as interprofessional care, involving interacting, communicating, and collaborating with all members of the health care team. Establishing working relationships within the team is instrumental in team collaboration and coordination.

Care coordination in *Closing the Quality Gap: A Critical Analysis of Quality Improvement Strategies* (Agency for Healthcare Research and Quality [AHRQ], 2007) is defined as the deliberate organization of patient care activities between two or more participants (including the patient) involved in a patient's care to facilitate the appropriate delivery of health care services. Organizing care involves assembling personnel and other resources needed to carry out all required patient care activities, and is often managed by the exchange of information among participants responsible for different aspects of care.

Group Process and Communication

Lack of team communication can lead to medical errors. In 1999, the Institute of Medicine's (IOM, 2010b) *To Err Is Human: Building a Safer Health System* reported between at least 44,000 and as many as 98,000 patients die every year in U.S. hospitals because of medical errors. Communication failures and absence of teamwork is a common cause of inadvertent patient harm (Leonard, Graham, & Bonacum, 2010, p. 85). The CNL directs group process and utilizes technology, and evidence-based research to strengthen practice.

Demonstrating critical listening is instrumental in a group process. Team coordination and effective communication is essential to the delivery of optimum patient care and outcomes. Are the messages of all group members being heard? A collaborative team may be formed for any number of reasons. Once a member of the interprofessional team identifies patient safety concerns, a clinical or systems issue affecting patient care, a team can be formed. The team coordinator is responsible for assessing solutions and implementing process changes to improve patient care. Members of the interprofessional team come to the table for diverse reasons. Individuals may come with enthusiasm and passion for a project, with goals to promote practice changes or a personal experience compelling them to seek change. At times, it is possible that team members may be assigned by management or leadership and have no desire to participate in the project. Individual motives for participation may have an overall effect on the group. When creating an interprofessional team, it is crucial to select members who are representative of different interprofessional teams.

A collaborative approach is a joint effort with a common goal identified to improve patient care outcomes. Tuckerman and Jensen (1977) identified five stages of group development (see Box 13.1).

The first stage is known as the forming stage. This stage involves the team coming together. Team members are looking to the team coordinator and CNL to set the mission and group expectations. Team members are forming relationships, identifying how they fit in, analyzing whether their goals mesh with the team goals, and exploring the team's expectations of themselves. The team members are seeking a safe and trusting environment, where they can feel comfortable expressing their ideas and concerns. The forming stage may produce uncomfortable silence, until members establish trust. According to the U.S. Office of Personnel Management (1997) building an effective collaborative team requires establishing a common goal, trust, respect, open communication, role clarity, appreciating diversity, and balancing the teams focus.

The second stage, storming, is the stage that is potentially tumultuous, one where conflict may occur. There may be a lack of unity, struggles over leadership, and power in the group. The team coordinator is responsible for keeping team members on track during this phase. Questions and concerns over the mission, goals, and the group's progress will come under fire. To be successful and

---

BOX 13.1
Five Stages of Group Development

- Forming
- Storming
- Norming
- Performing
- Adjourning/Mourning

progress to the next stage, the team members must grow together, being flexible and respectful in their views to meet the group's goals.

The third stage is called norming. The group is now established. The ground rules and agendas have been set and everyone is on the same page. Team members feel they are working in a safe environment, where everyone's opinions and ideas are shared openly and valued.

In the fourth stage, performing, is where tasks are being completed. Team members are working together or independently in their assigned roles collaboratively. The group has identified individual strengths and weaknesses of the project and are working together to manage and guide the outcomes. O'Daniel and Rosenstein (2008) find that "[u]nlike a multidisciplinary approach, each member is responsible only for the activities related to their own discipline, formulating separate goals." The team coordinator brings all expert professionals together to share their progress and successes of research in terms of meeting the team goals. Team members are focused on problem solving, seeking solutions, and on long-term outcomes. All members of the team are exhibiting responsibility and accountability for the project or team objectives during this stage.

The final stage is identified as adjourning or mourning. Team members have achieved the group's mission or goals that were set forth. This stage involves termination of the group. Some team members may feel a sense of loss after working so closely for many hours on a project. It is important for the group to have a final meeting that includes time for goodbyes and includes recognition to all team members for their hard work.

The IOM (2003) reports the need to "Cooperate, collaborate, communicate, and integrate care in teams to ensure that care is continuous and reliable." The CNL is continuously assessing how teams are operating in the dynamic care environment. Are team members participating and engaging fully with new and innovative strategies and ideas? Are roles with the team clarified? What characteristics does the team coordinator envision in the team members? Are there personality conflicts between team members, or, possibly, time management issues? Do team members communicate openly and effectively? Are team members exhibiting responsibility and accountability for the project or team objectives? What are the goals or strategic initiatives the team is challenged with reaching? What barriers exist in terms of accomplishing the team's goals? Are completion time frames being met?

Handling Difficult People and Conflict

Conflict occurs in teams and between individuals when there is a disagreement over views or goals. If a conflict occurs, immediate and swift resolution and actions are needed to deffuse the situation. Handling difficult situations requires enhanced communication skills. As a team coordinator, the CNL must demonstrate effective leadership qualities, including proficient communication skills. Communication is the number one means in which health care professionals, patients, and caregivers interact. The CNL is aware of the verbal, nonverbal, and written messages that are being portrayed to the team members. Difficult situations may arise at any time or place in the health care environment. Interprofessional team members are confronted not only with difficult patients, caregivers, and families; they require the skill to communicate effectively with other members of the health care team. Highly effective communication skills will promote a transparent and positive work environment that will build trust and a culture of retention for the interprofessional team (Box 13.2).

Interprofessional Team Collaboration

The foundation of the CNL was based on a concept of interdisciplinary or interprofessional collaboration. The AACN White Paper clearly delineates the CNL as a key figure in the support of safe and patient-centered care from all professional groups. This concept has gained tremendous attention in health care recently, from training professionals in an interprofessional format to training of practicing care providers in the importance of team collaboration to provide a safe environment. This recent awareness identifying the critical role of interprofessional teams has led to the emerging resources now available. From leading government health care agencies to private consulting firms, this topic has clearly gained national attention. Innovative strategies such as simulation are being utilized in supporting safe communication of team members and may play a pivotal role in the future of how students and practicing professionals develop the skill necessary for high-functioning teams. Resources highlighting interprofessional education and team coordination may be useful to CNL students, practicing CNLs, and all professionals interacting with, and leading teams.

Professional health care organizations are also supporting interprofessional collaboration by establishing competencies for interprofessional collaboration as part of formal education. This report is inspired by a vision of interprofessional collaborative practice as key to the safe, high-quality, accessible, patient-centered care desired by all (AACN, 2011). Imagine a health care team that has strong understanding and respect for team collaboration upon entering their chosen field! Achieving that vision for the future requires the continuous development of interprofessional competencies by health professions students as part of the learning process, so that they enter the workforce ready to practice effective teamwork and team-based care (AACN, 2011). This restructuring of professional education can only enhance the patient-centered care teams in which the CNL functions.

BOX 13.2
Resources for Interprofessional Team Collaboration

http://simcenter.duke.edu/3Dteams

http://www.aacn.nche.edu/education-resources/ipecreport.pdf

http://www.IHI.org

http://collaborate.uw.edu

http://www.saferpatients.com

http://teamstepps.ahrq.gov

http://www.ahrq.gov

Conclusion

The AACN White Paper (2007) states,

> The CNL is responsible for the clinical management of comprehensive client care, for individuals and clinical populations, along the continuum of care and in multiple settings, including virtual settings. The CNL is responsible for planning a client's contact with the health care system. The CNL also is responsible for the coordination and planning of team activities and functions. In order to impact care, the CNL has the knowledge and authority to delegate tasks to other health care personnel, as well as supervise and evaluate these personnel and the outcomes of care. Along with the authority, autonomy and initiative to design and implement care, the CNL is accountable for improving individual care outcomes and care processes in a quality, cost-effective manner.

In 2010, the World Health Organization (WHO) published a framework for action on interprofessional education and collaborative practice. CNLs are coordinators of care in the health care team. "Collaborative practice happens when multiple health workers from different professional backgrounds work together with patients, families, careers and communities to deliver the highest quality of care" (WHO, 2010, p.13). Research shows that teams working collaboratively improve patient care outcomes. CNLs are at the forefront of implementing change in the health care setting, with the education and knowledge to promote collaborative practice. The CNL certification exam covers many aspects of team coordination that are critical to supporting positive change (Table 13.1). Collaboration should occur within and across settings, following patients throughout the health care system.

TABLE 13.1 Team Coordination

CATEGORY	WEIGHT
A. Team Coordination	**6%**
1. Supervises, educates, delegates, and performs nursing procedures in the context of safety	
2. Demonstrates critical listening, verbal, nonverbal, and written communication skills	
3. Demonstrates skills necessary to interact and collaborate with other members of the interdisciplinary health care team	
4. Incorporates principles of lateral integration	
5. Establishes and maintains working relationships within an interdisciplinary team	
6. Facilitates group processes to achieve care objectives	
7. Utilizes conflict resolution skills	
8. Promotes a positive work environment and a culture of retention	
9. Designs, coordinates, and evaluates plans of care incorporating client, family, and team member input	
10. Leads gap analysis to create cohesive health care team	

Used with permission from the Commission on Nurse Certification.

Resources

Agency for Healthcare Research and Quality. (2007). Closing the Quality Gap: A critical analysis of quality improvement strategies. Vol. 7: No 9.7. *Care Coordination. Technical Reviews*. Rockville (MD): Retrieved from http://www.ncbi.nlm.nih.gov/books/NBK44012

American Association of Colleges of Nursing. (2007). *White paper. Education and role of the clinical nurse leader*. Retrieved from http://www.aacn.nche.edu/publications/white-papers/cnl

American Association of Colleges of Nursing. (2011). *Core competencies for interprofessional collaborative practice*. Retrieved from http://www.aacn.nche.edu/education-resources/ipecreport.pdf

Coordination. (2011). *Dorland's medical dictionary for health consumers*. Retrieved from http://medical-dictionary.thefreedictionary.com/coordination

Institute of Medicine. (2003). *Health professions education: A bridge to quality*. Washington, DC: National Academy Press. Retrieved from http://www.nap.edu/openbook.php?record_id=10681&page=45

Institute of Medicine. (2010a). *The future of nursing: Leading change, advancing health*. Washington, DC: National Academies Press. Retrieved from http://www.rwjf.org/files/research/Future%20of%20Nursing_Leading%20Change%20Advancing%20Health.pdf

Institute of Medicine. (2010b). *To err is human: Building a safer health system*. Washington, DC: National Academy Press. Retrieved from http://www.iom.edu/Reports/1999/To-Err-is-Human-Building-A-Safer-Health-System.aspx

Leonard, M., Graham, S., & Bonacum, D. (2010).The human factor: The critical importance of effective teamwork and communication in providing safe care. *Quality Safety Health Care*. Doi: 10.1136/qshc.2004.010033

O'Daniel, M., & Rosenstein, A. H. (2008). *Patient safety and quality: An evidence-based handbook for nurses* (Chapter 33). Rockville, MD: Agency for Healthcare Research and Quality (US).

Tuckman, B., & Jensen, M. (1977). Stages of small group development. *Group and Organizational Studies, 2*, 419–427.

U.S. Office of Personnel Management. (1997). Building a collaborative team environment. *Work Performance Newsletter*. Retrieved from www.opm.gov/perform/articles/072.asp

World Health Organization. (2010). *Framework for action on interprofessional education and collaborative practice*. Geneva, Switzerland: World Health Organization. Retrieved from http://www.who.int/hrh/resources/framework_action/en

14

Economics and Finance
for the Clinical Nurse Leader

E. Carol Polifroni and Denise M. Bourassa

As the role of the clinical nurse leader (CNL) develops, the individual must be aware of the environment in which he or she works, the economic climate of the environment, the specific fiscal details related to the nurses (and ancillary personnel), the supplies used for care delivery, and the reimbursement expected for this care delivered. This economic lens is a challenge for most nurses, as they typically view the care they give as being separate from finance.

As the average age of the nurse is well over 45 years, many practicing nurses began work at a time when costs were not discussed or not even known. The philosophy that guided patient care delivery was "whatever the patient needs." Individuals remained in acute care facilities for weeks on end, neither short-term rehabilitation nor subacute facilities existed, and how much something cost was not a known variable. The world of retrospective payment existed for the institution and the nurse practiced within that environment.

In 2012, all that has changed. Economics are at the forefront. It is impossible to watch the evening news without reference to the gross domestic product, the ever-escalating costs of health care, and the increasing percentage of every American dollar spent on health care. Depending on the reference used, current health care costs range from 15% to 19% of the annual gross domestic product in the United States. This means that for every dollar spent, 15 to 19 cents of that dollar goes toward health care costs in this country. Are the outcomes expected with such an expenditure delivered? The obvious answer is no. Not when we live in an industrialized nation. Yet the Centers for Disease Control and Prevention (CDC) estimates that approximately 50,000 people are newly infected with AIDS a year (cdc.gov, 2011). In 2005 the United States ranked 30th in infant mortality, behind most European countries—Canada, Australia, New Zealand, Hong Kong, Singapore, Japan, and Israel (MacDorman & Mathews, 2009). And lastly, in 2009, the top four leading causes of death were heart disease, malignant neoplasms, chronic lower respiratory disease, and cerebrovascular diseases. These indicators are a reflection of lifestyle as much as they are of economics, and we continue to push death away as far as it will go (National Vital Statistics Report, 2011).

Thus, the context for our discussion and review is that, in the United States, we spend up to 18 or more cents of every dollar on health care. This is in comparison with per capita spending in other countries as noted in Figure 14.1.

In a recent study (Kwok et al., 2011) it was noted that nearly a third of elderly Americans had a surgical intervention during the last year of life, and most of these procedures occurred in the month before death. The culture of the United States is such that we aim to push death away and to avoid it at all possible costs. Regardless of your beliefs on death with dignity and a rational and dignified end to life, or the need to avoid death no matter what, the costs of such a belief need to be known and addressed (Kelly, 2011).

Is it right and is it just for finite dollars to be spent at the end of life, or is it more right and more just to spend those dollars at an earlier time in the health care cycle or on something altogether different? This chapter does not aim to answer these questions, but makes readers aware of the question and the components within the question, so that they understand economics and finance as they relate to health care.

In addition to the aforementioned statistics, total health spending is projected to comprise 18.7% of the gross domestic product by 2014 (Heffler et al., 2005). As a response to this, the CNL is called to make adjustments in practice that answer to reimbursement changes, staffing shortages, the increasing rate of uninsured Americans, and mandates that link quality and outcomes to reimbursement. Areas of direct potential impact that the CNL, at the frontline of health care delivery, can influence is in the area of cost/financial outcomes, specifically in the areas of length of stay, readmission rates, patient flow, and quality/internal process outcomes (Ott et al., 2009). As patients more often are becoming consumers and the health care industry is expected to perform in a fiscally prudent manner, it is important that the registered nurse of the future understand how finance and economics impact the care he or she gives at the bedside.

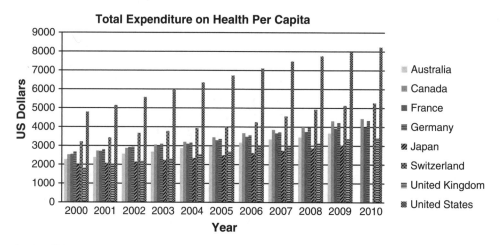

Source: OECD Health Data 2012.

FIGURE 14-1 Total expenditure on health per capita.

Cost Reduction and Standardization

Cost reduction for care delivery is a focus of a recent issue of *Hospitals & Health Network*'s (October 2011) financial fitness series. Moss advises that cost reduction be addressed in four phases. The first "is reducing variation by standardizing protocols. . . . Second is removing unnecessary care, including provider errors, preventable readmissions, avoidable conditions and unnecessary diagnostic tests. Third is cost restructuring to use the lowest cost setting and provider possible for each service. . . . The fourth is adopting a system of care strategy . . . such as medical homes and disease management . . . " (*H&HN*, October 2011, p. 30). There is a component of the CNL role in each of the four areas. Cost reduction is not the sole focus of the CNL, but as the CNL is the system's bridge between administration and the point of care, every strategy suggested has a component for the CNL role.

It is essential to note that the CNL must work toward standardizing protocols within his or her span of control. Within the hospital setting, the CNL needs to bring the need for standardized protocols to the attention of management and to facilitate committee activity from planning through the evaluation of the protocols. In an outpatient setting, protocols will drive services provided and costs. The CNL must educate the staff about the value of protocols and what it brings to them, as well as what it adds to the patient care. Reduction of provider errors is a key component of the CNL role, as he or she creates systems of care delivery that address ease of access, accuracy of use, and appropriate charging of cost to the right individual or center. The attention to preventable readmissions and unnecessary diagnostic tests is a key reason why the CNL is prepared with coursework and practice in assessment, pathophysiology, and pharmacology. They all relate to the cost of care provided in a very direct manner. Assigning the appropriate provider to care for a patient, in an inpatient or outpatient setting, also has a correlation to costs. Thus, the CNL must be keenly aware of which level of personnel/provider can do the job and be aware of the skill level of each individual within a role category. The last element that Moss addresses is disease management and the concept of the "medical home," a term for primary contact among multiple providers. Again, these are key roles of the CNL as they directly relate to cost and financial management within whatever type of setting the CNL is employed. Before we proceed further into this review, it is time to define terms that are imperative for the CNL to know (see Box 14.1).

BOX 14.1
Definition of Terms

Acuity: Level of intensity of care required by patients
Case mix: The mix (variety) of patients for whom care is delivered organized by specified characteristics (e.g., gender, DRG, payer)

(continued)

(*continued*)

Cost center: A microsystem responsible for providing services and monitoring the costs associated with such service provision

Diagnosis-Related Group (DRG): Group used by Medicare and other payers to determine reimbursement to organizations and providers

Direct costs: Costs that are directly related to the provision of a service; the cost can be specifically identified for an individual patient or activity

Expenses: Dollars owed as a result of both services delivered and organizational costs incurred in the delivery

First-party payers: Individual responsible for payment for services rendered

Gross domestic product: Market value of all goods and services produced (created) within a country in a specific period (www.en.wikipedia.org/wiki/Gross_domestic_product)

ICD-9-CM: International Classification of Diseases, Ninth Revision, Clinical Manifestations; used for documentation of diagnoses and procedures; in turn, used to assign a DRG and create patient charges

Indirect costs: Those costs of doing business that are not directly related to a specific individual, such as heat, electricity, overhead, water, and some administrative personnel

Length of stay: Time spent (number of days) in an organization receiving health care services

Medicaid: A program sponsored by states and federal government for low income and/or disabled individuals; services and payment are provided

Medical home: A concept initially designed in 1969 and now used to coordinate medical care among multiple providers

Medicare: A governmental program related to social security for the elderly

Outcome: The end product of an action

Private insurance: Third-party payers in the private marketplace not funded by government sources

Reimbursement: Dollars received by an organization or provider for services rendered

Revenue: Money received through the delivery of services

Retrospective/prospective payment: Prior to 1994, retrospective payment was a system used to reimburse hospitals for services delivered on the basis of cost without any foreknowledge; since 1994, prospective payment is a system wherein reimbursement to hospitals or other organizational entity is based on a DRG or ambulatory patient classification (APC)

Second-party payers: The agency providing the services also pays for the service

(*continued*)

Third-party payers: Governmental or private insurance entities who pay for all or some of the services provided

Volume: The number of beds occupied, procedures done, cases received, visits made, or other description of amount of services provided

Finances Within a Microsystem

The relevance of the terms found in Box 14.1 should be evident in their definition. Volume is the key factor in any discussion about inpatient or outpatient health care finance. Volume—the number of services provided, patients seen, or cases addressed—dictates the dollars available for care delivery. From these available dollars, revenue and all expenses incurred by the institution to deliver the care for a patient must be found. The revenue and expenses are typically assigned to an individual cost center for ease of monitoring and reporting. A cost center is a microsystem within the larger whole such as a unit (7 W), a service (outpatient cardiac rehab), or an entity. There are both direct and indirect costs associated with care. As noted, direct expenses are those directly related to care, such as the nurse caring for the patient, the supplies used for the needed dressing, food provided, and linen provided throughout the day. Indirect costs are still charged to the patient and they are those things that indirectly service the client, such as heat, water, physical space, aesthetics of the environment, and institution-wide electricity and equipment. Therefore, it is self-evident that the CNL must know the expected reimbursement, the planned length of stay on which the reimbursement is dependent, and the costs associated with the care provided.

In a direct relationship, the CNL is responsible and accountable for outcomes within the microsystem of care. Outcomes relate to conditions, incidence, and dollars as an end of the care delivered. The focus of this chapter is to achieve the desired clinical condition as an outcome within a defined dollar amount. The dollar amount is determined by the admitting diagnosis (DRG for patients for whom Medicare is the primary payer) and the length of stay associated with that DRG. Whether the length of stay for patient Y is less than the range provided, more than the range provided, or within the range provided, the reimbursement to the facility is the same. In other words, there is an incentive to the agency (not necessarily to the patient or the provider) for the individual to be discharged earlier than the defined range, or certainly within the defined range for which reimbursement will be provided. When the patient is discharged after the defined range without an approved comorbidity, no additional payments are made to the agency nor can the individual be charged a separate bill.

Thus, the key variables for the CNL are two: length of stay and utilization of services and supplies within that length of stay. These are two variables that the CNL must understand and influence. Variation may exist in how length of stay is managed and services allocated, but the purpose here is to know that this management is essential for cost-effective care delivery.

Within the supply component, it is imperative that the CNL know the costs of all supplies, those that are deemed direct, meaning they are then appropriately charged to the patient for whom the supplies are used, and the access to the supplies. The CNL needs to ensure that all users know how the charging system—bar code or otherwise—works, when charges are appropriate, and the relationship between the charge assigned to the correct payer and the financial solvency of the organization in which the care is provided. CNLs can also influence the correct use of these charging systems by being sure that they are user friendly to those responsible for charging the patient. The CNL cannot be responsible for every charge, as it is often incurred by the specific caregiver, but the CNL can design, or redesign, the system for ease of use, so that charges are appropriately made and not circumvented. Additionally, the CNL is responsible for educating the staff on system use, monitoring its utilization, and making changes as needed.

The indirect costs, while needing modest management, are typically outside the realm of responsibility for the CNL. Indirect costs are usually allocated to a cost center's operating budget on the basis of percentage, occupancy, or a simple mathematical formula created and monitored by the finance department of the agency. The CNL, however, is accountable for just utilization of the indirect costs.

Reimbursement

Within the reimbursement component, from which revenue is derived, the CNL needs to be aware of the payer mix of the patients. Payer mix, as noted earlier, is the specific payment mechanisms for all patients and when combined together is known as the case mix. The CNL needs to be aware of who the payer is; in most instances it will be a third-party payer of either the government (Medicare, Medicaid, VA benefit) or private insurance such as Anthem Blue Cross Blue Shield. As with indirect costs, the CNL will not be responsible for monitoring the payment but is accountable for the knowledge of which payer is involved, so that costs are appropriately allocated, length of stay is closely monitored within the expected range, and services are delivered consistent with payer expectations and requirements. In the instance that the patient's bill is going to be paid by himself or herself (first-party payer) or the organization (second-party payer), the CNL's accountabilities remain the same; namely knowing and implementing measures to monitor costs and utilization of services. When charitable care is provided by the agency delivering the care, this is known as second-party payer. Even though the agency is paying the bill for the care, the CNL must ensure that the care meets the required standards and can be defended fiscally.

In an outpatient setting, ICD 9 codes are used to track expenses and services provided. The CNL in these settings is responsible for educating the staff about the appropriate codes, monitoring the system for recording the codes, and auditing the code utilization as needed. These activities require diligence and a developed system to ensure that items are not missed, and teaching moments are seized.

Patient acuity is the transition between revenue/expenses and the discussion of staff to provide care to the patients. Acuity determines the amount of care required. There are varied patient classification systems with which the CNL needs to be familiar. The key to all systems is validity and reliability. An external system may be adopted in its entirety and the data benchmarked with institutions of like size and patient population. If it is an internal system, the limitation is that it cannot be benchmarked against like institutions. However, with a specialized patient population, an internal system may work best. A standardized product that has been tailored/individualized to an agency may be an option as well. With all systems, regardless of origin, they must be reliable and valid, and the role of the CNL is to contribute to this process. If not reliable, valid, and utilized for staffing purposes, the nurses, in particular, will not see the system as useful and may sabotage its reliability through inflated assessments. Therefore, the system needs to be reassessed for reliability and validity on a regular basis. Everyone must be confident that the numbers determined by the system reflect the needs of the patients for whom the care is being delivered. When the system is reliable and individuals have confidence in it, the acuity system can be used to allocate staff with confidence. However, numbers are only numbers and must be used only as a guide, and the role of the CNL is to use the numbers with reasoned judgment, knowing the context of the specific situation at hand.

The role of the CNL is to educate the staff on the system and its uses as well as how to implement the system. Within this discussion, the reliability and validity of the system must be addressed. When an effective patient classification for acuity determination is implemented, the staff and patients benefit alike. Another list of words is shared, as these definitions guide the next area of discussion (Box 14.2).

Staffing and Scheduling

The outcome of this effective system is the design of a staffing matrix. The matrix is determined by the number of hours of care per patient day delivered by the system,

---

BOX 14.2
Staffing Terms

FTE: Full-time equivalent based on a 40-hour work week for 2080 hours per year; expressed as a 1.0 or a fraction thereof; a .5 FTE is one-half of 2080 hours or coverage for 20 hours per week; an FTE is not an individual but a position with hours associated with it.

HCPPD: Hours of care per patient day; a numerical expression of the amount of care a type of patient receives in a 24-hour period.

Productivity: The work product of a unit or individual based on the amount of work required and the hours available to deliver that care.

Staffing matrix: The number of staff assigned to work on a given shift on a given day.

Staffing mix: The mixture of licensed and unlicensed staff as well as the type of license; a staffing mix may be 70% licensed and 30% unlicensed, with 80% of the licensed staff being RNs and the remaining 20% possessing an LPN license.

---

not by each individual nurse. Most inpatient settings operate on a 24-hour basis. Inherent in this perspective is care delivered over a 24-hour period. Thus, if a patient classification system determines a patient's acuity is a category "four," this, by a previous determination, translates to requiring 6 hours of care per day. If they are at a "three," the care hours required are 4, a classification of a "two" may be 3 hours of care, and a category "one" is 2 hours of inpatient care over a 24-hour period, and this patient is ready for transfer to another facility or to home! (see Box 14.3).

It is important to explain and appreciate that the hours of care required are on a per-patient basis and represent an average (Finkler, Kovner, & Jones, 2007). The categories of the classification system, as reliable and valid as they may be, are not able to capture every patient need. Thus, in a category 4 or any category, the individual patient may require a few less minutes or a few more minutes. This is one of the driving reasons that nursing care is not reimbursed on a per-nurse basis or per-treatment basis as is medical care for physician providers. Nursing care requires a holistic assessment and determination of need. The fact that an individual has a fractured hip repaired with a hemiarthro- plasty means that a certain number of hours of care are required. However, if the patient has a cardiac condition as a comorbidity, additional hours may be

---

BOX 14.3
Example of Staffing Determinants Based on a Classification System

Using this approach, let us say we have 24 patients; 6 in each category.
  Using a simple multiplication process, we determine:

- the six category-4 patients require 36 hours of patient care (6 × 6)
- the six category-3 patients require 24 hours (6 × 4) of care
- the six category-2 patients require 18 hours (6 × 3) of care
- the six category-1 patients require 12 hours (6 × 2) of care

  The total hours of care required for all 24 patients is 84 hours of care in a 24-hour period.

  The management of the unit has previously determined that there is a 70/30 mix of licensed to unlicensed staff. This means that 70% of the hours of nursing care required for all 24 patients must be delivered by a nurse with a license, and 30% can be delivered by a patient care assistant, a nurse's aide, or other title for an individual without a license. 70% of 84 is 58.8 hours.

  If each nurse works 7 hours after breaks are deducted, the CNL divides 7 into 60 and knows that 8.4 licensed nurses are needed to provide the nursing care, along with an additional 3.6 nursing assistants to provide the remaining 25.2 hours of care.

  For this example, the CNL knows that 12 people must be assigned to work over the 24-hour period, and the staffing mix must be a minimum of 8.4 nurses and 3.6 nursing assistants.

required if the patient experiences a dramatic decrease in blood pressure. There is no known system that can capture this nuance. However, it is understood that the number of nurses and aides available on a given shift determines the maximum hours of care that can be delivered. As the CNL understands this patient/staffing matrix as a frontline contributor, they can and should act as an advocate for patients and staff when ratios are inadequately represented, as they can be in the real world.

A productivity ratio may be calculated to determine effectiveness of care delivery in terms of staffing. This number is calculated as hours of care needed divided by hours of care available. Thus, if 84 hours are needed and 84 hours of care are available, the productivity is 100%. There is an inherent fallacy in productivity numbers when a clock is utilized in patient care delivery as it is. However, it is important to understand how hours are calculated so that the CNL can understand when presented with these data.

TABLE 14.1 Health Care Finance and Economics

CATEGORY	WEIGHT
C. Health Care Finance and Economics	**5%**

1. Identifies clinical and cost outcomes that improve safety, effectiveness, timeliness, efficiency, quality, and client-centered care

2. Serves as a steward of environmental, human, and material resources while coordinating client care

3. Anticipates risk and designs plans of care to improve outcomes

4. Develops and leverages human, environmental, and material resources

5. Demonstrates use of health care technologies to maximize health care outcomes

6. Understands the fiscal context in which practice occurs

7. Evaluates the use of products in the delivery of health care

8. Assumes accountability for the cost-effective and efficient use of human, environmental, and material resources within microsystems

9. Identifies and evaluates high-cost and high-volume activities

10. Applies basic business and economic principles and practices

11. Applies ethical principles regarding the delivery of health care in relation to health care financing and economics, including those that may create conflicts of interest

12. Identifies the impact of health care financial policies and economics on the delivery of health care and client outcomes

13. Interprets health care research, particularly cost and client outcomes, to policy makers, health care providers, and consumers

14. Interprets the impact of both public and private reimbursement policies and mechanisms on client care decisions

15. Evaluates the effect of health care financing on care access and patient outcomes

Used with permission from the Commission on Nurse Certification.

Conclusion

The CNL has a very powerful role to fill when it comes to economics and health care finance. While not the manager, the CNL must understand finance to make the most appropriate decisions in regard to services provided, by whom and for what length of time. The CNL is on the frontline at the point of care delivery and must recognize his or her role in educating staff about resource utilization, making recommendations to management and other providers about disease management and use of standardized protocols, ensuring the systems are in place to reduce system error and assisting environments to reduce human error, assigning the appropriate provider to care delivery, and ensuring that all charges incurred are assessed and tracked to the appropriate cost center. Each of these is an essential function within the CNL role and all are directly related to finance and economics. No one factor is more important than any other. When achieved in combination, financial solvency is not assured, but it is certainly on the path to achievement. The Commission on Nurse Certification includes many topics of economics and finance in the certification blueprint for CNLs (Table 14.1).

Resources

Cleverly, W., Song, P., & Cleverly, J. (2011). *Essentials of health care finance* (7th ed.). Sudbury, MA: Jones & Bartlett Learning.

Finkler, S., Kovner, C., & Jones, C. (2007). *Financial management for nurse managers and executives* (3rd ed.). St. Louis, MO: Saunders.

Harris, J., & Roussel, L. (2010). *Initiating and sustaining the clinical nurse leader role.* Sudbury: MA, Jones & Bartlett Learning.

Heffler, S., Smith, S., Keehan, S., Borger, C., Clemens, M., & Truffer, C. (2005). *U. S. health spending projections, 2004–2014.* content.healthaffairs.org/content/early/2005/02/23/hlthaff.w5.74.citation web exclusive retrieved October 21, 2011.

Kelly, A. (2011). Treatment intensity at end of life-time to act on the evidence. *The Lancet.* doi:10.1016/S0140-6736 (11)61420-7

Kocharek, M., Xu, J., Murphy, S., Minino, A., & Kung, H. (2011). Deaths: Prelimanry data for 2009. NVSR www.cdc.gov/nchs/data/nvsr/nvsr59/nvsr59_04.pc

Kwok, A., Semel, S., Lipsitz, S., Bader, A., Barnato, A., Gawande, A., & Jha, A. (2011). The intensity and variation of surgical care at the end of life: A retrospective cohort study. *The Lancet.* doi: 10.1016/S0140-6736(11)61268-3

Larkin, H. (2011). Cutting expenses. *Hospitals & Health Network, 28–32.*

MacDorman, M. F., & Mathews, T. J. (2009). Behind international rankings of infant mortality: How the United States compares with Europe. *NCHS Data Brief, No. 23, November 2009.*

OECD Health Data 2012: Health expenditure and financing. OECD Health Statistics (database). www.oecd.org/health/healthpoliciesanddata

Ott, K., Haddock, S., Fox, S., Shinn, J., Walters, S., Haridin, J., …, Harris, J. (2009). The clinical nurse leader: Impact on practice outcomes in the Veterans Health Administration. *Nursing Economics, 27(6), 363–370.*

15

Health Care Systems/Organizations

Dawn Marie Nair

The clinical nurse leader (CNL) practice model and role were developed and implemented in collaboration with leaders in nursing education and practice to address the current and future needs of the health care system and, most importantly, to provide quality patient care outcomes. This chapter will review the current state of health care systems, organizations, unit-level health care delivery, and microsystems CNL competencies in these areas.

Current State of Health Care Systems/Organizations

It is no secret that our current health care system is in chaos. Many people are involved with patient care but working in silos, all working hard but not efficiently and not always safely. According to Lee and Mongan (2009), who elaborate on chaos in health care in their book *Chaos and Organization in Healthcare,* the answer is organization. Yes, simply put, but not easily solved. We know additional spending in health care is not the answer, so where should we begin? Understanding where the center or nucleus of health care environment is located may be the best place to begin organizing care. In every instance, the core of care is with a single patient, group of patients, and populations of patients. It is here that change in the way we provide care will have the greatest impact in organizing the chaos.

A CNL is directly involved and responsible for many aspects of care in the health care environment. Being in a position to make necessary changes to improve care can be an enormous challenge. To fully assess the system or environment, a CNL must have a clear understanding of the structure, function, and goals that are in place, from the top of the organization to the bedside. The basic health care system can be broken down to gain perspective. First, the structure of our health care system is composed of three essential elements; the frontline clinical microsystems, mesosystems, and the all-encompassing macrosystems. According

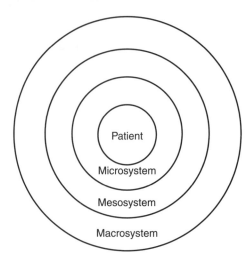

Source: Nelson et al. (2008, p. 371).

FIGURE 15.1   The structure of health care.

to Nelson et al. (2008), there are three fundamental assumptions in relation to these elements:

- Bigger systems (macrosystems) are made of smaller systems
- These smaller systems (microsystems) produce quality, safety, and cost outcomes at the frontline of care
- Ultimately, the outcomes of a macrosystem can be no better than the outcomes of the microsystems of which it is composed (Figure 15.1)

Leading Microsystems—A Role for the CNL

The term *microsystem* is used to describe the small, functional, frontline units that provide most health care to most people—and is essential to designing the most efficient, population-based services (Godfrey, Nelson, Wasson, Mohr, & Batalden, 2003). Clinical microsystems have become the focus for improvement of health care within our rapidly changing health care system/organizations. This approach can offer senior leaders a strategy and execution framework for competing in an increasingly competitive, data transparent, and value-seeking medical marketplace.

Why is the CNL a needed role in the health care system? First, it is a known fact that providing continuity of care to a complex and aging population is a challenge with no available silver-bullet solution. Breakdowns, as a result of fragmentations in care, medical errors associated with poor communication, confusion due to health professionals working in silos and not as a team cause unnecessary frustration, poor outcomes, and increased waste, which all contribute to the high cost of health care in this country. As a result, insurance companies are changing reimbursement policies for complications they deem to have resulted from poor or fragmented care. The CNL is therefore an intervention in changing the current model of health care that is driving up costs and waste by targeting patient care on the frontlines. The CNL will improve the current model through better control of resources, provide patient-focused care, and improve the outcomes with measurable goals. It is in achieving these goals that the CNL establishes the specific patient-focused solutions to the health care needs of patients and, simultaneously, decreases medical errors and length of stay, and increases patient satisfaction. The CNL relies on research as evidence for the patient-focused health care solutions that are implemented.

Understanding Complexity Theory

As far back as the 1960s, the view of health care systems was compared to being a machine, or, to be successful, a well-oiled machine. It followed traditional systems theory (Senge, 1990) that has roots in explaining the behavior of "dead" systems. This explains the closed system where individual organizations were not as dependent on the community. Today, health care organizations consist of multiple organizations dependent on each other within the system to survive. Open-ended systems have therefore taken over in health care with the newer metaphor of health care organizations being a living organism, not a machine. Such a metaphor is conveyed by the science of complex adaptive systems, which reformulates systems theory in a way that produces a "model" of the organization more closely related to reality.

Today's health care is an ever-changing entity. Complexity leadership is not just a new way to lead, but also a new way of thinking that is radically different from the linear, top-down approach many have experienced in health care (Crowell, 2011, p. 2). Complexity leadership is based on complexity science, the study of complex adaptive systems. It considers the pattern of relationships in the system, how they are sustained, how they self-regulate and self-organize, and how outcomes emerge (Crowell, 2011, p. 3). In this model, all things are connected and the systems thrive on this relationship (see Table 15.1).

When complexity theory is applied to today's nursing leadership, a model emerges and it draws structure from three key concepts. The complexity leadership model (Crowell, 2011, p. 4) emphasizes:

- Knowledge of complexity science and the application to the organization
- Leadership style that is transformational, self-reflective, collaborative, and relationship based
- Personal being and awareness utilizes self-care practices to sustain the personal strength and courage needed to lead in a complex environment

These key concepts prepare a health care leader to expect the unexpected and model of professional life of continued improvement. When one understands the enormity of the components making up the organization, in addition to the ever-changing external factors, one can learn to survive and thrive in the constant chaos. A leader who understands and appreciates the benefits of complex organization will also appreciate the benefits of this environment. Complex adaptive systems have the following key features (Crowell, 2011, p. 34):

- Diverse independent agents interact and adapt to change locally
- New behavior, ideas, patterns, and structure emerge from relationships
- Results are often nonlinear, unpredictable, and surprising
- Self-organization occurs with distributed leadership and simple rules

TABLE 15.1 Complexity Science Versus Established Science

COMPLEXITY SCIENCE	ESTABLISHED SCIENCE
Holism	Reductionism
Indeterminism	Determinism
Relationships among entities	Discrete entities
Nonlinear relationships	Linear relationships
Critical mass thresholds	Marginal increases
Quantum physics	Newtonian physics
Influence through iterative nonlinear feedback	Influence as direct result of force from one object to another
Expect novel and probabilistic world	Expect predictable world
Understanding; sensitivity analysis	Prediction
Focus on variation	Focus on averages
Local control	Global control
Behavior emerges from bottom up	Behavior specified from top down
Metaphor of morphogenesis	Metaphor of assembly

Source: Dent (1999).

Traditional Systems Thinking

For a CNL to understand how to emerge with complex adaption principles, it is first important to understand the results of traditional systems thinking. Traditional systems thinking has created a vicious cycle of (a) designing a system and (b) when the system does not act as predicted, redesigning the system. The assumption according to Begun, Zimmerman, and Dooley (2003) is that leaders can control the evolution of complex systems by intentions and clear thinking. Complexity science leads one to ask different questions. For example, when an intended intervention does not play out as predicted, how do things continue to function? The common result is that "things get done anyway." How do patients continue to get care, and clinicians provide care, despite the machinations of formal organizations? Complexity science focuses on how this "anyway" behavior unfolds through everyday interactions and in spite of the fact that leaders continue to focus on the "systems" that attempt to secure predicted changes. The challenge for the CNL is to stick with the lateral integration approach to overseeing patient care. The CNL can intervene, facilitate, or coordinate care for individual patients, groups of patients, and populations of patients in the community using complexity theory to identify areas in need of improvement.

It is through this research that service sector leaders were identified as the source of power and scope in the frontline interface that connected the organization's core competency with the needs of an individual customer. Here is the CNL's critical role; to lead the frontline staff in line with the organization's core competencies. How does this happen? The CNL can be guided by recent research by Donaldson and Mohr (2000a, 2000b), who identified eight dimensions that were associated with high quality in high-performing clinical microsystems:

- Constancy of purpose (goal is the same for all)
- Investment in improvement (dollars invested when needed)
- Alignment of role and training for efficiency and staff satisfaction (staff and other stakeholders give buy-in)
- Interdependence of care team to meet patient needs
- Inclusion of all members involved in the process of meeting the goal
- Integration of information and technology into workflow (utilizing benchmarks through statistics and data collection)
- Ongoing measurement of outcomes (real-time data to compare pre- and postinterventions)
- Supportiveness of the larger organization

Additionally, Nelson et al. (2008) surveyed 20 high-performing clinical microsystems (small groups of people who work together regularly to provide care to a discrete population of patients) and found that the microsystems shared a set of primary success characteristics that interacted with one another to produce a synergistic outcome:

- Leadership of microsystem
- Macrosystem support of microsystem
- Patient focus
- Staff focus
- Interdependence of care team
- Information and information technology
- Process improvement
- Performance result

Unit-Level Health Care Delivery/Microsystems of Care

Clinical microsystems can be reduced into smaller, more manageable pieces or units that can allow for rapid diffusion of change across the nursing division. In a unit where care is generally focused on a set of patients, a CNL can integrate emerging nursing science into practice and lead efforts to enhance patient care. The American Association of Colleges of Nursing (AACN) White Paper (2007) describes the competency that a CNL will execute through the following actions:

1. Accountable for health care outcomes within a unit and in line with the meso- and macrosystems goals
2. Assimilates and applies research-based information to design, implement, and evaluate the client plans of care

TABLE 15.2 Successful Characteristics of High-Performing Clinical Microsystems

CHARACTERISTIC	DEFINITION
Leadership	The role of leaders is to balance setting and reaching collective goals and to empower individual autonomy and accountability, through building knowledge, respectful action, reviewing, and reflecting
Organizational support	The larger organization looks for ways to support the work of the microsystem and coordinate the hand-offs between microsystems
Staff focus	There is selective hiring of the right kind of people. The orientation process is designed to fully integrate new staff into culture and work roles. Expectations of staff are high regarding performance, continuing education, professional growth, and networking.
Education and training	All clinical microsystems have responsibility for the ongoing education and training of staff and for aligning daily work roles with training competencies. Academic clinical microsystems have the additional responsibility of training students
Interdependence	The interaction of staff is characterized by trust, collaboration, willingness to help each other, appreciation of complementary roles, respect, and recognition that all contribute individually to a shared purpose
Patient focus	The primary concern is to meet all patient needs—caring, listening, educating and responding to special requests, innovating to meet patient needs, and smooth service flow
Community and market focus	The microsystem is a resource for the community; the community is a resource for the microsystem; the microsystem establishes excellent and innovative relationships with the community
Performance results	Performance focuses on patient outcomes, avoidable costs, streamlining delivery, using data feedback, promoting positive competition, and frank discussions about performance
Process improvement	An atmosphere for learning and redesign is supported by the continuous monitoring of care, use of benchmarking, frequent tests of change, and a staff that has been empowered to innovate
Information and information technology	Information is *the* connector—staff to patients, staff to staff, needs with actions to meet needs. Technology facilitates effective communication and multiple formal and informal channels are used to keep everyone informed all the time, listen to everyone's ideas and ensure that everyone is connected on important topics.

Source: Nelson et al. (2007, p. 21).

3. Synthesizes data, information, and knowledge to evaluate and achieve optimal client and care environment outcomes through measures of unit outcomes

4. Uses appropriate teaching/learning principles and strategies as well as current information, materials, and technologies to facilitate the learning of clients, groups, and other health care professionals

The CNL is positioned to mentor, coach, and lead multidisciplinary teams to evolve and sustain a culture of safety, utilizing evidence-based practices and quality improvement (Table 15.2). Nelson, Batalden, and Godfrey (2007) provide a series of questions and exercises for the CNL to incorporate in leading inter-disciplinary teams through a microsystem assessment. It is necessary to establish the condition of the microsystem (health), make obvious the areas requiring atten-tion (diagnosis) and the solutions (treatment) to be evaluated by the team. Here are sample questions for the CNL to answer in order to evaluate the microsystem and to develop goals in line with the macrosystem:

- What is the aim or purpose of the microsystem?
- Who is the small population of people who benefit from this aim?
- Whom do you work with daily (administratively, technically, and/or professionally)?
- What information and information technology is part of the daily work?
- How do you measure outcomes for the population?

Assessing the Microsystem

In order to assess in a systematic and thorough manner, a framework or tool is frequently employed, which makes the process more defined rather than ask-ing a group of random questions. One specific framework that offers a deliber-ate structure for CNLs to assess microsystems for quality improvement is the 5P (purpose, patients, professionals, processes, and patterns) framework. Each P has a definition associated with it, and these categories set a framework for the development of themes and aims (Nelson et al., 2007). When the 5Ps are reviewed and the team has chosen the area for improvement, it is essential to identify team roles, responsibilities, and ground rules. These then become the agreed-on guiding principles, rules, and accountabilities for each member of the team. When decided, a written agreement defining what the team goal is going to accomplish and how success will be measured is recorded in a team charter (Harris & Roussel, 2010). Templates and formats can be found on the Internet if none is available in the organization. Here are some general criteria found in a charter: project title, description of the project, scope of the project, specific problem to be addressed, criteria for success, time commitment, team member roles, process to be performed, decision-making process, conflict management process, communication plans, and expectations of team members (review of minutes, checking e-mail/voicemail, response and turnaround times, preparation prior to meetings, completing assignments).

In addition to identifying a project, there are several indirect key pieces to be considered for the project to be successful: starting with unit descriptors, skills, composition, and competence of the team members; presence of formal and infor-mal leaders; interdisciplinary team relationships and communication; accountabil-ity and control over practice; support for education; experience with the quality improvement processes and resources; and readiness for change. The latter is one of the most important factors to consider when evaluating a microsystem and the readiness for implementing changes within the microsystem. Every microsystem is part of the larger organization that needs to be taken into consideration as a CNL prepares for a microsystem assessment.

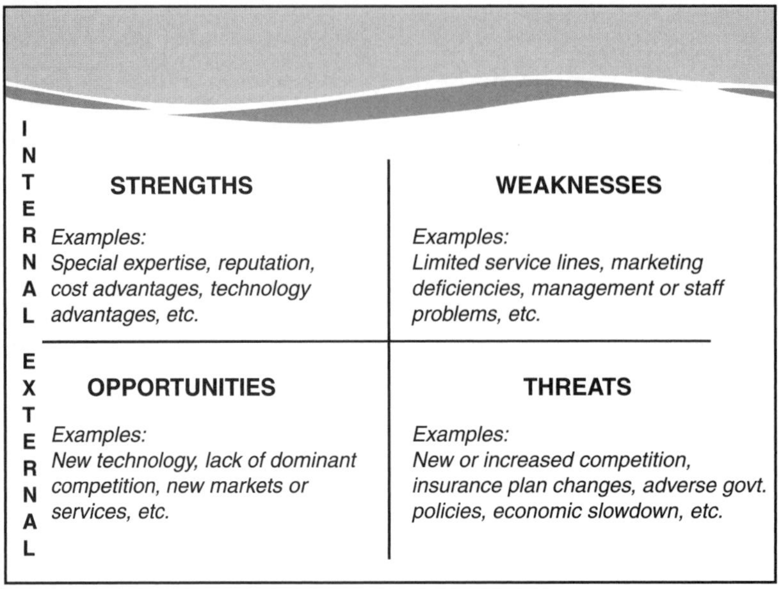

	STRENGTHS	WEAKNESSES
I N T E R N A L	**STRENGTHS** *Examples:* *Special expertise, reputation,* *cost advantages, technology* *advantages, etc.*	**WEAKNESSES** *Examples:* *Limited service lines, marketing* *deficiencies, management or staff* *problems, etc.*
E X T E R N A L	**OPPORTUNITIES** *Examples:* *New technology, lack of dominant* *competition, new markets or* *services, etc.*	**THREATS** *Examples:* *New or increased competition,* *insurance plan changes, adverse govt.* *policies, economic slowdown, etc.*

Source: http://www.healthcaresuccess.com/articles/swot.html

FIGURE 15.2   SWOT analysis.

CNL Assessing a Project Using SWOT

In order to identify aspects that may positively or negatively affect a project, the CNL will want to complete a SWOT assessment. This assessment is vital for the successful planning and implementation of a change in process or structure in a microsystem. A full SWOT assessment of the entire organization or health care system assists the team in developing strategies to deal with known forces, both internal and external, and to anticipate others. SWOT stands for strengths, weaknesses, opportunities, and threats, and a gap analysis of the three levels of the system: micro, meso, and macro. A SWOT analysis can take different forms, but it generally involves an objective view of internal processes and personnel (Figure 15.2).

A Model for Improvement

Microsystems are in need of continuous quality improvement. As new technology and knowledge enter into health care microsystems, the CNL will be a key leader in the achievement of quality indicators or measures. After microsystems are assessed and several areas or themes emerge that require change to meet quality and safety indicators, the CNL should utilize a model of improvement to establish a uniform method throughout the organization so that all CNLs in an organization have the ability to adapt changes that apply universally. In this highly critical role, it is essential to understand how using an established model of improvement can make a difficult task a smooth process. Nelson et al. presents a model for improvement referred to as the Deming cycle (Deming, 1986), which integrates the

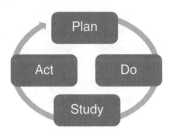

FIGURE 15.3 Continuous improvement model.

scientific process referred to as the plan-do-study-act (PDSA) method. This method is used repetitively to test changes in a disciplined and rapid fashion. This model was further adapted to include three key questions for leading change (Langley, Nolan, Norman, Provost, & Nolan, 1996) (see Figure 15.3).

1. **What are we trying to accomplish?**

   AIM: A specific, measurable, time-sensitive statement of expected results of an improvement process. A strong, clear aim gives necessary direction to improvement efforts. The four-step process can be repeated each time an adjustment is made to evaluate the change by studying the results. Refer to this website for details regarding the PDSA method of improvement www.hci.com.au/hcisite3/toolkit/pdcacycl.htm

   Plan—a specific planning phase

   Do—a time to try the change and observe what happens

   Study—an analysis of the results of the trial

   Act—devising next steps on the basis of analysis

2. **How will we know if the change is an improvement?**

   Measures are indicators of change. To answer this key question, several measures are usually required. These measures can also be used to monitor a system's performance over time. In PDSA cycles, measurement used immediately after an idea or change has been tested helps determine its effect.

3. **What change can be made that will result in an improvement?**

   Ideas for change or change concepts to be tested in a PDSA cycle can be derived from:

   a. Evidence or results of research/science

   b. Critical thinking or observation of the current system

   c. Creative thinking

   d. Theories, questions, hunches

   e. Extrapolations from other situations

After successful PDSA cycle experimentation, a change is reached that meets the aim or goal and comes standardization of the change throughout the microsystem. When the aim has been reached in the sample or pilot group, the adoption of this standard method is usually required throughout the microsystem.

This is called the standardize-do-study-act (SDSA) cycle. The purpose of the SDSA approach is to hold the gains that were made using the PDSA cycles and to standardize the process into daily work. Often, a new or better piece of equipment or technology can come along and cause the process to shift back to the PDSA cycle again. The PDSA and the SDSA are continuous processes. Once the PDSA cycle is complete, be prepared to move back to the SDSA to refine and standardize the process. In each stage, answer questions and follow the path.

Managing Change Theory

As a CNL gathers and organizes data, the one important consideration to whether a change will be successful or not is to assess the readiness for change within the microsystem. To assist a CNL in organizing data in a useful way to analyze readiness and plan effectively for changes, data collection points should be based on John Kotter's change theory (1996). Kotter's theory postulates that change does not occur without adequate time placed on establishing a sense of urgency, creating the guiding coalition, developing a vision, and communicating the vision. These first four steps in the change process are necessary to assist employees in recognizing the need for change and to embrace the process. To allow time for the CNL to enact the four steps and for the employees to embrace the change, outcome data for the 3 months' postimplementation should be included in the preimplementation analysis.

Kotter's Eight Stages of Change to Guide the CNL

1. Establishing a sense of urgency
2. Creating the guiding coalition
3. Developing a vision and strategy
4. Communicating the change vision
5. Empowering broad-based action
6. Generating short-term wins
7. Consolidating gains and producing more change
8. Anchoring new approaches in the culture (Kotter, 1996)

The Future of Microsystems With CNL Leadership

It is a known fact that the sickest 5% of patients account for about 50% of health care dollars according to Lee and Mongan (2009), with the vast majority having more than one medical issue. Cost does affect care and the ability to provide care. Microsystems are at the root of care and have therefore become the target for improving the care provided in a cost-effective way. Microsystems are currently disorganized, with providers working in silos. A potential solution is for more organized

TABLE 15.3 Health Care Systems

CATEGORY	WEIGHT
C. Health Care Systems	5%

1. Acquires knowledge to work in groups, manage change, and systems-level dissemination of knowledge

2. Applies evidence that challenges current policies and procedures in a practice environment

3. Implements strategies that lessen health care disparities

4. Advocates for the improvement in the health care system, policies, and nursing profession

5. Applies systems thinking (i.e., theories, models) to address problems and develop solutions

6. Collaborates with other health care professionals to manage the transition of clients across the health care continuum, ensuring patient safety and cost-effectiveness of care

7. Utilizes quality improvement methods in evaluating individual and aggregate client care

8. Understands how health care delivery systems are organized and financed and the effect on client care

9. Identifies the economic, legal, and political factors that influence health care delivery

Used with permission from the Commission on Nurse Certification.

providers working together in teams. CNLs can collaborate with a shared vision to create best practice with high-quality outcomes for patients. Within each microsystem, strong leadership will be provided by a CNL, who is the steward of the ship overseeing the many improvements needed in health care organizations. The CNL certification exam includes content related to general themes of health care systems that CNLs should be familiar with (Table 15.3).

Summary of Health Care Systems/Organizations

A CNL is a leader in every health care delivery setting. It is expected that the CNL will have an understanding of the economies of care, a basic understanding of business principles, and an understanding of how to work within and effect change in systems. The CNL assumes accountability for health care outcomes for a specific group of clients within a unit or setting through the assimilation and application of research-based information to design, implement, and evaluate client plans of care. PDSA and SWOT are useful tools for a CNL to incorporate an organized plan of care and successful implementation of new or evidenced-based interventions. Effective CNLs have the unique potential to create a new environment within the frontlines of patient care, including cost-effective, evidence-based, high-quality care within each individual microsystem.

Resources

American Association of Colleges of Nursing. (2007). *White paper on the education and role of the clinical nurse leader.* Washington, DC. Retrieved from http://www.aacn. nche.edu/publicaitons/Whitepapers/ClinicalNurseLeader07.pdf

Begun, J., Zimmerman, B., & Dooley, K. (2003). Health care organizations as complex adaptive systems. In S. M. Mick & M. Wyttenbach (Eds.), *Advances in health care organization theory* (pp. 253–288). San Francisco, CA: Jossey-Bass.

Crowell, D. (2011). *Complexity leadership.* Philadelphia, PA: F. A. Davis.

Deming, W. (1986). *Out of the crisis.* Cambridge, MA: MIT Center for Advanced Engineering Study.

Dent, E. B. (1999). Complexity science: A worldview shift. *Emergence, 1*(4), 5–19.

Donaldson, M., & Mohr, J. (2000a). *Exploring innovation and quality improvement in health care microsystems: A cross-case analysis. Technical Report for the Institute of Medicine Committee on Quality of Health Care in America.* Washington, DC: Institute of Medicine.

Donaldson, M., & Mohr, J. (2000b). *Improvement and innovation in health care microsystems. A technical report for the Institute of Medicine Committee on the quality of health care in America.* Princeton, NJ: Robert Wood Johnson Foundation.

Godfrey, M., Nelson, E., Wasson, J., Mohr, J., & Batalden, P. (2003). Microsystems in health care: Part 3. Planning patient-centered services. *The Joint Commission Journal on Quality and Patient Safety, 29*(4), 159–170.

Harris, J., & Roussel, L. (2010). *Initiating and sustaining the clinical nurse leader role.* Sudbury, MA: Jones & Bartlett Publishers.

Kotter, J. P. (1996). *Leading change.* Boston, MA: Harvard Business School Press.

Kouzes, J., & Posner, B. (2002). *The leadership challenge* (3rd ed.) San Francisco, CA: Jossey-Bass.

Langley, G., Nolan, K., Norman, C., Provost, L., & Nolan, T. (1996). *The improvement guide: A practical approach to enhancing organizational performance.* San Francisco, CA: Jossey-Bass.

Lee, T., & Mongan, J. (2009). *Chaos and organization in health care.* Cambridge, MA/ London, England: The MIT Press.

Nelson, E., Batalden, P., & Godfrey, M. (2007). *Quality by design: A clinical microsystems approach.* San Francisco, CA: Jossey-Bass.

Nelson, E., Godfrey, M., Bataladen, P., Berry, S., Bothe, A., McKinley, K., . . ., Nolan, T. W. (2008). Clinical microsystems, part 1: The building blocks of health systems. *The Joint Commission Journal on Quality and Patient Safety, 7*(34), 367–378.

Senge, P. (1990). *The fifth discipline: The art and practice of the learning organization.* New York, NY: Doubleday.

16

Health Care Policy

Catherine Winkler

Policy refers to standing decisions that serve as guidelines for action. Health policy generally denotes policy that impacts the health of the individual, or families, and communities through production, provision, and financing of health care services. In contrast, public health policy, although it intersects health policy, can be thought of as more comprehensive, with an impact on the general population by influencing actions, behaviors, and resources through legislative, executive, and judicial branches of the government (Porche, 2003). Health care policy over the past 50 years focused on the medical care model and biomedical research that "medicalized" health status problems. Through this lens, policymakers assumed that the primary solution to public health problems involved medical care, which focused on financial and geographic access to personal health services for vulnerable populations (Lantz, Lichtenstein, & Pollack, 2007). Today, the emphasis in health care policy is on public health and population health. Policy work that targeted only medical care and access missed important opportunities to address the larger issues of poverty, nutrition, education, housing, and security. Public health policy, which is focused on social and economic causes of health vulnerability and disparities, is a better way to influence the health of the nation rather than to wait until patients fall into the "safety net" of medical care. Clinical nurse leaders (CNLs) have the opportunity to dramatically impact the changing landscape of the nation's health care system by merging their clinical expertise with advocacy through participation in policy.

An emerging framework for health policy has expanded to population health with the goals of increasing the quality and years of a healthy life and elimination of health disparities (Healthy People, 2020) through the need to have a public health response to terrorism prompted by the September 11, 2001 terrorist attacks and the anthrax assaults that followed.

CNLs who use theory and research in coordinating care in an interdisciplinary health care team have the skill set to advise and develop policy that will be needed as the health care system evolves. A united voice, more strategic alliances, along with leadership, and added education in policy will be needed for CNLs to increase their influence in organizations, communities, and in national and international health care.

Health Care Policy Intentions

Policy is developed with specific intentions to regulate behaviors and actions and/ or allocate resources. A policy with regulatory intent proposes to prescribe and control the behavior of a particular population. A policy that is allocation focused aims to provide resources such as income, services, or goods to ensure implementation of a policy. The Patient Protection and Affordable Care Act (PPACA or ACA) P.L. 111-148 is an example of both, with the intent to improve access, decrease waste and costs, and support quality through process changes and improved outcomes. The principal stakeholders that affect policy decisions are consumers (patients and their families), providers (physicians, nurses, pharmacists, etc.), payers (employers, insurance companies), and regulatory bodies (Department of Public Health, Centers for Medicare and Medicaid Services [CMS], etc.). Policymaking is a complex, layered, and dynamic process that is influenced by the values of these stakeholders. The phases of the public policymaking process include:

- issue identification and agenda setting
- policy formulation
- policy adoption
- policy implementation
- policy evaluation
- policy revision or amendment

Medicare is an example of a federal program that was introduced as policy through the Social Security Act of 1965 that has been evaluated and amended more than 50 times since its inception (Social Security Bulletin Annual Statistical Supplement, 2000).

Policy and politics are interdependent, and this relationship is central to understanding their importance in health care delivery systems as well as their relevance to the nursing profession. Politics is a neutral term, although it raises negative connotations such as corruption, unethical compromises, and payoffs. Politics is actually the process of influencing the allocation of scarce resources and therefore, it is important in the process of policy development and implementation. Values are at the foundation of policy and politics. Consequently, CNLs need to be clear about the values that they hold and how they shape the policies and, political strategies in which they will engage in when working to improve conditions. Nursing has been voted as the most trusted profession in America for the 11th year (Jones, 2011) since added to the poll in 1999. All nurses inclusive of CNLs are in an excellent position to assume a leadership role in advancing the health care agenda because they are patient advocates, and the public has a high level of trust in the profession.

Policy is more important than politics, but politics were involved in health care reform. The present-day issue in the government is how to implement and finance the PPACA (P.L. 111-148) and the Health Care and Education Reconciliation Act (P.L. 111-152) signed into law in 2010. The combined legislation extends coverage to an estimated 30 million uninsured Americans. This overhaul of health care delivery, which started in 2010, will roll out over approximately 10 years and extend access to health care for most, though not all, Americans. It will cost the U.S. government an estimated $938 billion over the next decade while reducing the federal deficit by $143 billion, according to the Congressional Budget Office (2011). However, many Americans believe that the federal deficit and health care costs will skyrocket with the new law. Both doubters and supporters of the law will have time to assess it, as major provisions will not begin until 2014.

Becoming skilled at influencing the legislative processes as well as the regulatory processes is important. Legislation is a law proposed by a legislative body while a regulation is a specific requirement or rule within legislation. Legislation tends to be broad while the regulations reflect the details that are needed to give the law traction and allow it to be carried out. The ACA is an example of a law in effect through the legislation, but without full regulations in place yet to guide its implementation at the state and federal levels.

The process of policy development, analysis, and implementation occurs in the context of political diplomacy and negotiation. Once the problem is identified, an agenda set, and a proposal drafted, it will be introduced into the process through the executive branch, members of the legislative branch, and/or generated by citizens, organizations, or special interest groups that petition the government and elected officials. Once the bill becomes a law, it moves from policy formation to implementation with a proliferation of regulations followed by operationalization. During policy development, careful analysis is compulsory to promote policy success. Nurses are in the unique position of being particularly effective in policymaking because it is a natural extension of their role as an advocate and an educator in their practice. Health service's research unites with policy analysis and, again, nurses inclusive of CNLs are well positioned to systematically analyze the issues and develop strategies for advancing their agenda. As Leavitt, Chaffee, and Vance (2011) state, nurses bring value to the discussions of any health policy issue because they understand how such policies affect the delivery of care and patient outcomes and can anticipate unintended consequences. Any political analysis analogous to a clinical assessment involves problem identification, a plan for possible solutions, an understanding of the history and previous attempts to correct the problem, and knowledge of the stakeholders, values, and, finally, the resources required to secure the best outcome (Table 16.1).

Health Care Delivery System

The U.S. health care system is complex, involving patients, providers, and payers. It is also a mix of private and public initiatives with institutions that employ millions of workers in multiple settings to deliver health care services to a diverse population. The price tag was estimated to be 17.7% of the gross domestic product in 2011(Altarum Institute's Center for Studying Health Spending, 2011). Health insurance is provided through the private insurance industry and by the government, with approximately 60% of health care financed by Medicare, Medicaid, TRICARE, the Children's Health Insurance Program, and the Veterans Health Administration (Kaiser Commission on Medicaid and the Uninsured, 2009). Most of the health

TABLE 16.1 Political Analysis and Clinical Assessment Parallels

STEPS	POLITICAL ANALYSIS	CLINICAL ASSESSMENT
Problem identification	Heart failure program needed	Diagnosis of heart failure
Possible solutions	Assemble team Contact experts Develop program	Symptom management Education Goal setting
History	Poor transition in care Patients readmitted often Long length of stay Frequent readmission	Problem with fluid overload Confused about medicines
Stakeholders	Patient Family Health care professionals	Patient Family Health care professionals
Values	Cost-effective Decrease readmission rates Increase access	Enhanced quality of life Independence Cost-effective care
Resources needed	Time Money Staff Literature Chronic bundle checklist	Affordable medicines Clear direction for symptom management Transportation Diet assistance
Outcomes	Decrease readmissions to 10%	Improved quality of life

care dollars spent goes to hospitals (31%) and physicians (21%), with the balance of spending to pharmaceutical (10%), extended care facilities (6%), dental (4%), home health care (3%), other clinical services, and administrative overhead (CMS, Office of the Actuary, National Health Statistics Group, 2011).

The health care delivery system is disjointed with incentives misaligned, competing priorities, and many Americans uninsured or underinsured. An example of a misaligned incentive is in the hospital setting, where reimbursement is based on capitated payments made by Medicare called DRGs (diagnosis-related groups) and case rates preestablished by insurance companies. The practice of sending patients home quickly to maximize reimbursement through a shortened length of stay has an unintended consequence. Discharged patients who are still acutely ill or not fully recovered require a readmission to the hospital. In the past the hospital had received an additional fee for the new inpatient stay. Now, there is a disincentive or financial penalty that hospitals will incur if patients are readmitted within 30 days of discharge. This new policy will be a challenge because, although hospitals will be able to manage those patients who were perhaps sent home too soon, it will be quite another thing to prevent a readmission for patients who need hospitalization for another medical reason, have broader social issues such as poverty (cannot afford medications), transportation limits (cannot make follow-up appointments), and lack the knowledge to self-manage (complexity of illness or medical regimen). Beginning in 2012, CMS carefully examined the readmissions of those patients who are diagnosed with heart failure, acute myocardial infarction, and pneumonia within 30 days of discharge. Interdisciplinary teams together with CNLs will need to carefully plan each discharge. Patients may need to stay longer in the hospital setting to begin with, require follow-up assessment and education in their home or rehabilitation facility immediately, and have continuous communication with all health care professionals to avoid a readmission. However, even with intensive observation and care tracked and moving with the patient to the outpatient setting, some will be readmitted because of the often unavoidable disease trajectory.

The health care system has to deliver care on many fronts and often fails to manage the challenging needs of emergency care, urgent care, preventive care, chronic care, acute care, extended care, and home care. Each care setting, although related to each other in an episode of care, is separated financially, through payments made to each individual organization, and clinically, through breaks in communication during a transition of care period. Symptom management difficulties, complications, and readmissions follow when there is a break in the continuum of care. These two factors contribute to less efficient, more expensive care being rendered to our patients in the best-case scenario and potential harm in the worst-case scenario. CNLs need to actively engage in systems of care improvements and follow the idea that "form follows function." The form that the health care system takes will be the healthiest if it follows the functions or set of actions that factor in when we actively try to make a patient well. CNLs can be the catalyst of change by connecting care for the patient being discharged via comprehensive W10 forms, follow-up phone calls, and very clear medication reconciliation lists.

The traditional medical model involved complex hospital systems that focused on "sick care" with a plethora of technology. The health care system of the future needs to address the continuum of care that ranges from prevention services to hospice care over multiple settings, with more targeted use of technology. Accordingly, reimbursement is moving in this direction with new incentives that promote accountable care organizations (ACOs) in which physicians and hospitals work together to improve outcomes and share in cost savings, likewise to medical homes that tightly coordinate a patient's care within the system. Communication will be critical, whether it is between caregivers when transitioning patients across levels of care or through electronic medical records that are seamless and timely. Organizational and systems theory relates effectiveness of a system with the ability to adapt to internal and external factors to remain relevant and to survive (Chuang & Inder, 2009). The typical hierarchy in health care today begins with the patients and community at the base, the hospital-level health care system layered next, followed by standard-setting, accreditation, quality measurement and reporting systems with government and regulation at the top (Chuang & Inder). In 1996, Venegoni realized that change was coming in the delivery of services and identified five significant factors that would transform the health care system. Many of the proposed changes have occurred. The first, the site of delivery, has changed from, predominately, the hospital to other settings, including the home environment, outpatient clinics, and rehabilitation centers. The second involves diverse types of people who receive care with needs that vary in kind and intensity of care: from being well but needing a physical exam, to acutely ill requiring extensive diagnostic and therapeutic interventions. The other factor related to the second is the shift from illness to wellness care aimed at averting costs that can occur because of lack of early identification and intervention in a disease process.

Quality and customer satisfaction are also significant elements in today's health care climate. Value-based purchasing, the method of payment by CMS for in-hospital stays, which began in 2012, pays on the basis of hospital scores in processes and outcomes, such as core measures and patient experience ratings known as Hospital Consumer Assessment of Healthcare Providers and Systems (HCAHPS). Process, the last aspect in the model, involves modern technology, which is ever present through the introduction of electronic medical records and the ability to send and store diagnostic testing data (Table 16.2). Changes will continue to occur as the system expands to involve other entities contingent on the model of care that is adopted by a community, state, or government.

With the prospects of a capitated method of payment for an episode of care, the reimbursement period might be grouped. It could include a visit to a clinic, a brief hospital stay if the patient's condition worsens, and a follow-up home visit by a visiting nurse. All of this care would need to be coupled with planned communication between all caregivers.

To achieve the aim of evaluating the health care system, there needs to be a better integration of patient safety and quality into the system, which has established links between the layers with good control and communication (Chuang & Inder, 2009). It is commonplace today to evaluate health care systems on the basis of how well they provide safe and effective care at a cost that is reasonable and evenly disseminated in access, quality, and cost (Russell, 2011). However, such measures remain elusive because of fragmented care that lacks synergy between the principals (patients, health care professionals, and payers), the organizations (hospitals, extended care facilities, physician offices, etc.), and the payers (Medicare, Medicaid, private insurance, etc.). Of course, there are many entities

TABLE 16.2 Five Factors of Change Underway in Health Care Delivery

FACTOR	CURRENT	CHANGE
Site of care	Hospital	Extended care facility Home Rehabilitation center Rural clinic Medical home
Type of patient	Homogenous and ill	Heterogeneous and either well or ill
Health care model/focus	Sickness model of care Acute care	Wellness model of care Acute and chronic
Quality	Uncoupled with reimbursement	Linked to reimbursement—value-based purchasing
Technology processes	High-tech interventions	High- and low-tech interventions Electronic medical records E-mail between health care professional and patient

that evaluate health care systems at a global level, such as the World Health Organization (WHO); on a private level, such as The Joint Commission; and on a state level, such as the Department of Public Health. Other professional organizations, such as the American College of Surgeons, will evaluate care for trauma designation, or the American Nurses Credentialing Center will evaluate hospitals for Magnet status. Nevertheless, refining the delivery of care requires daily process improvements in practice to facilitate systemic progress in any health care organization. CNLs stand at the crossing where the patient enters the system needing direct care and within the system itself, which is a matter of public interest.

Economic, legal, and political factors that affect health care are the reasons that brought the American government and its citizens to the table to negotiate for a better future. We needed to decide whether health care was a human right, much in the same way that we, as a country, decided that education was a right many years ago. Although this issue may remain in part, many Americans do believe that health care is a human right. As such, financing, accessing, and restructuring health care to improve quality and safety while gaining in efficiency has begun.

Thus, as of 2012, the ACA requires any new federal health program to collect and report racial, ethnic, and language data to identify and reduce disparities in pursuit of better health outcomes.

Health Care Economics

Over the next 5 to 10 years, there will be a significant shift in health plan enrollment. Fewer people will be covered by profitable private plans, while more will join the deficit-generating government-sponsored programs, according to Kaufman (2011). Expanded coverage for the uninsured who will need to obtain insurance through state exchanges may not be enough to offset the growing number of Medicare and Medicaid beneficiaries. For many years, the hospital industry had subsidized losses incurred by Medicare and Medicaid by demanding higher premiums from commercial payers. It was estimated that aggregate payment-to-cost ratio from Medicare was 90.9%; from Medicaid, 88.7%; and from commercial payers, 123% (American Hospital Association [AHA], 2010). Cost shifting will diminish as a result of the ACA, the aging population, ongoing compression of government and private reimbursement, and increased patient responsibility (Kaufman, 2011). It is estimated that this will require most health care systems to reduce their current operating budgets by 10% to 15%, according to Kaufman (2011). Since cost shifting will not occur as it does today, more patients need to be prepared to pay a percentage of their health care costs. Inevitably, this will result in bad debt and lowered utilization of health services. Currently, many health insurance companies have raised their rates; sometimes the percentage of increase is double-digit. This change caused a number of states to enact legislation to block or reduce premium increases. In addition, the federal government through Health and Human Services (HHS) just recently spent $150 million to regulate the insurance industry to prevent excessive rate increases.

The cost of physician integration into an ACO will most likely increase the cost of care because the associated infrastructure costs can be very high. Nonetheless, hospitals are acquiring physician practices to secure patient volumes. The ACA states that the ACO will only be rewarded for improving quality and increasing cost savings. This will undoubtedly be done through reducing specialty consultations, high-tech procedures, and hospital admissions. The difficult problem with this model is that there is no evidence or previous experience with it to know if shared savings from working together will be enough to balance the loss in volume and revenue or the political capital invested in the effort.

CNLs and administration will be critically important influences in the system for setting the course and holding all staff accountable for performance-based budgets based on best practice. Services that do not generate a profit or reduce expenses will be under consideration for discontinuation, and workforce reductions can only be avoided through work redesign efforts to eliminate waste and inconsistencies in care. In addition, a programmatic approach to chronic illnesses such as heart failure and diabetes must be taken to address the complications and comorbidities associated with these illnesses. The complexity of these chronic conditions with the education requirements to keep these patients well is in line with the CNL's role to promote health and reduce risk.

Since there are limited resources in health care, it is necessary to continually evaluate the intervention options. By applying six techniques to clinical decisions, it is possible to decide on the best approach in terms of priority level to treatment, intervention, and outcome (Box 16.1). When looking at the cost of illness, investigators are comparing one or more illnesses to determine the primacy of the condition. Cost identification and minimization compare the expenditures and, once determined, selects a condition where reducing expense might be possible through the intervention type. Cost-consequence and -effectiveness analysis as well as cost-benefit analysis help to measure the pros and cons of competing interventions. As an example, pilot projects are now underway through the ACA to determine the best model for health care service delivery models. Rural health care clinics and medical homes are also currently funded projects seeking to determine their effectiveness in delivering care to segments of the population. Grant funding is available to investigate the application of navigator services to coordinate care and demonstration programs for chronically ill Medicare beneficiaries, using home-based teams as well.

In addition to a macroeconomic perspective of health care, CNLs are charged with integrating this knowledge into unit-level and patient-level budgeting. All

---

BOX 16.1
Techniques for Health Care Economic Decision Making

Cost of illness—total expenses related to care
Cost identification—summary of each expense
Cost minimization—analysis of costs and possible reductions
Cost-consequence analysis—expense associated with illness beyond care
Cost-effectiveness analysis—comparing two types of possible intervention
Cost-benefit analysis—comparing intervention versus not using it

too often in hospitals and health care organizations, budgeting, cost accounting, strategic planning, and financial and clinical analytics are disconnected—making budgeting and staffing to meet patient needs all but impossible. The case-mix, census, and length of stay are a few of the variables that need to be considered when staffing a unit 24 hours a day, 7 days a week. Staffing a unit is dependent on the level of practitioner that is assigned as well as support staff, transporters, aides, and technicians. The acuity and the activity of the unit are variables that should be considered too. A unit with very acute patients or one that has a large number of admissions and discharges will need the staff to flex to meet one-to-one direct care and/or the many admission orders and discharge instructions on any given shift. Databanks to help with calculating staffing ratios are available through the National Database for Nursing Quality Indicators with oversight by the American Nurses Association (ANA, 2011).

Health Care Policy and Professional Ethics

To frame a discussion of health care, policy involves consideration of professional ethics. Ethics broadly has to do with right and wrong and adherence to principles. Politics, which influences the allocation of scarce resources, balances power, human rights, and integrity and equality, is involved when there is an occasion involving justice in the distribution of social goods, fairness and equity in relationships, and access to education, health care, and assistance. Professional ethics has to do with how personal norms apply or conflict with the promises and duties of one's profession (Curtain, 2012). As Curtain outlines, professional ethics is composed of its purpose or responsibility to meet society's needs, the conduct expected of the professional, and the skills and expected outcomes in professional practice. Society demands that professionals such as nurses uphold an elevated moral standard because their clinical decisions can and do have a significant impact on the lives of others. Curtain lists the following areas where ethics come into play: human rights and the degree to which the patient exercises them; when technical options are available and choice is possible; the extent of research and learning on people; resource allocation in situations of scarcity; in futile care and patient's autonomy; in self-interest when exposed to hazards, biologic, or otherwise; and with law and regulations. When considering the areas where ethics factor into clinical care, it is important to note that this too translates into policy in the exploration of public initiatives that target broad public health concerns, such as better environmental conditions, nutrition, education, and economic viability.

The most common principles encountered in ethics are beneficence (weighing benefit versus risk of an action), nonmaleficence (doing no harm), justice, and autonomy. Values clarification is a process used to promote clarity regarding personal and professional values that will intersect thoughts and actions in relation to policy and politics (Porche, 2012). CNLs who are familiar with clarification of values and the ethical decision-making process will recognize that the same practice is required in the political process to avoid a conflict of interest, to problem-solve, and to promote public trust.

Quality and Safety in Health Care

Quality of care is the extent to which health care services for individuals and the population increases the likelihood of preferred outcomes that are consistent with current knowledge (Russell, 2012). Dimensions of the health care system are outlined in the landmark report *Crossing the Quality Chasm: A New Health System for the 21st Century* by the Institute of Medicine (IOM, 2001). The dimensions listed are safety, effectiveness, timeliness, efficiency, equity, and patient-centeredness. Bridge to Quality (IOM, 2003), a follow-up to the initial recommendation for change, provides direction related to oversight, training, research, public reporting, and leadership. In the United States, we continue to spend more health dollars than any other nation, yet spending amounts and quality seem ever far apart. When the United States is compared with other industrialized nations on equity, efficiency, and healthy life years, our scores are surprisingly poor. In 2000, the WHO survey ranked the U.S. health care system 37th in the world; 24th in attaining health; 32nd in terms of equity of health outcomes across the population; and 54th in terms of financial contributions toward health care (Russell, 2011). By translating research into practice, developing patient-specific evidence for effectiveness of care, and promoting needed policy change, CNLs will contribute to public health improvements.

In 2005, the Patient Safety and Quality Improvement Act was enacted to increase protection for those who reported errors. The intention of this act is to encourage reporting of medical errors to enable health care professionals to become more aware of problems, trend issues, and work to make system and process changes quickly to avoid error recurrence. Although there has been a shift from fear to accountability, health care professionals still struggle with reporting medical errors because of liability concerns or loss of work and the associated shame. Patient safety is the freedom from harm while receiving health care. Preventing avoidable harm is really the first level of quality. Institutions that demonstrate a culture of safety often have daily unit-based safety committees or huddles that serve as a forum for communication to avoid errors and secure safety. Hudson, Sexton, Thomas, and Berenholtz (2009) outline three distinct dimensions of safety that overlap to generate a safety profile for a unit. These dimensions are safety climate (compliance with rules and no-fault error reporting), teamwork climate (collaboration and communication), and positive perceptions of management (working conditions, opinions of management) (Hudson et al., 2009). The safety culture with reliability and team training efforts as well as staffing and scheduling are part of the day-to-day work for many CNLs.

The federal government continues to put a high priority on quality through funding and has placed legislation with the Recovery and Reinvestment Act, which allocates $1.1 billion for comparative effectiveness research. This type of research evaluates the impact of intervention options available for treating specific conditions in a particular group of patients. This research is in response to the ongoing variability that we continue to see in clinical practice as well as the concern over health care costs. Some see this type of research as timely, given the current depressed economic climate, while others worry that this will lead to fixed coverage benefits and rationing of care.

Typically report cards measure outcomes, while hospital performance and quality measures for specific indicators relate to processes. There is a current problem with the lack of standardization and regulation when it comes to quality and performance reports. The public uses them to make health care decisions. Still, public disclosure is generally viewed as positive because of transparency and purported accountability associated with this action. Associated ethical implications, due to lack of standardization, have led to an absence of control for data integrity, quality, or timeliness, or for the motivation and bias of quality and performance reports that are purchased by the hospital for hospital consumption (Suchy, 2010). Richard, Rawel, and Martin (2005) propose a framework for report card development and dissemination that incorporates the principles of legitimacy, unbiased data, enhanced transparency, consumer education, equitable information that is offered free of charge, and secure and private reporting of health care data. These activities are collaborative in nature with accountability and continuous improvement built into them. Agencies that lead the way in quality measures include National Quality Forum, Agency for Healthcare Research and Quality, American Nurses Association, the American Medical Association, and regulatory groups such as The Joint Commission and CMS. Several other respected organizations such as the WHO, the IOM, and the Commonwealth Fund evaluate quality, access, and costs when they evaluate a health care system.

The contribution of nurses and CNLs to the quality of care and safety of patients is significant although it is in the context of a system that is very large and where there are many moving parts that factor into the health care equation. Value-driven health care with nurse-sensitive indicators will be an area where nursing contributions can be noted and appreciated distinctly from the other dynamics. CNLs as information managers and system analysts can work at the unit level to sort out the actions that are needed to comply with HCAHPs, core measures, and other scoring procedures.

Health Services Research: Translating Research Into Practice

Health care research is very important to raise awareness about important health care issues, mobilize communities to action, and influence and inform public policy. Research can be used most effectively when it is relevant to a particular policy and local in its significance to the issue because it helps to make the community or state official more accountable to their constituent base. Policy makers also need a reasonable solution to the problem that does not necessarily need to include the results from a robust, randomized clinical study, but they would recognize the value of surveys and pilot studies. A strong, simple message needs to be developed to communicate the problem, the effect, and the policy solution to the public and the legislators so that it can be prioritized and addressed by the right people. The relationship between the researcher and the advocate should be balanced to avoid conflict when analyzing the information and promoting a particular solution. The reason that this affiliation requires a thoughtful approach is to avoid working at cross purposes. At times the researcher will work to maintain objectivity, taking time to describe the strengths and limitations of the research, whereas the advocate might subjectively summarize the data to get to the heart of the problem as quickly as possible and to advance the issue with a solution (Goldstein, 2009). As Philpott, Mahur, and GrossKurth (2002) state, "when researchers and policy makers form strategic alliances it is possible to shift policy." It works best when the relationship is started early, the data is in a form that is easy to understand, and the environment is conducive to obtaining credible results (Philpott et al., 2002).

Research can be used as a political instrument. However, translating public health and clinical science evidence into not only practice but policy requires a strategy. In an example, Ryan, Card-Higginson, McCarthy, Justus, and Thompson (2006) were able to translate research into a policy to fight childhood obesity. This work required a four-step framework that included assessing the problem, implementing individual- and population-level interventions, and conducting surveillance to monitor progress (Ryan et al., 2006).

In a policy roundtable report published in *Health Services Research* in 2005, Mitch Greenlick, PhD, also a Democratic representative from Oregon, indicated that it was important to develop the answer years before the question is asked. As he points out, often the questions are the same ones asked years before that had been

---

BOX 16.2
Examples of Resource Reference in Health Policy for the CNL

POLICY INSTITUTES

Brookings Institute

The Commonwealth Fund

Kaiser Family Foundation

Institute for Higher Education

Robert Wood Johnson

Institute of Medicine

POLICY RESOURCES

Centers for Disease Control and Prevention: www.cdc.gov

Healthy Persons 2020: www.healthypeople.gov

The Joint Commission: jointcommisssion.org

Department of Health and Human Services: www.hhs.gov

Centers for Medicare and Medicaid Services: www.cms.gov

U.S. Congressional Budget Office: www.cbo.gov

POLICY JOURNALS

Health Affairs

Journal of Public Health

Journal of Health Care Management

left unsolved even though they were important. He also indicated that there is a difference between a policy expert and an advocate because a researcher needs to be careful not to wrap science in values or in the position that one is advocating. Subsequently, it is important to know the difference between a point estimate and a confidence interval and that it is not the details of the sample size or confidence interval that are needed or even wanted, but rather a solid estimate so that focus can move off of the data and onto the solution to the problem (Foltz, 2005).

CNLs who use evidence-based research to inform their practice should use this same approach when participating in public health policy and health services research. In health services research, where the emphasis is on controlling costs, increasing efficiencies, expanding access to care, and improving quality and safety, CNLs who are familiar with qualitative and quantitative research methods and publically available datasets (U.S. Department of Health and Human Services, Centers for Disease Control, American Hospital Association, American Nurses Association, etc.,) are very competent in conducting research and addressing health care problems. Box 16.2 includes a list of policy institutes, resources, and journals that are helpful for health care policy research.

TABLE 16.3 Health Policy Certification Exam Content

CATEGORY	WEIGHT
D. Health Care Policy	**4%**

1. Acknowledges multiple perspectives when analyzing health care policy

2. Recognizes the effect of health care policy on health promotion, risk reduction, and disease and injury prevention in vulnerable populations

3. Influences regulatory, legislative, and public policy in private and public arenas to promote and preserve healthy communities

4. Understands the interactive effect of health policy and health care economics and national and international health and health outcomes

5. Accesses, critiques, and analyzes information sources

6. Incorporates standards of care and full scope of practice

7. Articulates the interaction between regulatory controls and quality control within the health care delivery system

8. Creates a professional ethic related to client care and health policy

9. Understands the political and regulatory processes defining health care delivery and systems of care

10. Evaluates local, state, and national socioeconomic and health policy issues and trends as they relate to the delivery of health care

11. Participates in political processes and grassroots legislative efforts to influence health care policy on behalf of clients and the profession

12. Understands global health care issues (e.g., immigration patterns, pandemics, access to care)

13. Understands the effect of legal and regulatory processes on nursing practice

Used with permission from the Commission on Nurse Certification.

Conclusion

Rising health care costs and patients who present with several comorbidities will need care that the CNL is responsible for, and able to deliver across the practice settings. The CNL who bridges the gap between the world of clinical care and that of health policy will be able to navigate patients and other stakeholders such as physicians, hospital administration, and members of the team through tumultuous times. Educating themselves and their patients about important health system issues and participating in health care reform processes are central CNL responsibilities. The system desperately needs CNLs in all practice settings to educate and involve patients in their own care, to coordinate clinical needs, to communicate effectively with professional colleagues, and assess and monitor changes in the health care delivery system. The certification exam covers a broad range of health care policy concepts that reflect the diverse role of CNLs in this area (Table 16.3).

Resources

Altarum Institute's Center for Studying Health Spending. (2011). Retrieved from http://www.altarum.org/about-altarum-nonprofit-research-institute

American Hospital Association. (2010). Retrieved from http://www.aha.org

American Nurses Association. (2011). Retrieved from http://www.nursingworld.org

Centers for Medicare and Medicaid Services. (2011). Retrieved from https://www.cms.gov/cmsleadership/09_office_oact.asp

Congressional Budget Office. (2011). Retrieved from http://www.cbo.gov

Chuang, S., & Inder, K. (2009). An effectiveness analysis of healthcare systems using a systems theoretic approach. *BMC Health Services Research, 9*(195), 1–11.

Curtain, L. L. (2012). Health policy, politics, and professional ethics. In D. J. Mason, J. L. Leavitt, & M. W. Chaffee (Eds.), *Policy and politics: In nursing and health care* (pp.77–87). St. Louis, MO: Elsevier.

Folz, C. E. (2005). Health policy roundtable. View from the state legislature: Translating research into policy. *Health Services Research, 40*(2), 337–346.

Goldstein, H. (2009). Translating research into public policy. Commentary. *Journal of Public Health Policy, 30,* S16–S20.

Hudson, D. W., Sexton, J. B., Thomas, E. J., & Berenholtz, S. M. (2009). A safety culture primer for the critical care clinician: The role of culture in patient safety and quality improvement. *Contemporary Critical Care, 7*(5), 1–13.

Institute of Medicine. (2001). Crossing the quality chasm (Executive Summary).

Institute of Medicine. (2003). Bridge to Quality. Retrieved from http://www.iom.edu/Reports/2003/Health-Professions-Education-A-Bridge to Quality.aspx

Jones, J. M. (2011). Nurses top honesty and ethics list for 11th year. *Gallup Poll.* Retrieved from http://www.gallup.com/poll/145043/nurses-top-honesty-ethics-list-11-year.aspx

Kaiser Family Foundation. (2009). Bridge to Quality Retrieved from http://www.kff.org/about/kcmu.cfm\

Kaufman, N. S. (2011). Changing economics in an era of healthcare reform. *Journal of Healthcare Management, 56*(1), 9–13.

Lantz, P. M., Lichtenstein, R. L., & Pollack, H. A. (2007). Health policy approaches to population health: The limits of medicalization. *Health Affairs, 26*(5), 1253–1257.

Leavitt, J. K., Chaffee, M. W., & Vance, C. (2012). Learning the ropes of policy, politics, and advocacy. In D. J. Mason, J .L. Leavitt, & M. W. Chaffee (Eds.), *Policy and politics: In nursing and health care* (pp.19–28). St. Louis, MO: Elsevier.

Philpott, A., Maher, D., & GrossKurth, H. (2002). Translating HIV/AIDS research findings into policy: Lessons from a case study of "the Mwanza trial." *Health Policy and Planning, 17*(20), 196–201.

Porche, D. J. (2012). *Health policy: Application for nurses and other healthcare professionals.* Sudbury, MA: Jones & Bartlett Publishers.

Richard, S. A., Rawel, S., & Martin, D. K. (2005). An ethical framework for cardiac report cards: A qualitative study. *BMC Medical Ethics, 6*(1), 3–13.

Russell, G. E. (2011). The United States healthcare system. In D. J. Mason, J. L. Leavitt, & M. W. Chaffee (Eds.), *Policy and politics: In nursing and health care* (pp. 122–134). St. Louis, MO: Elsevier.

Ryan, K. W., Card-Higginson, P., McCarthy, S. G., Justus, M. B., & Thompson, J. W. (2006). Arkansas fights fat: Translating research into policy to combat childhood and adolescent obesity. *Health Affairs, 25*(4), 992–1004.

Social Security Annual Statistical Bulletin Supplement. (2000). Social Security Act of 1965. Retrieved from http://www.ssa.gov/history/pdf/hlth_care.pdf

Suchy, K. (2010). A lack of standardization: The basis for ethical issues surrounding quality and performance reports. *Journal of Healthcare Management, 55*(4), 241–251.

Venegoni, S. L. (1996). Changing environment of healthcare. In J. V. Hickey, R. M., Ouimette, & S. L. Venegoni (Eds.), *Advanced practice nursing: Changing roles and clinical applications* (pp. 77–90). Philadelphia, PA: Lippincott Williams & Wilkins.

17

Quality Improvement, Risk Reduction, and Patient Safety

Kathryn B. Reid

Quality improvement, risk reduction, and patient safety clinical nurse leader (CNL) role functions provide the basis for point-of-care clinical leadership. Advanced knowledge of quality-safety principles and methodologies is core to CNL practice. This chapter reviews the underpinnings of the role of the CNL with respect to quality improvement, risk reduction, and patient safety. Environmental factors that support quality and safety are identified, and key terms are defined. Measures of quality and safety, including nurse-sensitive, safety, and core measure indicators, are described. Evidence-based quality improvement, risk reduction, and patient safety strategies are highlighted. The use of informatics and a dashboard in relation to quality and safety outcomes management is discussed. Some of the key terms and concepts covered in this chapter will include:

- Clinical audit
- Core measures
- Culture of safety
- Failure mode effects analysis (FMEA)
- Healthy work environment (HWE)
- High-risk cohorts
- High-risk patients
- Microsystem assessment (5Ps)
- National patient safety goals (NPSG)
- National quality forum (NQF)
- Nurse quality indicators

- Nurse sensitive indicators
- Patient safety
- Plan-do-study-act (PDSA) and standardize-do-study-act (SDSA)
- Quality
- Quality and Safety in Education for Nurses (QSEN)
- Quality dashboard
- Quality improvement
- Quality improvement methodologies: six sigma, lean, total quality management
- Risk reduction
- Root cause analysis (RCA)
- The Joint Commission

Background

National mandates emphasize the need for advanced nurses who are skilled in point-of-care clinical leadership to address critical problems in patient safety and quality care delivery. These include the following:

- *To Err Is Human: Building a Safer Health System* (Institute of Medicine [IOM], 1999), which estimated between 44,000 and 98,000 Americans die each year as a result of medical errors, and that medical errors lead to $17 billion to $29 billion in extra costs
- *Crossing the Quality Chasm* (IOM, 2001), which calls for professionals and organizations to promote health care that is safe, effective, client-centered, timely, efficient, and equitable (p. 6)
- *Health Professions Education: A Bridge to Quality* (IOM, 2003), which states, "All health professionals should be educated to deliver patient-centered care as members of an interdisciplinary team, emphasizing evidence-based practice, quality improvement approaches, and informatics" (p. 3)

In response to these broad mandates for health care delivery reforms, the role of the CNL, an advanced master's-prepared nurse, was envisioned by key stakeholders within the nursing profession. "The nursing profession must produce quality graduates who, among other things, are prepared to implement outcomes-based practice and quality improvement strategies" (AACN, CNL White Paper, 2007, p.1). The focus of the CNL as a frontline leader at the point of care (microsystem) fulfills critical gaps necessary to re-engineer health care delivery systems to improve quality and safety in today's complex care environments. A core role competency of the CNL is that of a "Systems Analyst/Risk Anticipator" who participates in system reviews to evaluate/anticipate client risks to improve patient safety (AACN, 2007). The Quality Improvement Task Elements in the CNL role are delineated in Box 17.1 (Tan, CNL Job Analysis Report, 2011).

BOX 17.1
Quality Improvement Task Elements in the CNL Role

1. Evaluates the health care outcomes through the acquisition of data and the questioning of inconsistencies

2. Leads the redesign of client care after RCA of sentinel events

3. Gathers, analyzes, and synthesizes data related to risk reduction and patient safety

4. Analyzes systems and outcome datasets to anticipate individual client risk and improve quality care

5. Understands economies of care, cost-effectiveness, resource utilization, and effecting change in systems

6. Evaluates the environmental impact on health care outcomes

7. Collaborates and consults with other health professionals to design, coordinate, and evaluate client care outcomes

8. Evaluates the quality and use of products in the delivery of health care

9. Identifies opportunities for quality improvement and leads improvement activities utilizing evidence-based models

Source: *AACN Clinical Nurse Leader Job Analysis Report* (2011, p. 38).

Environmental Factors Supporting Quality and Safety

The CNL fulfills critically important linkages between the larger organization's quality-safety initiatives and implementation of these initiatives at the point of care (unit or microsystem). Several key factors provide the basis for effective quality improvement and maintenance of safe care environments at the unit level. These include concepts related to an HWE, described in Box 17.2, and a culture of safety, described in Table 17.1. The American Nurses Association's (ANA) National Center for Nursing Quality provides resources related to quality professional practice and health care delivery environments. More information can be accessed at www.nursingworld.org/MainMenuCategories/ThePracticeofProfessionalNursing/PatientSafetyQuality. Additional information about the National Center for Nursing Quality is discussed later in this chapter. Through advocacy for the professional practice environment itself, the CNL advances quality-safety initiatives designed for continuous outcome improvement.

Measures of Quality and Safety

Indicators of quality and safety that fall within the scope of CNL practice and oversight include safety measures, nurse-sensitive quality and safety indicators, and disease-specific core measures. The Joint Commission provides national direction for major patient safety issues through the NPSG, which are updated annually

BOX 17.2

Hallmarks of a HWE (AACN STANDARDS FOR ESTABLISHING AND SUSTAINING HWE, AACN, 2005)

- Skilled communication
- True collaboration
- Effective decision making
- Appropriate staffing
- Meaningful recognition
- Authentic leadership

TABLE 17. 1 Subcultures Present in a Culture of Safety (Sammer, 2010) and Related CNL Role Competencies

CNL ROLE FUNCTION	CNL COMPETENCIES	SAFETY SUBCULTURE CONTRIBUTION
Advocate	Effects change through advocacy for the profession, interdisciplinary health care team, and the client	*Leadership*
	Communicates effectively to achieve quality client outcomes and lateral integration of care for a cohort of clients	*Just*
		Leadership
		Teamwork
		Communication
		Patient centered
Member of a profession	Actively pursues new knowledge and skills as the CNL role, needs of clients, and the health care system evolve	*Leadership*
		Learning
Team manager	Properly delegates and utilizes the nursing team resources (human and fiscal) and serves as a leader and partner in the interdisciplinary health care team	*Leadership*
	Identifies clinical and cost outcomes that improve safety, effectiveness, timeliness, efficiency, quality, and the degree to which they are client centered	*Teamwork*
		Communication
		Learning
		Patient centered
Information manager	Uses information systems and technology at the point of care to improve health care outcomes	*Evidence based*
		Communication

(continued)

TABLE 17.1 *(continued)*

CNL ROLE FUNCTION	CNL COMPETENCIES	SAFETY SUBCULTURE CONTRIBUTION
Systems analyst/risk anticipator	Participates in systems review to critically evaluate and anticipate risks to client safety to improve quality of client care delivery	*Communication* *Learning*
Clinician	Assumes accountability for health care outcomes for a specific group of clients within a unit or setting recognizing the influence of the meso- and macrosystems on the microsystem	*Patient centered*
	Assimilates and applies research-based information to design, implement, and evaluate client plans of care	*Evidence based* *Learning*
Outcomes manager	Synthesizes data, information, and knowledge to evaluate and achieve optimal client and care environment outcomes	*Evidence based*
		Learning
		Patient centered
Educator	Uses appropriate teaching/learning principles and strategies as well as current information, materials, and technologies to facilitate the learning of clients, groups, and other health care professionals	*Leadership* *Teamwork* *Communication*

Source: Reid & Dennison (2011)

(www.jointcommission.org/standards_information/npsgs.aspx). The NPSG for 2012 are listed in Box 17.3. The NQF provides national leadership to establish national priorities and goals for ensuring that health care delivery is safe, effective, patient centered, timely, efficient, and equitable. The NQF establishes standards for measurement and reporting and provides education and outreach to drive continuous quality improvement in the nation's health care system. More information, including the complete quality standards information, is available through the NQF website at www.qualityforum.org/Home.aspx. The Centers for Medicare and Medicaid Services (CMS) also advances national quality initiatives through various mechanisms, such as the Hospital Quality Initiative (HQA). The ANA, in conjunction with the University of Kansas, maintains the National Database for Nursing Quality Indicators (NDNQI), and these indicators are listed in Box 17.4 (ANA, 2012). Many of these indicators are also endorsed by the NQF (as noted in the box).

Processes Used for Quality and Safety Improvement

With the CNL focus on point-of-care leadership, the use of a microsystem framework provides a valuable organizing framework. Microsystem improvement processes center on a comprehensive microsystem assessment using the "5Ps" approach

BOX 17.3
NPSG for 2012

Improve accuracy of patient identification.

• Use at least two patient identifiers when providing care, treatment, and services.

• Eliminate transfusion errors related to patient misidentification.

Improve the effectiveness of communication among caregivers.

• Report critical results of tests and diagnostic procedures on a timely basis.

Improve the safety of using medications.

• Label all medications, medication containers, and other solutions on and off the sterile field in perioperative and other procedural settings.

• Reduce the likelihood of patient harm associated with the use of anticoagulant therapy.

• Maintain and communicate accurate patient medication information.

Reduce the risk of health care-associated infections.

• Comply with either the current Centers for Disease Control and Prevention (CDC) hand hygiene guidelines or the current World Health Organization (WHO) hand hygiene guidelines.

• Implement evidence-based practices to prevent health care-associated infections due to multidrug-resistant organisms in acute care hospitals.

• Implement evidence-based practices to prevent central line-associated bloodstream infections.

• Implement evidence-based practices for preventing surgical site infections.

• Implement evidence-based practices to prevent indwelling catheter-associated urinary tract infections (CAUTI).

Reduce the risk of patient harm resulting from falls.

Prevent health care-associated pressure ulcers (decubitus ulcers).

The organization identifies safety risks inherent in its patient population.

• Identify patients at risk for suicide.

• Identify risks associated with home oxygen therapy, such as home fires.

Universal Protocol for Preventing Wrong Site, Wrong Procedure, Wrong Person Surgery™

• Conduct a preprocedure verification process.

• Mark the procedure site

• A time-out is performed before the procedure

Source: The Joint Commission, 2012.

BOX 17.4
National Database of Nursing Quality Indicators (NDNQI)

1. *Patient falls**
2. *Patient fall with injury**
3. *Pressure ulcers*
   a. *Community*
   b. *Hospital-acquired**
   c. *Unit-acquired*
4. Skill mix*
5. Nursing hours per patient day*
6. *RN surveys*
   a. *Job satisfaction*
   b. *Practice environment scale**
7. RN education and certification
8. *Pediatric pain assessment cycle*
9. *Pediatric IV infiltration rate*
10. *Psychiatric patient assault rate*
11. *Restraints prevalence**
12. *Nurse turnover**
13. *Hospital-acquired infection (HAI)*
    a. *Ventilator-associated pneumonia (VAP)**
    b. *Central line-associated bloodstream infection (CLABSI)**
    c. *Catheter-associated urinary tract infection (CAUTI)**

*NQF-endorsed standard.
The text in italics shows an indicator within CNL role focus.

Source: American Nurses Association, 2012.

(Box 17.5), followed by careful analysis of the "metrics that matter," as already described. Processes used for point-of-care quality and safety improvement include application of a systematic methodology. Eight common steps in quality improvement are listed in Box 17.6 (Harris & Roussel, 2010). Other commonly used quality improvement methodologies include "PDSA," Lean, and Six Sigma. Continuous quality improvement processes are enhanced through the use of a quality-safety dashboard system, in which the CNL accesses, tracks, and monitors quality-safety data on a regular basis to help inform staff and drive change.

BOX 17.5
Microsystem Assessment: The "5Ps"

1. Purpose: What is the purpose or overall mission of the setting?
2. Patients: What are the characteristics of the patients served by the setting?
3. Professionals: Who are the individuals involved in delivery care in the setting?
4. Processes: What are the processes involved in delivering care?
5. Patterns: What are the patterns observed in care delivery?

BOX 17.6
Eight Common Steps in Quality Improvement

1. Establish a clear and defined aim or purpose
2. Review the literature
3. Examine current resources available to facilitate quality improvement
4. Map current processes
5. Analyze root cause
6. Select appropriate tools for process analysis
7. Select measures and metrics (baseline and outcome)
8. Conduct rapid cyclical review of the plan, data, interventions, and outcomes

Source: McLaughlin & Kaluzny; Newhouse, 2006; Harris & Roussel, 2010.

The New Age of Quality Improvement and Patient Safety

In the past, there have been many internal and external drivers for organizations to pursue optimal outcomes for consumers of health care in many settings. Recent implications of pay-for-performance initiatives have put new and urgent focus on quality, safety, and risk reduction, which has a direct impact on CNLs. Unlike some quality programs that identify nursing quality indicators, the implications of health care reform have a compelling financial impact on organizations and are truly associated with all disciplines. The implications for the CNL are many. The CNL competencies related to a culture of safety (Table 17.1) are perfectly suited to enable CNLs to lead or significantly contribute to the emerging role of interdisciplinary improvement teams.

Let us take, for example, the issue of avoidable rehospitalizations. The CMS has identified this topic as one of the first areas to implement pay-for-performance mandates for Medicare patients. The rationale for this prioritization stems from data that indicate up to 20% of Medicare patients discharged from hospitals are readmitted within 30 days, and of those readmissions, up to 76% are potentially avoidable (Hackbarth, Reischaucer, & Miller, 2007). Health care systems across the country are addressing this issue with renewed enthusiasm, knowing that this is only the beginning of a new era of quality outcomes that impact the organization's bottom line.

Based on the academic preparation of a CNL coupled with the clinical expertise of this master's prepared generalist, many skills and talents can be utilized in the team approach to reducing readmissions. To begin with, the CNL is well acquainted with the benefits and challenges of working with an interdisciplinary team. The CNL can utilize and develop leadership skills to cultivate a highly functional team of professionals, in which all voices are valued, but the top priorities of the team are addressed. A topic such as readmission of patients requires an understanding of the larger system as well as the smaller microsystems where patients receive care. A structured process of improvement should be utilized, that is, PDSA. In addition, global and specific aims of the group as well as a timeline should be established.

One of the key elements to any quality improvement initiatives is the establishment of metrics to measure the success of the initiative. Vast amounts of data are collected in today's health care world based on the use of electronic medical records and other informatics advances. Although the CNL is not required to be the expert on all data, he or she should be sure to include a data and informatics expert on the team and utilize the skill and knowledge of that individual to support the team's knowledge of metrics involved. The role of informatics is exploding in today's health care and all disciplines benefit from working closely to understand the complicated world of health care technology. In the future of pay for performance, there is a greater responsibility of informatics, electronic medical record, and compliance with accepted standards of practice. The CNL should be continually expanding on this knowledge and facilitating increased knowledge to nursing and nonnursing disciplines.

Once a group of professionals has been assembled and common professional aims established for the improvement initiative, how do you tackle the vastness of a topic such as hospital readmissions? The area of quality improvement has many tools that the CNL can utilize in supporting the team to examine the task at hand. A flowchart could help map a patient's care from the primary care setting to the emergency department (or other inpatient access point) to the inpatient areas and back to the discharge destination. A Pareto chart could help identify top readmission rates and guide the group in a focus on the top readmission issues. Cause and effect diagrams may aid in the analysis of particular problems that are identified to categorize them and address such categories. RCA can be a tool to identify a particular situation and determine what happened, how it happened, and why it happened, with the goal of making changes to prevent future events. Many options are available for groups, but the knowledge of a CNL can lead the group to make the best use of time and stay focused on the aims of the group.

We often hear the term "let's not reinvent the wheel." There are many areas of quality, safety, and risk reduction that have comprehensive, scholarly, and interdisciplinary work available to interested organizations. Publications regarding quality improvement, evidence-based practice, and improving patient safety are available. The CNL should conduct or contribute to a literature search in the area of interest. Many professional organizations have been mentioned in this chapter as excellent resources for quality work. In many cases there may be an abundance of resources, and the CNL should work with other group members to identify the most useful and highly regarded materials. Even publications of initiatives that did not lead to improved metrics by a particular group can be valuable to a team. Again, the role of the CNL and others to critically review available resources is critical. On the topic of hospital readmissions, the Institute for Healthcare Improvement (IHI) has extensive resources on this topic in the form of a "how-to guide." Improving transitions from the hospital to the clinical office practice to reduce avoidable rehospitalizations (IHI, 2011) is a comprehensive, interdisciplinary body of work. A work of this kind could be a critical component to a time-efficient, productive team. The example provided here, which utilizes common practices of quality improvement as listed in Box 17.6, will eventually inform a structured plan of action. For more information on the resources to prevent readmissions, visit www.IHI.org.

The example of preventing hospital readmissions illustrates the value of the CNL in the first phases of an improvement team and continues through the team's process. Just a few elements of that value have been described in terms of getting the improvement team started in the right direction. CNLs have had academic and clinical preparation to support the success of such groups through each phase of the project and also on the critical role of sustainability. A key element of quality and safety is the ongoing presence of the CNL in the clinical setting; supporting direct care members not only to improve outcomes but also to sustain multiple initiatives. This vital link of information from various sources to the frontline caregivers is critical to a culture of safety.

Conclusion

There is a wonderful and important synergy between the CNL and the new era of quality and safety. The master's-prepared clinical expert is perfectly equipped to be a driving force, facilitator, and valued team member in the work that is to be done. Even in the few years since the CNL was envisioned and became a reality, major changes to health care and financial implications of quality have created a new world of opportunities for CNLs to be the link between the front line of care and the chief officers of the organization. CNLs will impact quality and safety in every health care setting and support safe and patient-focused transitions of care. The certification exam for CNLs covers many aspects of quality improvement and the various competencies involved in improved outcomes for patients (Table 17.2).

TABLE 17.2 Quality Management

CATEGORY	WEIGHT
E. Quality Improvement	**6%**

1. Evaluates health care outcomes through the acquisition of data and the questioning of inconsistencies

2. Leads the redesign of client care following RCA of sentinel events

3. Gathers, analyzes, and synthesizes data related to risk reduction and patient safety

4. Analyzes systems and outcome datasets to anticipate individual client risk and improve quality care

5. Understands economies of care, cost-effectiveness, resource utilization, and effecting change in systems

6. Evaluates the environmental impact on health care outcomes

7. Collaborates and consults with other health professionals to design, coordinate, and evaluate client care outcomes

8. Evaluates the quality and use of products in the delivery of health care

9. Identifies opportunities for quality improvement and leads improvement activities utilizing evidence-based models

Used with permission from the Commission on Nurse Certification.

Resources

American Association of Colleges of Nursing. (2007). *White paper on the education and role of the clinical nurse leader*. Retrieved March 20, 2008, from http://www.aacn.nche.edu

Hackbarth, G., Reischaucer, R., & Miller, M. (2007). *Report to congress: Medicare payment policy*. Washington, DC: Medicare Payment Advisory Committee.

Harris, J., & Roussel, L. (2010). *Initiating and sustaining the clinical nurse leader role: A practical guide*. Sudbury, MA: Jones & Bartlett Publishers.

Institute for Healthcare Improvement. (2011). *How-to guide: Improving transitions from the hospital to the clinical office practice to reduce avoidable rehospitalizations*. Retrieved May 25, 2012, from www.IHI.org

Institute of Medicine. (1999). *To err is human*. Washington, DC: The National Academies Press.

Institute of Medicine. (2001). *Crossing the quality chasm: A new health system for the 21st century*. Washington, DC: The National Academies Press.

Institute of Medicine. (2003). *Health professions education: A bridge to quality*. Washington, DC: The National Academies Press.

National Association of Clinical Nurse Specialists (2008a). *National Association of Clinical Nurse Specialists update on the clinical nurse leader. September 2005*. Retrieved March 20, 2008, from http://www.nacns.org

National Association of Clinical Nurse Specialists (2008b). *National Association of Clinical Nurse Specialists position statement on the clinical nurse leader. March 2004*. Retrieved March 20, 2008, from http://www.nacns.org

Reid, K., & Dennison, P. (2011). The clinical nurse leader (CNL)®: Point-of-care safety clinician. *Online Journal of Issues in Nursing, 16*(3), 4.

Sammer, C. E, Lykens, K., Singh, K., Mains, D. A., & Lackan, N. A. (2010). What is a patient safety culture? A review of literature. *Journal of Nursing Scholarship, 42*(2), 156–165.

Tan, R. (2011). *CNL Job Analysis Report, 2011*.Schroeder Measurement Technologies, Inc. Retrieved January 31, 2012, from http://www.aacn.nche.edu/cnl/Job-Analysis-Report.pdf

18

Health Care Informatics

Carol Fackler

Never before has the utilization of health care information technology been so important to the delivery of safe, quality care to the citizens of the United States. Since the groundbreaking report *To Err Is Human* (Institute of Medicine [IOM], 1999), highlighting 98,000 medical errors annually in the United States, stakeholders in health care from clinicians to policymakers have focused on designing better systems to measure the delivery of quality care and evaluate the outcomes of that care in ways that lead to improvement. The six aims of quality care proposed by the IOM in their report *Crossing the Quality Chasm: A New Health Care System for the 21st Century* (2001) provide a blueprint for improvement. These six aims are safe, timely, patient-centered, effective, efficient, and equitable. Implementation of the clinical nurse leader (CNL) role is one way to provide the clinical expertise needed to address the ability to achieve these aims. With the CNL's focus on quality, safety, monitoring, and evaluating the processes and outcomes of health care delivery, a nurse in this leadership role may serve as both a facilitator and a catalyst in improving quality care and ensuring client safety.

As we begin the second decade of the 21st century, the confluence of health care information technology utilization with the work of the CNL positions nursing as a key player in how technology is developed, implemented, and evaluated. Health information technology is not new to the nursing profession; nursing has been involved with informatics in health care for a long time. As early as the 1970s, nurses were involved in interdisciplinary work developing technology to assist in the delivery of health care (Ozbolt & Saba, 2008). Nurses' involvement in defining nurses' work in ways that could be documented and evaluated with a variety of technology tools led to the creation of a nursing minimum data set (NMDS) (Ozbolt & Saba, 2008). Other explication of nursing work resulted in nursing diagnoses developed by the North American Nursing Diagnosis Association (NANDA) and the development of the Nursing Interventions Classification (NIC), the Nursing Outcomes Classification (NOC), and the National Database for Nursing Quality Indicators. Despite challenges in standardizing the language defining nursing work and operationalizing data elements for input into computer software, nurses have moved forward both nationally and internationally in becoming involved in explicating nursing nomenclature in ways that capture the important role that nurses play in promoting quality health care and client safety.

The federal government is currently taking a lead role in coordinating major efforts to implement the use of electronic health records (EHRs) across the health care delivery system. These efforts require the expertise of informaticists, engineers, computer specialists, health care administrators, and nursing leaders such as the CNL. Now more than ever, the CNL is in a position to influence what information technology is implemented as well as its ongoing evaluation. The availability of an increasing number of technological tools with which to assess, monitor, implement, and evaluate the care of clients enhances the CNL's ability to effect changes in clinical care processes to improve client outcomes.

The purpose of this chapter is to examine the ways by which the CNL should approach the use of health care information technology; these include but are not limited to:

- assessing and monitoring clients
- planning and delivering care
- evaluating outcomes of care
- disseminating health care information among team members
- safeguarding the privacy and confidentiality of client information
- meeting the needs of geographically remote clients
- recognizing the advantages and challenges of consumer use of health technology
- analyzing existing systems to identify supports and gaps
- participating in the development of new technologies

The CNL and the Role of Informatics

In order to serve clients in today's health care system, the use of information technology is essential. Today's CNL may work alongside many others with expertise in information systems, including nurse informaticists. As a specialty, nurse informaticists' work is based on the integration of nursing science, information science, and computer science (Mastrian & McGonigle, 2012). While this specialty of nurses with expertise in health care information technology is emerging, there are many settings where nurse informaticists are not employed. In the absence of a nurse informaticist, it is up to the CNL to have knowledge of and become involved with available health care information technology. The CNL should be aware of what the American Nurses Association (ANA), in its *Scope and Standards of Practice for Nursing Informatics* (2008), notes is the responsibility of the informatics nurse specialists (INS):

> . . . the INS must navigate the complex relationships between the following elements and understand how they facilitate decision making:
> - Data, information, knowledge, and wisdom
> - Nursing science, information science, computer science, cognitive science and other sciences of interest

- Nurse, person, health, and environment
- Information structures, information technology, management and communication of information (p. 13)

Because the use of health care information technology is becoming more prevalent, it is also important for the CNL to be knowledgeable about resources that provide ongoing updates of the state of the science in this discipline. Therefore, in addition to reading this chapter, prospective CNLs are encouraged to read the references cited here and refer to the web-based resources referenced in this chapter. These resources are a source of helpful information about the state of the current efforts in bringing this country's health care information technology into the 21st century.

Setting the Stage: The Current Climate in Health Information Technology

Since 2009, with the passage of the American Recovery and Reinvestment Act (ARRA) (Pub.L. 111-5), there has been increasing attention to how the country's providers of health care use health information technology. Under ARRA, monies available through the Health Information Technology for Economic and Clinical Health (HITECH) Act are earmarked for the development of the EHR. Regional Extension Centers across the country, coordinated by the Office of the National Coordinator for Health Information Technology (ONC) (www.hhs.gov/healthit), are assisting health care providers in the implementation of certified EHRs.

Following the passage of ARRA, the Centers for Medicare and Medicaid Services (CMS; www.cms.gov) developed an incentive program to encourage the adoption of the EHR by critical access hospitals (CAHs), community hospitals, and primary care practice providers. Educational resources helpful to implement EHRs, in ways that meet federal certification guidelines, are available for both institutions and individual providers from a number of sources. For example, the ONC coordinates and supports a number of initiatives that support not only EHR development and implementation, but also other aspects of health IT (www.hhs.gov/healthit). These include initiatives related to clinical decision support (CDS), cyber security, rural health IT, and state-level health initiatives for health information exchange (HIE). The Healthcare Information and Management Systems Society (HIMSS), a global nonprofit organization with a majority of its 44,000 individual members working in health care, promotes the optimal use of information technology and management systems through its content expertise, professional development, research initiatives, and media vehicles (www.himss.org).

The importance of delivering health care using evidence-based practice makes other health care information technology such as clinical decision support (CDS) essential as institutions and providers work to comply with governmental guidelines and professional practice standards. Current federal guidelines require that clinical information systems be interoperable; for example, clinical decision support systems (CDSS) developed today must be capable of being embedded into any EHR. The goal is to have all health care information tools be able to "talk" to each other.

HIEs are organizational or geographical entities that manage health care information electronically across organizations or regions (McGonigle & Mastrian, 2012). Organizational and/or regional management of protected health information (PHI) makes it possible for the information to reside in one central location, available to all providers of care requesting that information at any point in time. Before a scheduled visit or at the time of an unscheduled visit, the patient gives consent for health care providers to access PHI or to send PHI to the exchange.

It is incumbent upon the CNL to remain informed of the ever-changing climate in health information technology, one that is evolving as new technologies, new applications of current technologies, and increasing consumer use of information systems emerge. One example of the explosion of new health care technology applications is consumers' utilization of telehealth to share subjective and objective data with health care providers from the comfort of their homes and in situations when access to providers is limited by distance, lack of transportation, or other factors. Telehealth technologies and the emerging use of mobile applications such as smartphones represent exciting possibilities for health care delivery to remote populations by addressing issues related to access to care, chronic care management, and client satisfaction.

Assessing and Monitoring Clients

The integration of clinical data into computer systems allows for the input and retrieval of large amounts of data on clients. That data, viewed in the context of the environment in which care is delivered, yields important information about processes and outcomes involving clients. Just a few years ago, much of the information collected on clients in any health care delivery system reflected only demographic, scheduling, and billing information. Today, health information technology includes the input, management, and retrieval of clinically important data. Large health care systems have created data repositories, called data warehouses, from which important clinical indices can be retrieved to examine the processes and outcomes associated with care delivery. One notable example of such a system is the U.S. Department of Veterans Affairs Clinical Case Registries (CCR), a program that supports the delivery and evaluation of care for thousands of clients in this large national health care delivery system (Backus et al., 2009). Lessons learned from managing registries of clinical data from clients with HIV and hepatitis C virus (HCV) include the need for manual confirmation of electronic data, for updating software to reflect changes in clinical diagnostic and laboratory test coding, and for monitoring updated software for missing critical data elements (Backus et al., 2009). The experience of the Department of Veterans Affairs in maintaining their clinical registries underscores the significance of the human—computer interface in managing electronic information.

Access to clinical data stored in data warehouses also allows large health care systems to conduct rigorous research related to processes and outcomes; one example is the work of Intermountain Healthcare of Salt Lake City. Working with data collected from multiple facilities in its large network, this health care system has been able to examine processes such as the relationship between the amount of nursing care clients receive and client outcomes (Hall et al., 2009).

The meaningfulness of clinical data is recognized in the development, adoption, and implementation of the EHR. Meaningful use is the term used to denote the standards defining what meaningful data should be included in the EHR; however, challenges exist related to how to make clinically relevant data available for collection, management, and retrieval within the EHR. Data reflecting nursing care remains some of the most difficult data to capture. How to embed language reflective of nursing care into the EHR continues to be a challenge. What data should be collected has been informed by efforts such as the development of the Systematic Nomenclature of Medicine (SNOMED) (www.ihtsdo.org), the Nursing Minimum Data Set (NMDS), the Nursing Interventions Classification (NIC) (www.nursing.uiowa.edu), and the Nursing Outcomes Classification (NOC) (www.nursing.uiowa.edu) and by organizations such as the North American Nursing Diagnosis Association (NANDA) (www.nanda.org).

The CNL, in managing the care of a subpopulation of clients, should play an active role in decision making about what clinical data should be collected in and from the EHR and other technology tools, how that data should be managed, and who should have access to the data for the purpose of analyzing and improving care delivery processes and client outcomes. The CNL also needs to be vocal about the importance of standardizing nursing terminology in health care information technology. In the absence of such standardization, data that could be meaningfully related to nurses' contribution to quality, safe health care may be lost. As Ozbolt and Saba (2008) explain:

> Faced with the bewildering array of choices and the licensing fees required for the use of NANDA, NIC, NOC, and SNOMED, many health care organizations adopting nursing information systems opted to use their own or vendor-provided, non-standard terms. This approach allowed entry of data via familiar terms, but because the terms were not consistent in definition or usage, investigators could not retrieve meaningful data to analyze for quality improvement or research. (p. 202)

Planning and Delivering Care

The process of delivering safe, quality care requires ongoing collection, management, and analysis of clinically relevant data. The CNL may have data requiring analysis from a number of sources, including individual paper medical records, unit-based computerized reports, or aggregate data from a data warehouse. In addition, nationally benchmarked data analysis may be available from recognized sources such as the National Database of Nursing Quality Indicators (NDNQI) (www.nursingquality.org) and Press Ganey (www.pressganey.com).

Once data analysis is complete, the CNL can then share the results with the unit's interdisciplinary team, encourage feedback, and involve those on the team in decision making about change that positively impacts client outcomes. That change may come in the form of alterations in processes to deliver care or the development of new processes to address a clinical problem. Recognized approaches to implementing change may include quality improvement processes such as continuous quality improvement with its plan-do-study-act (PDSA) process.

In the delivery of health care to clients, health care information technology itself offers a number of modalities with which to prevent errors in real time. Computerized physician order entry (CPOE) is a feature of the EHR that assures standardized, legible communication of the medical plan of care to other members of the health care team. Clinical decision support systems (CDSS) may be embedded in the EHR, prompting clinicians in their assessment and ongoing monitoring of clients to address deficits in documentation; to consider potential outcomes related to their decision making (e.g., drug–drug interactions); or as reminders to order, for example, standard screening tests for clients. This CDS may be passive, consisting of pop-up reminders or alerts on the computer screen, or it may be more active. In an active system, the clinician is not only reminded of a drug–drug interaction, but also advised by the system about what to monitor and what other care to consider when two interacting drugs are being utilized simultaneously.

Evaluating and Improving Outcomes of Care

Evaluating outcomes of care requires an interdisciplinary approach. The CNL is in a key position to orchestrate the evaluation process because he or she is in constant interaction with the health care team at the point of patient care. Evaluation of unexpected outcomes may use processes such as root cause analysis (RCA). Analyses resulting from such processes result in identification of changes needed to improve outcomes of care.

The CNL can foster both collaborative and collegial approaches to the delivery of safe, quality care to patients. Educated as a nurse, the CNL's educational background includes a holistic approach to care, reflecting knowledge from multiple disciplines including medical science, psychology, public health, nutrition, and information technology. Additional graduate preparation as a CNL affords further opportunities for exposure to principles underlying clinical microsystems, leadership, and the change process. This background provides the CNL with the knowledge and skills needed to identify problems, analyze data, communicate findings to other health care team members, and lead the change process. Only through an educated, systematic approach to addressing deficiencies in the delivery of client care can the health care team improve processes and outcomes.

Disseminating Health Care Information Among Team Members

A nurse who is effective in the role of a CNL brings together the health care team to assess, implement, and evaluate initiatives aimed at delivery of safe, quality care to a subpopulation of clients. The CNL has an obligation and is accountable for timely dissemination of the analysis of client data to members of the health care team. That analysis may include frequency distribution of data, trends in the clinical data, probability statistics, and the interpretation of run and control charts. In addition to the dissemination of client care data and analysis for the particular subset of clients with whom the CNL is working, this nursing leader also has an obligation to remain current with the peer-reviewed published literature on quality, safety, and health care outcomes. The CNL should be an active member of organizations that examine and monitor quality outcomes in health care and keep the health care team abreast of new developments, current research, and nationally recognized guidelines.

CNLs should remain informed about the work of such organizations as:

- Agency for Healthcare Research and Quality (AHRQ) (www.ahrq.gov)
- National Quality Forum (NQF) (www.qualityforum.org)
- Institute of Medicine (IOM) (www.iom.edu)
- Quality and Safety Education for Nurses (QSEN) (www.qsen.org)

Safeguarding Privacy and Confidentiality of Client Information

Both clients and health care providers are understandably concerned about how the privacy and confidentiality of clients' PHI will be assured as more and more technology is utilized to collect and manage data, as well as use data to evaluate health care processes and outcomes. Assurances from the federal government are not enough. There must be a commitment by those interacting directly with clients to safeguard client information, making it available on a need-to-know basis only.

The development of HIEs has elevated the level of concern of both clients and providers. HIEs allow for multiple health care organizations serving a client to share health information across electronic networks. This has the potential to contribute to continuity of care and client satisfaction. The exchange of information addresses the IOM aims of timeliness, effectiveness, and efficiency. The electronic transmission of client information from one organization to another is more timely than the transfer of paper records. The receiving provider has faster access to information with which to plan care and make decisions; this timeliness may therefore achieve greater benefit (effectiveness). Having timely access to client information also avoids unnecessary retesting, thereby enhancing efficiency. The sharing of client information, however, requires a level of electronic encryption to assure the security necessary to avoid breaches in confidentiality. It demands a level of trust in information technology experts that leads clients and clinicians to feel assured that privacy and confidentiality are being maintained.

According to one nurse scholar, nurses involved in the development, use, and evaluation of information systems in health care should be guided by nursing theoretical frameworks, principles, and concepts when expressing their thoughts about the ethical issues related to the privacy and confidentiality of PHI (Milton, 2009). Others will look to nurses, placing their trust in the input nurses have in this important area of concern around the use and potential abuse of information available as a result of health care information technology.

Meeting the Needs of Geographically Remote Clients

As the country embraces the increased use of health information technology, no longer will the issue of access be so dramatically affected by the lack of geographic proximity to large health care institutions. With the advent of telehealth technologies, clients can now be cared for without needing to be face-to-face with a clinician. Across the continuum of wellness to illness and recognizing especially the needs of those with chronic illnesses, remote assessment, monitoring, and decision making are now possible through the use of technology.

In rural communities, where expertise in critical care medicine and nursing may be concentrated in metropolitan areas far removed, the ability to remotely monitor critically ill clients through live streaming video has enabled clinicians to have available 24-hour consultation with critical care specialists in the care of those clients. Furthermore, where a shortage of clinicians exists in more remote areas of the country, having the ability to remotely monitor very ill clients on the "off shift" in small hospitals has been invaluable to critical care nurses at the bedside during those times. This remote monitoring is called the electronic ICU or E-ICU.

In managing subpopulations of chronically ill patients, today's technology makes it possible for at-home clients to communicate with clinicians and for clinicians to assess clients through live video viewing. If managing a large cohort of clients with chronic illness, computer systems have the ability, when programmed, to triage incoming data from clients so that clinicians have a prioritized list of clients to contact. By redefining the location of care using health care information technology, programs such as the Department of Veteran Affairs' Care Coordination/ Home Telehealth (CCHT) program have reported that benefits of such a program include the reduction in the numbers of hospital admissions, reduction in the number of hospital bed days of care, and improvement in veterans' satisfaction with services (Darkins et al., 2008).

Advantages and Disadvantages of Consumer Use of Health Technology

Consumers today are active users of technology, both in their workplace and in their personal lives. It is not surprising that consumers are increasingly turning to the Internet for health care information. There are a number of applications consumers may use in accessing computers for their health care needs, and there are many reasons consumers choose to use web-based resources; these include information-seeking, communication and support, the maintenance of personal health records, decision support, and disease management (Zielstorff & Frink, 2012). In a review of 12 studies on health care consumers' experiences with health care information technology, Akesson, Saveman, and Nilsson (2007) found that consumers were empowered by the perceived knowledge and support they gained in using technology. The ONC agrees, making consumer access to timely summaries of health care visits and other health care information part of the "meaningful use" criteria that must be met in adopting EHR technology.

There are, however, issues of concern regarding consumers' use of computers for health. These include, but are not limited to, the issues of variability in quality of available information, privacy and security of data on the Internet; the digital divide; educational, ethnic, and cultural barriers; physical and cognitive disabilities; and the impact on consumers' relationships with health care providers (Zielstorff & Frink, 2012). The digital divide may reflect both access to and comfort with computer use. Educational and literacy barriers associated with the ability to use computers need to be areas of focus for intervention and research as we move forward as a nation toward a more fully computerized health care delivery system.

Analyzing Systems to Identify Supports and Gaps

As health care institutions examine their existing health technology products to assess whether they meet national standards, the CNL has the opportunity to provide input on how those products might best meet the need for quality improvement and control. Using the standards set by the federal government and available on the website of the ONC (www.hhs.gov/healthit), the CNL is in a position to assess whether the organization's EHR meets the standards set for a comprehensive quality-outcome-driven electronic portal. Also in need of evaluation is whether clinical decision support systems in use in the organization reflect the application of evidence-based clinical practice in the delivery of quality care. If not already embedded as part of the EHR, CDS should be interoperable with the existing EHR. For ongoing monitoring or follow up of patients with chronic disease, telemedicine in the form of remote monitoring and mobile applications for ongoing assessment should also be considered by the organization for delivering comprehensive, patient-centered care.

Improvements in quality and safety related to client outcomes can be achieved with health information technology if human–technology interfaces are effective (Effken, 2012). Human factors that influence the performance of clinicians within the human–machine system include human capabilities and the environment (Alexander, 2012). Human capabilities include physical and sensory characteristics, including functions such as attention, perception, learning, memory, recall, reasoning, making decisions, and transmitting information (Alexander, 2012). The environment includes organizational structures and processes, tasks (cognitive and physical), and feedback mechanisms (Alexander, 2012).

The CNL plays a role as an advocate for user involvement early in the design and implementation of technology, with particular attention to human–technology interfaces. The CNL is also in a position to prevent workarounds by being involved as a coach and cheerleader for members of the multidisciplinary team. Aware of the human factors that might impede successful implementation and consistent use of technology, this involvement may include orientation to the technologies, continuing education, and other methods of achieving and maintaining "buy-in" from colleagues.

Development of New Technologies

The recent IOM report, *The Future of Nursing: Leading Change, Advancing Health* (2010), highlights the role nursing must play in the current and future health care delivery system. One of the IOM's key messages is that nurses "should be full partners, with physicians and other health professionals, in redesigning health care in the United States" (IOM, 2010, p. 4). Much of that change is now integrated with industry-wide efforts to incorporate information technology into all aspects of client care. In order to remain current with all the new developments in the field of electronic assessment, management, and outcome evaluation of the country's health, it is incumbent upon the CNL to be an active member in ongoing development, implementation, and evaluation of health care information technologies. This includes participation in research.

CNLs are encouraged to participate in the information technology-oriented organizations that currently exist to educate, support, and provide leadership opportunities for its members. These organizations include, but are not limited to, the American Nursing Informatics Association—Caring (www.ania-caring.org) and the Health Information and Management Systems Society (www.himss.org). Participating in the TIGER Initiative (www.tigerinitiative.org) also affords a way to remain current with what nurses are doing to educate health care professionals about health care information technology. TIGER, which is the acronym for Technology Informatics Guiding Education Reform, was formed by a group of nurses who believe in the importance of nursing's role in the implementation of information technology. TIGER's mission is to help develop the nursing workforce's capabilities in the utilization of EHRs, to engage clinicians in the development of the national health care information technology infrastructure, and to assist in accelerating the interdisciplinary adoption of technologies that will improve and enhance the delivery of safe, timely, efficient, and accessible health care (www.tigerinitiative.org).

The CNL should also embrace and be engaged in assisting nurse researchers and others involved in information technology research in addressing important issues related to the use of health care information technology. Bakken, Stone, and Larson (2012), evaluating what needs to be done related to research in this area, propose a research agenda for nurses:

> A nursing informatics agenda for 2008–2018 must expand users of interest to include interdisciplinary researchers; build upon the knowledge gained in nursing concept representation to address genomic and environmental data; guide the reengineering of nursing practice; harness new technologies to empower patients and their caregivers for collaborative knowledge development; develop user-configurable software approaches that support complex data visualization, analysis and predictive modeling; facilitate the development of middle-range nursing informatics theories; and encourage innovative evaluation methodologies that attend to human-computer interface factors and organizational context. (p. 286)

TABLE 18.1 Health Care Informatics

CATEGORY	WEIGHT
F. Health Care Informatics	**4%**

1. Analyzes systems to identify strengths, gaps, and opportunities

2. Applies data from systems in planning and delivering care

3. Evaluates clinical information systems using select criteria

4. Incorporates ethical principles in the use of information systems

5. Evaluates impact of new technologies on clients, families, and systems

6. Assesses and evaluates the use of technology in the delivery of client care

7. Validates accuracy of consumer-provided information on health issues from the Internet and other sources

8. Synthesizes health care information for client-specific problems

9. Refers clients to culturally relevant health information

10. Demonstrates proficiency in the use of innovations such as the electronic record for documenting and analyzing clinical data

11. Individualizes interventions using technologies

12. Identifies and promotes an environment that safeguards the privacy and confidentiality of patients and families

13. Leads the quality improvement team and engages in designing and implementing a process for improving client safety

14. Utilizes information and communication technologies to document, access, and monitor client care; advance client education; and enhance the accessibility of care

15. Aligns interdisciplinary team documentation to improve accessibility of data

Used with permission from the Commission on Nurse Certification.

Conclusion

There has never been a better time for the CNL to be engaged in the development, implementation, and evaluation of health care information technology. Experts at multiple levels of intersecting sciences are moving at an exhilarating pace to bring our health care delivery system into the 21st century with regard to the use of information technology. As knowledgeable, skillful, and trusted members of the health care team, CNLs have the opportunity to drive important change, keeping in mind the issues of access, support, education, and confidentiality. Since the middle of the last century, nurses have worked to highlight the importance of capturing the delivery of nursing care as health care information technologies have been designed. This nursing care data, carefully collected and analyzed, holds the key to improving the quality and safety of the care we deliver. There is no better leader to continue this important work than the CNL. The certification exam blueprint lists a number of concepts related to informatics in relation to the CNL role (Table 18.1)

BOX 18.1
CNL Resources Related to Informatics

- American Nursing Informatics Association—Caring (www.ania-caring.org)
- Health Information and Management Systems Society (www.himss.org)
- TIGER Initiative (www.tigerinitiative.org)
- Office of the National Coordinator for Health Information Technology (ONC) (www.hhs.gov/healthit)
- Systematic Nomenclature of Medicine (SNOMED) (www.ihtsdo.org)
- Nursing Interventions Classification (NIC) (www.nursing.uiowa.edu)
- Nursing Outcomes Classification (NOC) (www.nursing.uiowa.edu)
- North American Nursing Diagnosis Association (NANDA) (www.nanda.org)

There is also a wide range of resources and organizations available to support knowledge in this complex area (see Box 18.1).

Resources

Akesson, K. M., Saveman, B-I., & Nilsson, G. (2007). Health care consumers' experiences of information communication technology—A summary of literature. *International Journal of Medical Informatics, 76*, 633–645. doi: 10.1016/j.ijmedinf.2006.07.001

Alexander, G. L. (2012). Human factors. In V. K. Saba & K. A. McCormick (Eds.), *Essentials of nursing informatics* (5th ed., pp. 119–132). New York, NY: McGraw Hill.

American Nurses Association. (2008). *Nursing informatics: Scope and standards of practice.* Silver Springs, MD: author.

Backus, L. I., Gavrilov, S., Loomis, T. P., Halloran, J. P., Phillips, B. R., Belperio, P. S., & Mole, L. A. (2009). Clinical case registries: Simultaneous local and national disease registries for population quality management. *Journal of the American Medical Informatics Association, 16*, 775–783. doi: 10.1197/jamia.M3203

Bakken, S., Stone, P. W., & Larson, E. L. (2012). A nursing informatics research agenda for 2008-2018: Contextual influences and key components. *Nursing Outlook, 60(5)*, 280–290. http://dx.doi.org/10.1016/j.outlook.2012.06.001

Darkins, A., Ryan, P., Kobb, R., Foster, L., Edmonson, E., Wakefield, B., & Lancaster, A. (2008). Care Coordination/Home Telehealth: The systematic implementation of health informatics, home telehealth, and disease management to support the care of veteran patients with chronic conditions. *Telemedicine and e-Health, 14*(10), 1118–1126. doi: 10.1089/tmj.2008.0021

Effken, J. A. (2012). Improving the human-technology interface. In D. McGonigle & K. G. Mastrian (Eds.), *Nursing informatics and the foundation of knowledge* (2nd ed., pp. 232–242). Burlington, MA: Jones & Bartlett Learning, LLC.

Hall, E. S., Poynton, M. R., Narus, S. P., Jones, S. S., Evans, R. S., Varner, M. W., & Thornton, S. N. (2009). Patient-level analysis of outcomes using structured labor and delivery data. *Journal of Biomedical Informatics, 42,* 702–709. doi: 10.1016./j.jbi.2009.01.008

Institute of Medicine. (1999). *To err is human: Building a safer health system.* Washington, DC: National Academies Press.

Institute of Medicine. (2001). *Crossing the quality chasm: A new health system for the 21st century.* Washington, DC: National Academies Press.

Institute of Medicine. (2010). *The future of nursing: Leading change, advancing health.* Washington, DC: National Academies Press.

Mastrian, K. G., & McGonigle, D. (2012). Nursing science and the foundation of knowledge. In D. McGonigle & K. G. Mastrian (Eds.), *Nursing informatics and the foundation of knowledge* (2nd ed., p. 5). Burlington, MA: Jones & Bartlett Learning, LLC.

McGonigle, D., & Mastrian, K. G. (2012). *Nursing informatics and the foundation of knowledge* (2nd ed.) Burlington, MA: Jones & Bartlett Learning, LLC.

Milton, C. L. (2009). Information sharing: Transparency, nursing ethics, and practice implications with electronic health records. *Nursing Science Quarterly, 22*(3), 214–219. doi: 10.1177/0894318409337026

Ozbolt, J. G. & Saba, V. K. (2008). A brief history of nursing informatics in the United States of America. *Nursing Outlook, 56,* 199–205.

Zielstorff, R. D., & Frink, B. B. (2012). Consumer and patient use of computers for health. In V. K. Saba & K. A. McCormick (Eds.), *Essentials of nursing informatics* (5th ed.). New York, NY: McGraw Hill.

19

Ethical Considerations for Clinical Nurse Leaders

Sally O'Toole Gerard

There is a long history of ethical concerns with life, a history that dates back to biblical times and the origins of human life. The ethical dilemmas and challenges of each time period may have commonality with the essence of humanness or may be very specific to the circumstances of the day. Contemporary nurses have a unique set of ethical and moral issues, a result of rapidly changing health care policies, technology explosions, and increases in longevity.

Modern nursing stems from the work of Florence Nightingale (1820–1910) who focused on responsible obedience to physicians. The American Nurses Association (ANA) first published a code of ethics for nurses in the 1950s, a model that addressed collaborative relationships with members of the health professions and other citizens in order to meet the needs of the public. Accountability and professional responsibilities have received more emphasis in the most recently revised document. *The Code of Ethics for Nurses with Interpretive Statements* (ANA, 2001) has nine provisions regarding the professional practice of nursing and serves the following purpose: It is a succinct statement of the ethical obligations and duties of every individual who enters the nursing profession, it is the profession's nonnegotiable ethical standard, and it is an expression of nursing's own understanding and commitment to society (Guido, 2010).

The clinical nurse leader (CNL) has a unique opportunity to model ethical professionalism, support the ethical challenges of direct care nurses, raise ethical concerns in the care of patients, and influence ethical practices on an organizational level. The CNL, as a highly educated, expert clinician intimately involved with patient care, has been named as a guardian of the nursing profession (American Association of Colleges of Nursing [AACN], 2007). This guardianship considers the intentions of Florence Nightingale, the ANA, and others who consider nursing to be a profession with profound respect for patients and their complex needs. The CNL has specific charge to identify actual and potential ethical issues arising from practice and to help address such issues (AACN, 2007). For this reason, the CNL must have knowledge of ethical issues, decision making, organizational perspectives of ethical considerations, legal guidelines, advocacy, and conflict resolution.

A good place to begin is with a review of terms related to this content:

- Ethics—involves the principles or assumptions underpinning the way individuals or groups should conduct themselves and is concerned with motives and attitudes and the relationship of these attitudes to the individual
- Values—personal beliefs about the truths and worth of thoughts, objects, or behavior
- Autonomy—personal freedom and self-determination
- Beneficence—supporting actions that promote good
- Nonmaleficence—the concept that one should not do harm
- Justice—the concept that all people should be treated fairly
- Respect for others—acknowledgment of the rights of individuals to make decisions and live or die on the basis of those decisions
- Codes of ethics—formal statements that serve to articulate the values and beliefs of a given discipline, serving as a standard for professional actions and reflecting the ethical principles shared by its members

Personal and Organizational Decision Making

There is no better way to consider ethical issues than in practice. Here is a scenario.

Sue is a senior charge nurse assigned to a surgical unit. She is waiting to care for Mr. L, who is about to come back from the post-anesthesia care unit after vascular bypass surgery. Claire is a newer nurse on the unit, who observes charge nurse Sue draw up morphine, stating it is for Mr. L when he arrives. Ten minutes later the newer nurse observes Sue return to the medication room to discard an empty syringe, stating she had injected the patient when he arrived. Confused, Claire went to the room, which confirmed her suspicion that the patient had not yet arrived.

Many ethical concerns are raised in the day-to-day practice of nursing. Some involve patients, families, colleagues, and organizations. The desire to maintain an ethical perspective in all areas of practice includes the examination of our duties, obligations, or responsibilities to other health care professionals and staff. But how do we make decisions about ethical concerns? In daily life an individual draws on knowledge, life experience, values, and a variety of circumstances to arrive at a decision. When it comes to decisions on complex ethical decisions, many decision-making frameworks have been described. When making ethical decisions, nurses need to combine all the elements using an orderly, systematic, and objective method (Guido, 2010). One such model that describes this process is the MORAL model most recently applied to nursing by Halloran (1982).

- M—Massage the dilemma. Identify and define issues in the dilemma. Consider the opinions of other players as well as their value system.
- O—Outline the options. Examine all options full, including less realistic and conflicting ones. Make a list of pros and cons.
- R—Resolve the dilemma. Review the issues and options, applying basic ethical principles to each option. Decide the best option based on the views of those concerned in the dilemma.

- A—Act by applying the chosen option. This step is usually the most difficult because it requires actual implementation versus dialogue and discussion.
- L—Look back and evaluate the entire process, including the implementation. No process is complete without a thorough evaluation.

A process allows time for a deeper understanding of the issue, related issues, and considerations of others who may be involved in the situation. Some issues are easier to reach than others and it is important to allow sufficient time to allow for a supportable option to be reached (Guido, 2010).

Health care, by virtue of the complexity of caring for human life, may benefit from a model of decision making adapted to the environment. Thompson and Thompson (1981) describe a *bioethical decision* model of using a 10-step process:

Step 1:   Review the situation to determine health problems, decision needed, ethical components, and key individuals

Step 2:   Gather additional information to clarify the situation

Step 3:   Identify the ethical issues in the situation

Step 4:   Define personal and professional moral positions

Step 5:   Identify moral positions of key individuals involved

Step 6:   Identify value conflicts, if any

Step 7:   Determine who should make the decision

Step 8:   Identify range of actions with anticipated outcomes

Step 9:   Decide on a course of action and carry it out

Step 10:   Evaluate/review results of decision/action

There are an infinite number of ethical dilemmas that can occur in health care, some mildly complex and some profoundly complex. Nurses need to realize the need for process to allow for inquiry, reasoning, and thoughtful consideration of the multiple aspects involved in a particular situation. The CNL can support nurses of varied levels of experience to recognize their important role in assuring ethical care in all health care settings. A CNL can also support nurses who face moral distress, confusion, and professional fear when dealing with issues that present themselves daily in our health care system.

Health care organizations put many systems into place to maintain proper care that adheres to governing laws, standards of best practice, regulations of the health department, and a plethora of human resource policies to ensure just treatment of patients and employees. The legal system is founded on rules and regulations, whereas ethics are subject to philosophical, moral, and individual interpretations (Guido, 2010). Ethics committees are common in health care organizations as a mechanism to address and process the inevitable issues that arise. Ethics committees can provide structure and guidelines for potential problems, serve as an open forum for discussion, and function as a true patient advocate (Guido, 2010). Despite the existence of ethics committees in many organizations, staff nurses may not have access to these meetings or even know they exist. In many settings, any member of the health care team can request an ethics review of a case. This is a valuable resource to nurses that many may be unaware of. The CNL, as an advanced generalist who is very involved with supporting direct care nurses, can make this resource available to nurses.

Advocacy and the CNL

The AACN specifically describes the CNL as an advocate. The CNL advocates to ensure that clients, families, and communities are well informed and included in planning of care (AACN, 2007). The CNL also ensures that the voice of the vulnerable, frail, inexperienced, and incapacitated is represented throughout the life span. Although all persons have the ability to advocate for a cause or another individual, the nurse is uniquely suited to guard the standards of the profession to ensure ethical care. The CNL plays a natural role of advocate in the spectrum of health care and especially for direct care nurses served by the CNL. Perhaps never before has this CNL support of direct care nurses been so necessary as now, in an age of rapid change.

CASE STUDY: Missy is an RN who has been working on a surgical unit for 2 years. She is caring for Mrs. Brown, who has just returned from surgery to remove an abdominal mass. Mrs. Brown's family has been waiting in the room for her to return and is very happy to have the surgery over and to sit with Mrs. Brown in the room as she sleeps. After about 1 hour, the family shares with the nurses that they had expected the surgeon to have been in to tell them the outcome of the surgery. After the second inquiry from the family, the nurse phones the surgeon and inquires about his plans to see the family. The surgeon states that he spoke to Mrs. Brown (the patient) in the recovery holding area and he did not plan to visit the family as he had left the hospital and was off duty. The nurse shares that she is quite confident the family was expecting to speak with him, but the physician is terse and ends the conversation. Missy speaks to a sleepy Mrs. Brown, who states she does not remember whether the physician spoke to her or not. The family is very upset and not consoled by the news that the surgical resident would be seeing Mrs. Brown that evening on rounds. Missy does her best to support the family but feels a significant deal of distress in the poor communication that this family has received. Missy contemplates providing the family with the physician's personal phone number, to which the charge nurse has access.

Why is advocacy so important? What more could Missy do for the Brown family and for her own sense of wrongdoing? Without advocacy and effective protection of rights, there are no rights. The nurse carries the role of securing the patient's interests by every means at her disposal. The nurse understands that the advocacy role promotes, protects, and makes every effort to promote healing. This healing extends to families. Situations in which nurses are advocates in subtle and deliberate ways for patients and families happen daily. It is the cumulative effect of these many battles that can diminish a nurse's personal and professional satisfaction. The CNL can help to protect the direct care nurse by supporting the moral stress encountered. *Moral stress* most often occurs when faced with the situations in which two ethical principles compete (Guido, 2010). The CNL can be supportive by assisting the nurse to approach ethical decisions and situations in a thoughtful and knowledgeable manner. Utilizing one of the models previously mentioned could support a best outcome to the situation.

In addition to supporting the use of a decision-making model, the CNL can also model the guidelines for acting as a patient advocate or provide them directly to nurses at appropriate times. Guido (2010) shares five guidelines for acting as a patient advocate:

1. Nurses should be aware of hospital policies and protocols, as well as acceptable standards of care. They should question physician orders when they are contrary to accepted standards of care or when they believe the order could harm the patient. They should not be intimidated into following orders but use professional and independent judgments. If physicians persist or refuse to change orders, they should consult a nursing supervisor.

2. In emergency situations in which the nurse believes that following the physician's order could result in harm to the patient, the nurse should refuse to follow the order, ensure patient safety and appropriate care, and notify the nursing supervisor and administrators.

3. If the patient is prescribed care that could cause direct harm, voice your concern to the physician and nursing supervisor.

4. In transitioning from one area of care to another, the patient/family should be fully informed, prepared, and educated to the situation. Patient teaching and discharge teaching are often a primary responsibility of nurses and they should prepare patients with sufficient teaching regarding symptoms and complication and provide adequate resources/instruction. If the nurse feels the patient is not being safely transitioned from the area of care, she should notify the physician and supervisor.

5. The patient is your priority concern, and nurses have an affirmative duty to serve as patient advocates.

CASE STUDY FOLLOW-UP: The CNL on Missy's floor overhears her vent her frustration over what she feels is poor treatment of this patient/family and also that she is spending so much time and energy trying to console this family's anxiety. Missy states, "I don't care if they fire me; I'm going to give them the surgeon's cell phone number." The CNL speaks to Missy to review the details of the situation. The CNL supports Missy's moral stress and offers the following input: "Why don't we call the nursing supervisor and explain the situation, and provide her with the surgeon's cell phone number so that she can call him and request a call to the family as soon as possible. In the meantime, let's call the surgical resident and request that she come see the family at the beginning of her evening rounds to review how the surgery went and the next steps."

End-of-Life Care Decisions

Nurses are so often a critical factor in the ethical treatment of people at the end of their life. End-of-life care is a general term that refers to the medical and mental care given in the advanced or terminal stages of illness. Choices regarding invasive treatments, resuscitation, hydration, nutrition, and so on are often left to emotionally charged relatives if specific planning has not been put into place. Conversations about end-of-life choice are often some of the most difficult for families and caregivers. Mentoring of a CNL can support care that is patient centered, holistic, and humane.

Advance directives are a valuable tool in the planning of end-of-life care. Advance directives are a way for patients to communicate their wishes to family, friends, and health care professionals, but they are often misunderstood. Some patients may be fearful of creating a living will, thinking it will give permission to potentially "pull the plug" at a premature time in the illness. Landmark cases of end-of-life controversies can make national headlines and often provide a forum for discussion in many circles, both professional and private citizens. Often confusion and uncertainty surface in these complex situations. Nonetheless, professionals understand the importance of considering patient preferences in clinical decision making and often must advocate with patients, families, and professional colleagues.

Advance directives are legal documents, such as a living will, durable power of attorney, and health care proxy. These documents allow people to convey their decisions about end-of-life care. Advance directives are a way for patients to communicate their wishes to family, friends, and health care professionals. The use of these documents can help avoid confusion, turmoil, and guilt and promote a person's choices for care. They are often developed with an attorney and can be modified as a patient's situation changes. Unfortunately, these critical documents often do not exist or are misunderstood by patients and families.

The federal Patient Self-Determination Act of 1991 supported the patient's right to determine the medical care he or she receives. The law requires hospitals to provide information about advance directives to adult patients on admission for any condition (Tiden et al., 2010). Although this law supported the integration of advance directives into hospital care, these documents continue to be underutilized, misunderstood, and possibly feared by some. The American Academy of Nursing issued a policy calling for advance care planning as an urgent public health concern. With the aging American population and misunderstandings about advance care planning in the health care reform debates, this organization has made a strong call for attention to this issue (Tiden et al., 2010). The organization has put forth recommendations as a part of this statement to support advance care planning, which is holistic and patient centered. The following four recommendations of Tiden and colleagues (2010) are:

1. The time invested in advance care planning by qualified health professionals for patients with life-limiting illness should be reimbursed by all payers.

2. Health information technology offers promise for documenting advance directives care planning and making such information more readily available with and between patients' care settings. As electronic medical records (EMRs) are developed, the approach to documenting advance care planning, advance care, and advance directives must be built into electronic systems so that this information is prominent and readily available for use in care decisions.

3. The 1991 Patient Self-Determination Act should be updated and expanded beyond the clerical function of providing forms to patients on hospital admission.

Expanded requirements upon hospital admission should facilitate the components of advance care planning to include initiating conversations, providing information and assistance to patients, and facilitating patients' determination of their preferences.

4. Health professions education and training are critical to the knowledge, skills, and attitudes that future clinicians bring to the clinical care of patients with life-limiting conditions. Health professionals' education programs must include content on advance care planning.

So why is this area of care so fraught with conflict and turmoil and why must the CNL be knowledgeable about the major concepts involved? This area of health care offers some of the most challenging clinical situations and also some of the most rewarding opportunities. Hopefully, every experienced nurse can recall one example of supporting a patient in a peaceful, holistic death where the patient's wishes were known, respected, and communicated to family members. This can be one of the most satisfying and profound experiences, and for newer nurses, it can be a surprise that, although entering a profession to support healing, a peaceful death can be a proud component of a nursing career. Unfortunately, these situations are sometimes less common and the end-of-life path can be filled with conflict and confusion.

Addressing the issue of end-of life choices requires a person to consider their own mortality. The spectrum of how individuals respond to this is as varied as human beings. Some people want to assure from a young age and with no immediate health concerns that legal documents are in order. Some people at advanced ages and with serious medical conditions refuse to address these issues. The timing of developing these documents is also complex. Those who are healthy do not feel the need or urgency to develop them. Those who are older or sick may be upset or emotional to consider this topic for fear it will make some impact on their current health situation. Ideally, advance care planning among clinicians, patients, and patients' families has occurred over time; patients have expressed and clarified their preferences verbally and in writing (Tiden et al., 2010). A lack of this preparation often causes great conflict, anxiety, and turmoil for families when an individual can no longer express them. Siblings, especially, can have significant guilt and conflict when they are trying to come to a consensus on emotionally charged issues.

Living wills, in particular, are valuable documents but are misunderstood and woefully underutilized. A majority of adults do not have living wills, and if they have one in which a surrogate has been designated, often the surrogate is not aware of having been designated as a decision maker (Mahon, 2010). Although it seems logical to discuss one's wishes, the emotional, spiritual, religious, and psychological responses to this topic are powerful. Many patients have not acclimated to being asked questions about advance directives on admission to hospitals, and despite the illness at hand, it is often not seriously contemplated.

Misinformation about advance directives is an excellent opportunity for CNLs to support patients, families, and direct care nurses. A knowledge of hospital policies, state laws, and resources is key for CNLs and nursing staff. As stated above, based on legal changes in 1991 and the Patient Self-Determination Act, adults entering the hospital must be asked for such documents and have information about these documents available for health care personnel. Without attention to detail and tracking by organizations, these documents, if not available on admission, may not be followed up on. Many systems may also need to have patients bring the document with each admission to the organization to guard against changes that may have been made to these documents. Patients would often not understand the logic or importance of providing these documents with each admission. Some patients are naïve with regard to the complexity of modern health care may feel: "My doctor knows I don't want any of those machines to keep me alive." They do not realize that full resuscitation will routinely take place on any individual who does not have specific orders to the contrary.

A key misunderstanding around living wills is when they become effective. Patients may not understand that these documents do not come into play until they have become unable to make a decision for themselves and are deemed to be in a terminal condition. This judgment of terminal illness can be subjective and controversial among families and caregivers. Many nurses have worked with professionals treating terminal patients, but the provider communications to families are focused on continued medical treatment, interventions, and seemingly unnecessary suffering. This is often an ethical dilemma for staff nurses and requires a level of advocacy that can be supported by the CNL.

> **SCENARIO:** A patient with advanced Alzheimer's disease is brought to the emergency department from a nursing home with fever and dyspnea. A chest x-ray confirms severe pneumonia, which will require antibiotics, oxygen therapy, and possibly mechanical ventilation. The patient has an advance directive that indicates that she does not want intubation if she is in a terminal condition. The nurses share with the physician the existence of the living will and the patient's wishes. The physician responds that pneumonia is not a terminal condition and therefore the advance directive does not come into effect. The nurse is surprised and distressed at this response as she cares for the demented and agitated patient. The patient is already being physically restrained to protect the intravenous line, and the nurse is morally distressed at the thought of intubating this patient with limited cognitive function.

Patients and families face difficult decisions across the course of a lifetime, and especially in a time of illness. Many factors affect these decisions such as understanding of the disease, experiences, hopes and goals, the desire to please health care providers, family support, beliefs about quality of life, religious or spiritual beliefs, practicalities of daily living, and more (Mahon, 2010). The following four dimensions of decision making have been proposed: medical indications, patient preferences, quality of life, and contextual features (Jonsen, Siegler, & Winslade, 2006). At times, caregivers impart their own values and beliefs into patient/family discussions. This is usually quite unintentional. One approach to this level of communication seeks to keep the information from caregivers factual and objective. This decision making describes the health care team as bringing the raw data of the situation and the patient/family adding the meaning and values around the choices and consequences of the decision (Jonsen et al., 2006).

Palliative Care

Palliative care is an interdisciplinary approach to care in which nursing is the core discipline. Palliative care is a field of nursing that is unique in its approach, focus, and goals of patient interaction. This approach to care concerns patients whose diseases are not responsive to curative treatment, where control of pain, symptoms, psychological distress, and spiritual distress is paramount (Kuebler, Berry, & Heidrich, 2002). This model is the ultimate in patient-centered care and places additional emphasis on family support. The palliative care nurse frequently cares for patients experiencing major stressors: physical, psychological, and spiritual. Many of these patients recognize themselves as dying, and it is the role of a palliative care nurse to maximize all resources to support this process.

CNLs can assist patients and staff nurses by having a solid knowledge of what is palliative care, what are the resources in the care setting, and when to encourage conversations around this program of care. Because hospice may equate to death for some patients and family, these are often difficult conversations for health care members to initiate. The national Hospice and Palliative Care Organization (1999) describes hospice in the following way:

> Hospice provides support and care for persons in the last phases of incurable illness so that they may live as fully and comfortably as possible. Hospice affirms life and neither hastens nor postpones death. Hospice exists in the hope and belief that through appropriate care and the promotion of a caring community sensitive to their needs, that individuals and their families may be free to attain a degree of satisfaction in preparation for death. Hospice programs provide state-of-the-art palliative care and supportive services to individuals at the end of their lives, their family members, and significant others, 24 hours a day, 7 days a week, in both the home and facility-based care settings.

Many organizations also have palliative care advanced practice registered nurses (APRNs) who specialize in supporting the appropriate and holistic care at the end of life. CNLs with access to this type of professional are wise to collaborate as often as possible. CNLs can model therapeutic communication with patients and families around this topic as well as advocacy for patients in leading the interdisciplinary team to focus on patient choice and preference.

Pain assessment and management can be a significant consideration in all patient care but especially in end-of life care. CNLs can support nursing in a variety of ways, such as proper assessment of pain, knowledge of pharmaceutical and nonpharmaceutical interventions, and knowledge of organizational resources and advocacy. There are a variety of barriers to optimal pain management that the CNL can support. These involve professional barriers, health care barriers, and patient/family and societal barriers. Support for nurses who are strong advocates of proper pain management is growing. Increasingly, feedback from patients regarding pain relief and assessment by health care organizations is gaining significance as a quality indicator of care. Organizational outcomes regarding quality indicators are becoming more transparent and accessible to the public via the Internet.

Additionally, these quality outcomes are being evaluated in relation to reimbursement in a new era of "pay for performance." This new approach to pain relief as a quality indicator of care should support those who advocate for comfortable and humane care, especially at the end of life.

Active knowledge of professional organizations that support the ethical health care of all persons is another resource for CNLs and staff nurses. In 2010, the ANA published a position statement onto support nurses, as a profession, who are supporting end-of-life care. The document was created to articulate the roles and responsibilities of registered nurses in providing expert end-of-life care and guidance to patients and families concerning treatment preferences and end-of-life decision making (American Nurses Association [ANA], 2010). This valuable document addresses practice issues, health care reform issues, and hospice and palliative care together with nurses' guidance and support of patients and families. Also included is specific mention of the advancing technology of health care and appropriate use of resources. The organization calls for reshaping and redirecting away from the overuse of technology-driven, acute, hospital-based services to a model of balance between high-tech treatment, community resources, and preventative services (ANA, 2010). The document can be accessed at www.gm6.nursingworld.org/MainMenuCategories/Policy-Advocacy/Positions-and-Resolutions/ANAPositionStatements/Position-Statements-Alphabetically/Nursess-Role-in-Ethics-and-Human-Rights.pdf.

Clearly, the support of professional organizations and nurse experts will be critical in the decades ahead, as the number of aging Americans grows along with technology focused on prolonging life. Who will help patients and families navigate the health care system, make informed choices, and address emotionally painful issues of illness? Nurses have and will continue to be an integral part of the team trusted with this responsibility. And how will the role of the CNL help to support, nurture, and model the professional finesse required to connect with patients at this difficult time? The emotional and spiritual toll of caring for patients, advocating for basic rights, and, at times, battling against colleagues can incapacitate our direct care nurses and drive them from the profession. The CNL has the opportunity to partner with these nurses, assure proper resources are considered, and support the development of moral courage.

The Ethical Considerations of Patient Safety

One of the most significant improvements in health care has been the prioritization of patient safety. It was this emphasis on patient safety, highlighted by publications of the Institute of Medicine and The Joint Commission, that spurred a national conversation and the advent of the CNL role. The complexity and fragmentation of the health care system have set the stage for patients to experience injury and possible death as a result of medical errors. The CNL is in a unique position to advocate for a safe environment that is supported by all members of the health care team.

Assessments of microsystems and macrosystems show that variation in best practice procedures can cause errors. Recent attention to measures that standardize care such as best practice order sets, procedural time-outs, and checklists has been implemented. Checklists, in particular, have received particular attention for success in reducing errors and infection rates and improving patient outcomes (Gawande, 2009). Although issues of patient safety and quality improvement are detailed in other chapters of this book, there is an ethical responsibility of all nurses, especially the CNL, to be instrumental in implementing these important initiatives and sustaining them over time.

Ethical considerations of health care can be illustrated in any setting. Nurses as a whole have a responsibility that includes protecting patients from falls, from injuring themselves, from abuse, medication-related safety and unsafe conditions, or treatment by members of health-related disciplines (Guido, 2010). National initiatives to motivate organizations to address these patient safety issues have spurred an onslaught of improvement initiatives. The CNL can be a model of ethical decision making and advocacy and can support the development of moral courage. By maintaining a patient/family focus, he or she can often direct the interdisciplinary team in a way that is congruent with the care we would all desire for our own family. Nationally, organizations are supporting a culture of safety and empowerment that encourages all members to speak up and have a voice when patient safety is being compromised. This change in culture will not come without conflict, the need for open communication, and leaders who set the tone for the patient as the highest priority. Opportunities for CNLs in this culture will be numerous, although not clear cut and not without controversy.

> **CNL SCENARIO:** One of the least experienced nurses in a busy surgical ICU has expressed distress to the unit's CNL regarding the behavior of some of the surgical residents. A checklist has been put into place for the insertion of central line catheters, and yet when the nurse attempts to incorporate the checklist into the care of the patient as she assists with the procedure, she is ignored. The following week in report the CNL learns that this nurse's patient will be having a central line catheter placed by the surgical service. The CNL discusses the issue with the young nurse, and they prepare the checklist for the procedure. Later that morning, the residents arrive to begin the procedure. The CNL accompanies the staff nurse into the room to prepare the patient and the necessary supplies. The CNL announces to the group assembled that all the supplies for the procedure are available, including the checklist for this procedure. The surgical resident makes a disparaging remark. After an attempt to remind the resident of best practice and hospital policies, he continues to refuse. The CNL discreetly shares that she and the staff nurse would not assist in this procedure and would be immediately contacting the hospital administrators. The shocked and angry surgical resident agrees to utilize the procedural checklist for the procedure.
>
> Following this exchange, the CNL and staff nurse debrief about the situation. They discuss the often difficult situations in which nurses must advocate for patients and the courage to find that voice. The CNL assures the newer nurse that almost all members of the health care team are very committed to a safe culture and would support the actions taken. The CNL also requests a meeting with the manager of the unit, medical director of the ICU, and the chief of surgery to discuss the bigger issue of patient safety, compliance with best practice initiatives, and the role of the staff nurse as a patient advocate despite objections of others.

The CNL can be a role model in advocating for the patient and the development of moral courage. Young nurses often struggle with their role in taking a stand against improper care and disregard for policies put in place to protect patients, staff, and the organization. The moral stress can result in moral distress when nurses are put in a painful state of imbalance when they are unable to implement a decision because of real or perceived institutional constraints (Guido, 2010). This moral distress can be generated by a wide variety of clinical and professional situations and can exact a toll on the individual. Is it acceptable for me to question more experienced health professionals? Is it acceptable for me to refuse to assist with this procedure that is not following the standards and policies of the organization? What will the repercussions be if I refuse? Will this person dislike me? Will my peers mock me? Finding the moral courage to stand up to professional issues is a development in the professional life of a nurse. A CNL can model, facilitate, and support the healthy decision making, coping skills, and often difficult communications that may be necessary to keep patients safe.

Ethical Considerations of Health Information

Advances in technology have made dramatic changes to the accumulation of health information and issues of access. Never before has so much information been available, and the future will continue to expand in this area in ways we can probably not imagine. Health information professionals, as a community, have an established code of ethics or code of conduct and cannot function in today's environment without a clear understanding of ethical principles (Harman, 2006). Many of the values of this industry's code of ethics can easily be shared with nursing and should be embraced. Those values include providing service, protecting medical/social information, promoting confidentiality, securing health information, promoting quality, reporting data with accuracy, and promoting interdisciplinary collaboration (Harmon, 2006).

The protection of patient information has long been a responsibility of nurses as well as all members of the team. Prior to the advent of the EMR, this issue may have been more clearly delineated. In today's world of electronic data, a patient's health information could be viewed by countless individuals at a variety of locations in one day. The development of these EMRs by information specialists have a clear connection to ethical principles of privacy and confidentiality. Likewise, nurses must approach the protection of a patient's privacy with a strong ethical regard and respect. As more and more data are collected on individuals over time, access to this information will take on greater significance and the protection of this information will become more challenging.

> **SCENARIO:** Lisa, a nurse on the telemetry unit, has a chronically ill father. Lisa's peers are all quite familiar with her father's long medical history and his general status, as they have provided emotional support for their friend over the last few years. This past week Lisa's father was admitted to the medical unit for treatment of a urinary tract infection. After morning report, the staff asks Lisa about her father's status. Lisa gives her colleagues

an update, including a summary of his lab results from that morning. It is clear to the CNL that Lisa is accessing the EMR to follow her father's care. Is this a problem? What should the CNL do?

Many protections can be put into place to help safeguard the EMR, and these safeguards will be of even greater significance as the technology continues to advance. Some of these securities include restricted access to health records based on security clearance and scope of practice, monitoring of EMR access by organizations to identify misuse and violations, high-level passwords changed on a regular basis, termination of access to EMRs when employment is terminated, and confidentiality statements signed by employees. Future security will most likely continue to be more sophisticated and focused on bioidentification, utilizing fingerprints or retinal images.

One of the most significant issues in health care information was the introduction of the Health Insurance Portability and Accountability Act (HIPAA) in 1996. This law provides for the portability of health care coverage, antifraud and abuse program, streamlining of the transfer of patient information between insurers and providers, incentives toward the acquisition of health insurance, and establishment of the federal government as a national health care regulator (Guido, 2010). All nurses working at this time saw significant changes in the practice environment in order to comply with this new law. Patient names could no longer be posted on the units for room assignments, clipboards used in everyday assignments needed to be altered, information sent to other agencies required cover sheets, and other provisions to protect patient information. Shredding of health information became the norm, as any information with patient information would no longer be placed in the traditional garbage. Organizations as a whole scrambled to reorganize systems to maintain patient confidentiality. Policies and procedures were created and implemented to integrate these new regulations into the practice environment from acute care to rehabilitation, homecare, and long-term care. Nurses and CNLs, especially, must be aware of the policies and procedures around health information, privacy issues, access issues, and all facets of protecting health care information. How does a CNL advise a nurse when a patient requests to see his or her medical record? What are the resources within the organization for questions related to privacy? Is there a privacy officer? Some issues of privacy are straightforward and some pose ethical concerns.

The age of information presents some unique challenges with the increasing use of e-mail, the Internet, and social media networks. This area can pose potential ethical and liability issues for organizations and nurses (Guido, 2010). With the advent of social networks, the Internet, and the majority of individuals having cellular telephones with picture-taking capabilities, the issues of privacy and patient information have taken on an added dimension. Most organizations have needed to introduce new policies regarding any reference to patients, patients' families, or patient information in these venues. One organization instituted a new social media policy after a patient's family complained that they recognized that nurses from the hospital were referring to their family member on a social media site, even though the patient's name was not used. Derogatory information about the patient and family were shared between nurses on the site, which was a clear violation of ethical care. Nurses and other health care workers may not recognize that ethical lines are being crossed, especially in a generation raised on sharing information on social media sites.

Without a code of ethics, issues of privacy, patient information, and patient rights can be obscure. A code of professional ethics supports beneficence, non-maleficence, and justice. A common respect for others should be the guide for all health care workers, but often that value of respect can be lost when workers become desensitized by their surroundings and the daily interactions of a health care environment. The CNL can help nurses develop a voice of advocacy for the proper treatment of patients and clearly can be a guardian of information, especially in a world of access to a plethora of information venues.

Resources for Ethical Concerns

Most organizations have a plethora of policies, procedures, and provisions of practice. Despite a system put in place to provide order, there will always be complex ethical situations that require support and reflection. Most health care organizations have established ethics committees to advise health care professionals when difficult decision points are reached. The ethics committee is usually an interdisciplinary team composed of physicians, nurses, ethicists, social workers, chaplains, dieticians, and others with experience with ethical deliberation in health care (Harmon, 2006). These groups are meant to be unbiased professionals who facilitate communication in emotionally charged issues (Harmon, 2006). Often, these groups will meet after a situation has occurred, as an opportunity to reflect and deliberate possible opportunities to provide the best possible care.

Many direct care nurses may not know that an ethics committee exists in their institution or that they can request an ethics consult by the team. A CNL is an excellent medium of making nurses aware of resources such as an ethics committee. Oftentimes, nurses will have lingering conflict and possible moral distress over a patient's or family's situation. An ethics committee can provide that support needed for frontline nurses to see the many complex dimensions of some patient situations. There may also be open ethics discussions or seminars at an organization, and the CNL can raise the awareness of staff nurses to the importance of understanding these resources and having a voice in the interdisciplinary team, in which nursing is a key member.

Other resources for ethical dilemmas and concerns can be supervisors, administrators, and advanced practice nurses. Many facilities have nurses who specialize in palliative care and pain management. These nurses can be a valuable resource of knowledge of clinical issues and facing issues of patient advocacy and ethical dilemmas. Some areas of health care are more prone to dilemmas and conflict, and it is critical for nurses to be aware of any support available for their professional development, rather than wrestle with moral conflict. These resources can often provide support for a direct care nurse who may make decisions solely on the basis of the needs of the patient but may not be popular with members of the health care team.

Conclusion

The care of complex human beings will never be without areas of ethical concern and conflict. As technology advances along with easy access to information through the EMR, Internet, and other avenues, nurses will have a critical role in protection and advocacy of patient care. End-of-life issues are common for nurses to encounter across the continuum of health care and will always have grey areas of providing care versus prolonging suffering. Despite a growing population of older adults, advance directives are often underutilized and misunderstood. A lack of clear planning and sharing of wishes in the event of a terminal illness can send families into a crisis. Regardless of what circumstances come together to cause this crisis, the nurse is often integrally involved. The CNL provides leadership, guidance, role modeling, and support for frontline nurses in this venture. Awareness of hospital policies, resources, and strategies that can optimize patient outcomes is essential. The Commission on Nurse Certification includes many ethical areas in the certification blueprint for CNLs (Table 19.1).

TABLE 19.1 Ethics

CATEGORY	WEIGHT
G. Ethics	**7%**

1. Evaluates ethical decision making from both a personal and an organizational perspective and develops an understanding of how these two perspectives may create conflicts of interest

2. Applies an ethical decision-making framework to clinical situations that incorporates moral concepts, professional ethics, and law and respects diverse values and beliefs

3. Applies legal and ethical guidelines to advocate for client well-being and preferences

4. Enables clients and families to make quality-of-life and end-of-life decisions and achieve a peaceful death

5. Identifies and analyzes common ethical dilemmas and the ways in which these dilemmas impact client care

6. Identifies areas in which a personal conflict of interest may arise and proposes resolutions or actions to resolve the conflict

Used with permission from the Commission on Nurse Certification.

Resources

American Association of Colleges of Nursing. (2007). *White paper on the education and role of the clinical nurse leader.* Washington, DC. Available at http://www.aacn.nche.edu/Publications/WhitePapers/ClinicalNurseLeader07.pdf

American Nurses Association. (2001). *Code of ethics for nurses with interpretive statements.* Retrieved from http://nursingworld.org/MainMenuCategories/EthicsStandards/Codeof EthicsforNurses/Code-of-Ethics.pdf

American Nurses Association. (2010). *Registered nurses' roles and responsibilities in providing expert care and counseling at the end of life.* Retrieved from http://gm6.nursingworld.org/MainMenuCategories/Policy-Advocacy/Positions-and-Resolutions/ANAPositionStatements/Position-Statements-Alphabetically/Nursess-Role-in-Ethics-and-Human-Rights.pdf

Gawande, A. (2009). *The Checklist Manifesto: How to get things right.* New York, NY: Henry Holt.

Guido, G. (2010). *Legal and ethical issues in nursing* (5th ed.). Upper Saddle River, NJ: Pearson Prentice Hall.

Halloran, M. (1982). Rational ethical judgments utilizing a decision-making tool. *Heart and Lung, 11*(6), 566–570.

Harmon, L. (2006). *Ethical challenges in the management of health information* (2nd ed.). Sudsbury, MA: Jones and Bartlett.

Jonsen, A., Siegler, M., & Winslade, W. (2006). *Clinical ethics: A practical guide to ethical decisions in clinical medicine* (6th ed.). New York, NY: McGraw-Hill.

Kuebler, K., Berry, P., & Heidrich, D. (2002). *End of life care. Clinical practice guidelines.* Philadelphia, PA: Springer.

Mahon, M. (2010). Clinical decision making in palliative care and end of life care. *Nursing Clinics of North America, 45,* 345–362.

National Hospice and Palliative Care Organization. (1999). Standards of accreditation committee, hospice standards of practice. Arlington, VA.

Thompson, J., & Thompson, H. (1981). *Ethics in nursing.* New York, NY: Macmillan.

Tilden, V., Corless, I., Dahlin, C., Ferrell, B., Gibson, R., & Lentz, J. (2011). Advance care planning as an urgent public health concern. *Nursing Outlook, 59,* 55-56.

Online Resources

American Nurses Association

http://www.ana.org

http://nursingworld.org/MainMenuCategories/EthicsStandards

http://nursingworld.org/MainMenuCategories/Policy-Advocacy/Positions-and-Resolutions

Center to Advance Palliative Care

http://www.capc.org/palliative-care-professional-development/Training

Compassion and Support at the End of Life

http://www.compassionandsupport.org

Hospice and Palliative Nurses Association

http://www.hpna.org

Pain Management Guidelines

http://www.guideline.gov/content.aspx?id=9744

Promoting Excellence: Advanced Practice Nursing: Pioneering Practices in Palliative Care

http://www.promotingexcellence.org/apn

The Center for Ethics and Advocacy in Healthcare

http://www.healthcare-ethics.org

The National Center for Ethics in Health Care

http://www.ethics.va.gov

APPENDIX A

Exam Content Outline

Overview of Exam Content

I. Nursing leadership 33%
- A. Horizontal leadership; weight 7% and 11 topics
- B. Interdisciplinary communication and collaboration skills; weight 7% and 16 topics
- C. Health care advocacy; weight 5% and 9 topics
- D. Integration of the CNL role; weight 8% and 15 topics
- E. Lateral integration of care services; weight 6% and 7 topics

II. Clinical outcomes management 30%
- A. Illness and disease management; weight 7% and 23 topics
- B. Knowledge management; weight 5% and 12 topics
- C. Health promotion and disease prevention management; weight 5% and 12 topics
- D. Evidence-based practice; weight 8% and 13 topics
- E. Advanced clinical assessment; weight 5% and 7 topics

III. Care environment management 37%
- A. Team coordination; weight 6% and 10 topics
- B. Health care finance and economics; weight 5% and 15 topics
- C. Health care systems; weight 5% and 9 topics
- D. Health care policy; weight 4% and 13 topics
- E. Quality improvement; weight 6% and 9 topics
- F. Health care informatics; weight 4% and 15 topics
- G. Ethics; weight 7% and 6 topics

TABLE A.1 Clinical Nurse Leader Certification Exam—Detailed Blueprint

I. Nursing Leadership	33%

A. Horizontal Leadership	7%

1. Applies theories and models (e.g., nursing, leadership, complexity, change) to practice

2. Applies evidence-based practice to make clinical decisions and assess outcomes

3. Understands microsystem functions and assumes accountability for health care outcomes

4. Designs, coordinates, and evaluates plans of care at an advanced level in conjunction with interdisciplinary team

5. Utilizes peer feedback for evaluation of self and others

6. Serves as a lateral integrator of the interdisciplinary health teamw

7. Leads group processes to meet care objectives

8. Coaches and mentors health care team serving as a role model

9. Utilizes an evidence-based approach to meet specific needs of individuals, clinical populations, or communities within the microsystem

10. Assumes responsibility for creating a culture of safe and ethical care

11. Provides leadership for changing practice on the basis of quality improvement methods and research findings

B. Interdisciplinary Communication and Collaboration Skills	7%

1. Establishes and maintains working relationships within an interdisciplinary team

2. Bases clinical decisions on multiple perspectives, including the client and/or family preferences

3. Negotiates in group interactions, particularly in task-oriented, convergent, and divergent group situations

4. Develops a therapeutic alliance with the client as an advanced generalist

5. Communicates with diverse groups and disciplines using a variety of strategies

6. Facilitates group processes to meet care objectives

7. Integrates concepts from behavioral, biological, and natural sciences in order to understand self and others

8. Interprets quantitative and qualitative data for the interdisciplinary team

9. Uses a scientific process as a basis for developing, implementing, and evaluating nursing interventions

10. Synthesizes information and knowledge as a key component of critical thinking and decision making

11. Bridges cultural and linguistic barriers

12. Understands clients' values and beliefs

13. Completes documentation as it relates to client care

14. Understands the roles of interdisciplinary team

15. Participates in conflict resolution within the health care team

16. Promotes a culture of accountability

C. Health Care Advocacy	**5%**

1. Interfaces between the client and the health care delivery system to protect the rights of clients

2. Ensures that clients, families, and communities are well informed and engaged in their plan of care

3. Ensures that systems meet the needs of the populations served and are culturally relevant

4. Articulates health care issues and concerns to officials and consumers

5. Assists consumers in informed decision making by interpreting health care research

6. Serves as a client advocate on health issues

7. Utilizes chain of command to influence care

8. Promotes fairness and nondiscrimination in the delivery of care

9. Advocates for improvement in the health care system and the nursing profession

D. Integration of the CNL Role	**8%**

1. Articulates the significance of the CNL role

2. Advocates for the CNL role

3. Assumes responsibility of own professional identity and practice

4. Maintains and enhances professional competencies

5. Assumes responsibility for lifelong learning and accountability for current practice and health care information and skills

6. Advocates for professional standards of practice using organizational and political processes

7. Understands the history, philosophy, and responsibilities of the nursing profession as it relates to the CNL

8. Understands scope of practice and adheres to licensure law and regulations

9. Articulates to the public the values of the profession as they relate to client welfare

10. Negotiates and advocates for the role of the professional nurse as a member of the interdisciplinary health care team

11. Develops personal goals for professional development and continuing education

12. Understands and supports agendas that enhance both high-quality, cost-effective health care and the advancement of the profession

13. Supports and mentors individuals entering into and training for professional nursing practice

14. Publishes and presents CNL impact and outcomes

15. Generates nursing research

E. Lateral Integration of Care Services	**6%**

1. Delivers and coordinates care using current technology

2. Coordinates the health care of clients across settings

3. Develops and monitors holistic plans of care

4. Fosters a multidisciplinary approach to attain health and maintain wellness

5. Performs risk analysis for client safety

6. Collaborates and consults with other health professionals in the design, coordination, and evaluation of client care outcomes

7. Disseminates health care information with health care providers to other disciplines

(continued)

II. Clinical Outcomes Management	**30%**
A. Illness and Disease Management	**7%**

1. Assumes responsibility for the provision and management of care at the point of care in and across all environments

2. Coordinates care at the point of service to individuals across the lifespan with particular emphasis on health promotion and risk reduction services

3. Identifies client problems that require intervention, with special focus on those problems amenable to nursing intervention

4. Designs and redesigns client care based on analysis of outcomes and evidence-based knowledge

5. Completes holistic assessments and directs care based on assessments

6. Applies theories of chronic illness care to clients and families

7. Integrates community resources, social networks, and decision support mechanisms into care management

8. Identifies patterns of illness symptoms and effects on clients' compliance and ongoing care

9. Educates clients, families, and care givers to monitor symptoms and take action

10. Utilizes advanced knowledge of pathophysiology and pharmacology to anticipate illness progression and response to therapy and to educate clients and families regarding care

11. Applies knowledge of reimbursement issues in planning care across the lifespan

12. Makes recommendations regarding readiness for discharge, having accurately assessed the client's level of health literacy and self-management

13. Applies research-based knowledge from nursing and the sciences as the foundation for evidence-based practice

14. Develops and facilitates evidence-based protocols and disseminates these among the multidisciplinary teams

15. Understands the role of palliative care and hospice as a disease management tool

16. Understands cultural relevance as it relates to health care

17. Educates clients about health care technologies using client-centered strategies

18. Synthesizes literature and research findings to design interventions for select problems

19. Monitors client satisfaction with disease action plans

20. Evaluates factors contributing to disease, including genetics

21. Designs and implements education and community programs for clients and health professionals

22. Applies principles of infection control, assessment of rates, and inclusion of infection control in plan of care

23. Integrates advanced clinical assessment

B. Knowledge Management	**5%**

1. Applies research-based information

2. Improves clinical and cost outcomes

3. Utilizes epidemiological methodology to collect data

4. Participates in disease surveillance

5. Evaluates and anticipates risks to client safety (e.g., new technology, medications, treatment regimens)

6. Applies tools for risk analysis

7. Uses institutional and unit data to compare against national benchmarks

8. Designs and implements measures to modify risks

9. Addresses variations in clinical outcomes

10. Synthesizes data, information, and knowledge to evaluate and achieve optimal client outcomes

11. Demonstrates accountability for processes for improvement of client outcomes

12. Evaluates effect of complementary therapies on health outcomes

C. Health Promotion and Disease Prevention Management   5%

1. Teaches direct care providers how to assist clients, families, and communities to be health literate and manage their own care

2. Applies research to resolve clinical problems and disseminate results

3. Engages clients in therapeutic partnerships with multidisciplinary team members

4. Applies evidence and data to identify and modify interventions to meet specific client needs

5. Counsels clients and families regarding behavior changes to achieve healthy lifestyles

6. Engages in culturally sensitive health promotion/disease prevention intervention to reduce health care risks in clients

7. Develops clinical and health promotion programs for individuals and groups

8. Designs and implements measures to modify risk factors and promote engagement in healthy lifestyles

9. Assesses protective and predictive (e.g., lifestyle, genetic) factors that influence the health of clients

10. Develops and monitors holistic plans of care that address the health promotion and disease prevention needs of client populations

11. Incorporates theories and research in generating teaching and support strategies to promote and preserve health and healthy lifestyles in client populations

12. Identifies strategies to optimize client's level of functioning

D. Evidence-Based Practice   8%

1. Communicates results in a collaborative manner with client and health care team

2. Uses measurement tools as foundation for assessments and clinical decisions

3. Applies clinical judgment and decision-making skills in designing, coordinating, implementing, and evaluating client-focused care

4. Selects sources of evidence to meet specific needs of individuals, clinical groups, or communities

5. Applies epidemiological, social, and environmental data

6. Reviews datasets to anticipate risk and evaluate care outcomes

7. Evaluates and applies information from various sources to guide client through the health care system

8. Interprets and applies quantitative and qualitative data

(*continued*)

9. Utilizes current health care research to improve client care

10. Accesses, critiques, and analyzes information sources

11. Provides leadership for changing practice on the basis of quality improvement methods and research findings

12. Identifies relevant outcomes and measurement strategies that will improve patient outcomes and promote cost-effective care

13. Synthesizes data, information, and knowledge to evaluate and achieve optimal client outcomes

E. Advanced Clinical Assessment	**5%**

1. Designs, coordinates, and evaluates plans of care

2. Develops a therapeutic alliance with the client as an advanced generalist

3. Identifies client problems that require intervention, with special focus on those problems amenable to nursing intervention

4. Performs holistic assessments across the lifespan and directs care based on findings

5. Applies advanced knowledge of pathophysiology, assessment, and pharmacology

6. Applies clinical judgment and decision-making skills in designing, coordinating, implementing, and evaluating client-focused care

7. Evaluates effectiveness of pharmacological and complementary therapies

III. Care Environment Management	**37%**
A. Team Coordination	**6%**

1. Supervises, educates, delegates, and performs nursing procedures in the context of safety

2. Demonstrates critical listening, verbal, nonverbal, and written communication skills

3. Demonstrates skills necessary to interact and collaborate with other members of the interdisciplinary health care team

4. Incorporates principles of lateral integration

5. Establishes and maintains working relationships within an interdisciplinary team

6. Facilitates group processes to achieve care objectives

7. Utilizes conflict resolution skills

8. Promotes a positive work environment and a culture of retention

9. Designs, coordinates, and evaluates plans of care incorporating client, family, and team member input

10. Leads gap analysis to create cohesive health care team

B. Health Care Finance and Economics	**5%**

1. Identifies clinical and cost outcomes that improve safety, effectiveness, timeliness, efficiency, quality, and client-centered care

2. Serves as a steward of environmental, human, and material resources while coordinating client care

3. Anticipates risk and designs plans of care to improve outcomes

4. Develops and leverages human, environmental, and material resources

5. Demonstrates use of health care technologies to maximize health care outcomes

6. Understands the fiscal context in which practice occurs

7. Evaluates the use of products in the delivery of health care

8. Assumes accountability for the cost-effective and efficient use of human, environmental, and material resources within microsystems

9. Identifies and evaluates high-cost and high-volume activities

10. Applies basic business and economic principles and practices

11. Applies ethical principles regarding the delivery of health care in relation to health care financing and economics including those that may create conflicts of interest

12. Identifies the impact of health care's financial policies and economics on the delivery of health care and client outcomes

13. Interprets health care research, particularly cost and client outcomes, to policy makers, health care providers, and consumers

14. Interprets the impact of both public and private reimbursement policies and mechanisms on client care decisions

15. Evaluates the effect of health care financing on care access and patient outcomes

C. Health Care Systems   **5%**

1. Acquires knowledge to work in groups, manage change, and systems-level dissemination of knowledge

2. Applies evidence that challenges current policies and procedures in a practice environment

3. Implements strategies that lessen health care disparities

4. Advocates for improvement in the health care system, policies, and nursing profession

5. Applies systems thinking (i.e., theories, models) to address problems and develop solutions

6. Collaborates with other health care professionals to manage the transition of clients across the health care continuum, ensuring patient safety and cost-effectiveness of care

7. Utilizes quality improvement methods in evaluating individual and aggregate client care

8. Understands how health care delivery systems are organized and financed and the effect on client care

9. Identifies the economic, legal, and political factors that influence health care delivery

D. Health Care Policy   **4%**

1. Acknowledges multiple perspectives when analyzing health care policy

2. Recognizes the effect of health care policy on health promotion, risk reduction, and disease and injury prevention in vulnerable populations

3. Influences regulatory, legislative, and public policy in private and public arenas to promote and preserve healthy communities

4. Understands the interactive effect of health policy and health care economics and national and international health and health outcomes

5. Accesses, critiques, and analyzes information sources

6. Incorporates standards of care and full scope of practice

(continued)

7. Articulates the interaction between regulatory controls and quality control within the health care delivery system

8. Creates a professional ethic related to client care and health policy

9. Understands the political and regulatory processes defining health care delivery and systems of care

10. Evaluates local, state, and national socioeconomic and health policy issues and trends as they relate to the delivery of health care

11. Participates in political processes and grass roots legislative efforts to influence health care policy on behalf of clients and the profession

12. Understands global health care issues (e.g., immigration patterns, pandemics, access to care)

13. Understands the effect of legal and regulatory processes on nursing practice

E. Quality Improvement   6%

1. Evaluates health care outcomes through the acquisition of data and the questioning of inconsistencies

2. Leads the redesign of client care following root cause analysis of sentinel events

3. Gathers, analyzes, and synthesizes data related to risk reduction and patient safety

4. Analyzes systems and outcome datasets to anticipate individual client risk and improve quality care

5. Understands economies of care, cost-effectiveness, resource utilization, and effecting change in systems

6. Evaluates the environmental impact on health care outcomes

7. Collaborates and consults with other health professionals to design, coordinate, and evaluate client care outcomes

8. Evaluates the quality and use of products in the delivery of health care

9. Identifies opportunities for quality improvement and leads improvement activities utilizing evidence-based models

F. Health Care Informatics   4%

1. Analyzes systems to identify strengths, gaps, and opportunities

2. Applies data from systems in planning and delivering care

3. Evaluates clinical information systems using select criteria

4. Incorporates ethical principles in the use of information systems

5. Evaluates impact of new technologies on clients, families, and systems\

6. Assesses and evaluates the use of technology in the delivery of client care

7. Validates accuracy of consumer-provided information on health issues from the Internet and other sources

8. Synthesizes health care information for client-specific problems

9. Refers clients to culturally relevant health information

10. Demonstrates proficiency in the use of innovations such as the electronic record for documenting and analyzing clinical data

11. Individualizes interventions using technologies

12. Identifies and promotes an environment that safeguards the privacy and confidentiality of patients and families

13. Leads quality improvement team and engages in designing and implementing a process for improving client safety

14. Utilizes information and communication technologies to document, access, and monitor client care; advance client education; and enhance the accessibility of care

15. Aligns interdisciplinary team documentation to improve accessibility of data

G. Ethics	**7%**

1. Evaluates ethical decision making from both a personal and an organizational perspective and develops an understanding of how these two perspectives may create conflicts of interest

2. Applies an ethical decision-making framework to clinical situations that incorporates moral concepts, professional ethics, and law and respects diverse values and beliefs

3. Applies legal and ethical guidelines to advocate for client well-being and preferences

4. Enables clients and families to make quality-of-life and end-of-life decisions and achieve a peaceful death

5. Identifies and analyzes common ethical dilemmas and the ways in which these dilemmas impact client care

6. Identifies areas in which a personal conflict of interest may arise and proposes resolutions or actions to resolve the conflict

Used with permission from the Commission on Nurse Certification (2012).

Resource

Commission on Nurse Certification. (2012). *Clinical nurse leader (CNL®) job analysis summary and certification exam blue print*. Washington, DC: Author. http://www.aacn.nche.edu/cnl/publications-resources

APPENDIX B

Reflection Questions for the Chapters

Chapter 3

1. How would you describe horizontal leadership?
2. How does horizontal leadership differ from other types of leadership?
3. Which of the change theories do you expect to use in your practice as a CNL?
4. What is the difference between coaching and mentoring, and how would you use them once you are a CNL?

Chapter 4

1. As a CNL what is your responsibility to your microsystem when change in practice becomes necessary to provide better patient care?
2. How do you see the role of CNL in your microsystem as it relates to interdisciplinary communication and patient outcomes?
3. How do you see the role of CNL in relation to bedside nursing and the therapeutic relationship with the client as an advanced generalist?
4. How will you use conflict resolution in your microsystem to facilitate effective communication between disciplines?

Chapter 5

While reflecting on a situation where you, as a CNL, had to act as the patient/family advocate:

1. What are the two ways CNLs incorporate social justice into practice?
2. Describe two ways that CNLs can advocate for nursing in general and, more specifically, two ways to advocate for CNLs.
3. What are other disciplines that CNLs can seek as resources for advocacy issues?
4. Why should patients be allowed to make changes or end health care treatments?

Chapter 6

1. Describe the eight aspects of the CNL role that a new CNL must integrate into practice.
2. Reflect on and describe a situation where a CNL is able to enhance both high-quality, cost-effective health care, and the advancement of the profession.
3. Identify two ways a CNL can help to integrate his or her role into the practice setting.
4. What resources might a CNL choose to help with the integration of his or her role into practice?

Chapter 7

1. Describe the role of the CNL called lateral integration.
2. What are the four components of lateral integration?
3. How can a CNL promote communication?
4. Who are some of the stakeholders who may be involved with the CNL in lateral integration, and how might they help?

Chapter 8

1. What are some of the prevalent illnesses and diseases in your specialty area? Are these diseases preventable? Are the illnesses and diseases amenable to nursing interventions?
2. What factors should be taken into account when assessing readiness for discharge to the next level of care?
3. What are some key aspects to consider when assessing an individual's level of pain?
4. What are some of the differences in individuals' responses to illness, considering their cultural, ethnic, socioeconomic, religious, and lifestyle preferences?

Chapter 9

1. Describe how a CNL might incorporate summaries of outcomes data to direct care givers into the routine operations of a microsystem.
2. The amount of knowledge required by all members of the health care team in today's work environment is overwhelming to many. Describe organizational resources a CNL might utilize to best plan a strategy for improving knowledge management in a microsystem.

3. Compare and contrast the role of a root cause analysis (RCA) and a failure mode effect analysis (FMEA), and how a CNL can maximize the use of these strategies.

4. Consider how the role of the CNL is key to prioritizing the communication of new knowledge to direct care givers.

Chapter 10

1. How could a CNL working on Mrs. Louis's unit initiate a change project related to her experience and the coordination of patient care?

2. What type of team would a CNL organize to make improvements?

3. What type of data and outcomes could be measured in the team's project?

4. How would the challenges of health promotion impact the work of the team, for example, health care literacy?

Chapter 11

1. What are key aspects of the definition of evidence-based practice (EBP) that the CNL can use to teach other professional nurses about this important topic?

2. Explain two ways that a CNL can implement EBP into the practice setting.

3. How does a CNL know what is the current best practice related to a clinical topic?

4. What are the two key databases or websites that a CNL might use to search for evidence to support practice?

Chapter 12

1. What are the important data that should be collected in an initial clinical assessment?

2. How can the CNL use the Healthy People 2020 Leading Health Indicators to coordinate client care?

3. Explain why a therapeutic relationship is important for the CNL in the clinical assessment process.

4. The mnemonic PQRSTU can also be used to organize the client's symptoms. What do the letters in the mnemonic stand for?

Chapter 13

1. At what stage of Tuckman and Jensen's group process may team members experience conflict and struggle over power in the group? How can a CNL support this phase of group development?

2. As a CNL you have identified an issue with near misses in patient home medication dosing and in hospital medication dosing. How would you go about building an effective team to address this issue? What interprofessional team members would you include when coordinating care?

3. Identify any reason a collaborative interprofessional team may be formed in your unique health care setting.

4. What resources can a CNL seek out to deal with conflict among teams? How can friction among a group impact the outcomes of the group in a negative and positive way?

Chapter 14

1. Describe the concept of patient volume and the related impact of this key variable on the financial structure of the microsystem.

2. Utilization of services and supplies has a great impact on the microsystem and also the mesosystem/organization as a whole. Consider multiple ways that the CNL can be a driving force in most efficient utilization of services and supplies.

3. Discuss how issues of staffing mix, productivity, and design of the staffing matrix impact the work of the CNL within the microsystem.

4. Why is it relevant for the CNL to understand factors related to staffing, budgets, and skill mix?

Chapter 15

1. The role of CNL was created to directly impact patient safety at the point of care. Describe how the CNL's knowledge of the health care system is integral to the success of CNL outcomes.

2. Apply elements of complexity theory to a current health care initiative that involves CNLs and interprofessional teams. Relate how the concepts of open-ended, adaptable systems play a role in the work of improvement teams.

3. Discuss the benefits of a thorough microsystem's assessment in relation to implementing care in a complex health care system.

4. Consider competencies of the CNL role that support the translation of emerging nursing science into the microsystem and throughout the complex health care system.

Chapter 16

1. What are the three things that would help CNLs increase their influence in organizations, communities, and in national and international health care?

2. How is a political analysis similar to a clinical assessment?

3. What skill sets do clinical nurses have that enable them to work at the unit level to sort out the actions that are needed to comply with HCAHPS, core measures, and other scoring procedures?

4. How do clinical nurse leaders use evidence-based research to inform their practice? What are some of the ways in which this same approach would apply in public health policy and health services research?

Chapter 17

1. Discuss the current and future role of frontline nurses in the rapidly advancing field of quality improvement. Consider the role of the CNL in supporting this engagement of nursing critical voice.

2. Develop a systematic process to organize the vast resources available on health care improvement topics.

3. How would you critically review publications, best practice guidelines, and related information on the topic and share it with the improvement team?

4. How does the CNL function as an integrator of lateral care in quality improvement and patient safety initiatives within a health care system?

Chapter 18

1. Consider those human factors that might impede the development of health information technologies in the workplace and address how you would manage those factors.

2. There are concerns about privacy and confidentiality in the use of health information exchanges. Knowing the definitions of privacy and confidentiality and anticipating resistance by both staff and patients on the basis of their concerns, make a case about why organizations and patients should embrace the use of HIEs—what is in it for them?

3. How might you encourage clinicians to become engaged in the development and implementation of clinical decision support systems, both passive and active, on the basis of current evidence and experiential knowledge?

4. Identify questions/problems related to health information technology that should be a priority for those developing information technology.

Chapter 19

1. How can the CNLs best equip themselves with the skills and knowledge needed to address ethical concerns in health care? Discuss general and specific strategies.

2. How can the CNL best support direct care nurses as they are confronted with moral stress?

3. What areas of health care have classically been associated with ethical challenges in patient care and what emerging issues are presenting ethical concerns?

4. Consider the varied work environments across the health care systems. Discuss ways that CNLs can help direct care givers to seek out support for appropriate resources when they feel a patient/family is being unjustly treated.

APPENDIX C

Multiple-Choice Questions and Case Studies

Kimberlee-Ann Bridges, MSN, RN, CNL
Care Coordinator
Western Health Network
Danbury, CT

Leah Ledford, MSN, RN, CNL, SANE
Clinical Nurse Leader
Carolinas Medical Center
Charlotte, NC

Marie D. Litzelman, MSN, RN, CMSRN, CNL
Clinical Nurse Leader
Carolinas Medical Center
Charlotte, NC

Danielle Morton, MSN, RN, CNL
Pediatric Nurse Educator
Yale New Haven Hospital
New Haven, CT

Sara Pratt, MSN, RN, CNL
Clinical Nurse Leader
Carolinas Medical Center
Charlotte, NC

Katarzyna A. Qutermous, MSN, RN, CNL
Clinical Nurse Leader
Carolinas Medical Center
Charlotte, NC

Josephine Ritchie, MSN, RN, CNL
Performance Improvement Manager
Norwalk Hospital, Norwalk, CT

Mary-Jo Smith MSN, RN, CNL
Patient Services Manager
Yale-New Haven Children's Hospital
New Haven, CT

Correspondence to:
Cynthia R. King, PhD, NP, MSN, CNL, FAAN
11313 Coreopsis Road
Charlotte, NC 28213
Cell phone: 336-416-8668
Home: 704-900-8097 answering machine
E-mail: Kingc@queens.edu

Sally O'Toole Gerard, DNP, CDE, RN, CDE, CNL
Assistant Professor
CNL Track Coordinator
Fairfield University
Fairfield, CT
sgerard@fairfield.edu

1. Patient satisfaction scores in the emergency department (ED) have shown a downward trend over the past three quarters. As a clinical nurse leader (CNL) in the ED, your focus is to:

   A. Create a script for the triage nurse in welcoming the patient

   B. Assign a volunteer to welcome patients to the hospital

   C. Compare desired outcomes with national and state standards

   D. Write a letter of apology to each dissatisfied patient

2. Which of the following actions illustrates the CNL professional value of altruism?

   A. Leading an interdisciplinary team looking at the remote cardiac monitoring process

   B. Sponsoring a meeting with the monitor technicians to understand their barriers in the cardiac monitoring process

   C. Flow mapping the admission process of the remote cardiac-monitored patient

   D. Editing the policy for the remote cardiac monitoring process

3. You are a CNL on the telemetry unit and orienting a newly graduated nurse. Critical thinking is best demonstrated when:

   A. The CNL discusses with the physician the rationale for discontinuing cardiac monitoring in the hospice patient

   B. Drawing the scheduled cardiac enzymes every 8 hours

   C. Reviewing the patient care guidelines and protocols related to hourly rounding

   D. The CNL balances both the charge role and the preceptor role simultaneously

4. You are a CNL selected to lead a team focused on implementing a multidisciplinary clinical pathway for acute ischemic stroke and transient ischemic attack. The risk assessment tool that you have adopted identifies all of the following as independent stroke risk factors except:

   A. Age

   B. Systolic blood pressure

   C. Liver dysfunction

   D. Current smoking

   E. Diabetes mellitus

5. A lack of compliance with deep vein thrombosis (DVT) prophylaxis has been identified in retrospective chart reviews of all ischemic stroke patients in your organization. As a CNL on the neurological unit, your primary goal will include:

   A. Challenging the guidelines on primary prevention of ischemic stroke written by the American Stroke Association

   B. Gaining an understanding of how DVT prophylaxis is initiated on each stroke patient on your unit

   C. Developing an organization-wide educational program on DVT prophylaxis

   D. Developing a unit-based team of nursing personnel to investigate the problem

6. You are working on improving the patient discharge process. Which of these targets would best reflect clinical microsystem outcomes?

   A. Hospital length of stay

   B. Time of discharge order for all medical patients to the actual time the patient left

   C. Number of discharge orders on your unit entered before 11 a.m.

   D. Total number of discharged patients leaving by 11 a.m.

7. Electronic nursing documentation has recently been instituted in your organization. Select a response that best defines a clinical decision support:

   A. A reminder to save and sign your admission assessment

   B. A visual red alert when a patient's potassium is 6.8 mEq/L

   C. A pop-up to initiate the discharge instruction sheet with every physician discharge order

   D. An electronic nursing care plan

In 2008, the Centers for Medicaid and Medicare Services (CMS) collaboratively with the Centers for Disease Control and Prevention enacted a new payment provision related to eight hospital-acquired conditions. Hospital falls and traumas occurring during a hospital stay will not receive CMS reimbursement. Health promotion, risk reduction, and disease prevention are core competencies of the clinical nurse leader. As a CNL on the telemetry unit, you have recognized the importance of this issue.

8. Which level within a system does this issue affect?

   A. Microsystem

   B. Mesosystem

   C. Macrosystem

   D. All of the above

9. Clinical nurse leaders focus on projects within a clinical microsystem. A clinical microsystem can be best described as:

   A. A department-wide program focused on improving continuity of care and patient satisfaction

   B. Trending the postoperative care on all surgical units

   C. The clinical and business processes of a single unit within an organization

   D. All medical and surgical units guided by a chief nursing officer

10. All are part of the data necessary for a CNL to fully understand and assess his or her clinical unit except:

    A. The organization financial statement

    B. The target population and age distribution

    C. The percentage of full-time equivalents (FTEs)

    D. Rate of nosocomial infections

    E. Fall rates

11. The results of a quarterly report identify an increase in patient falls on the telemetry unit. Your first action will be to:

    A. Implement hourly rounding

    B. Gain an understanding of patient care practices on the telemetry unit

    C. Assign patient personal alarms to all patients at risk

    D. Revise the current fall risk documentation form

12. You have been asked to lead the telemetry fall prevention committee. Which combination of team members would best suit the initial phase of this group?

    A. A behavioral health APRN

    B. A staff nurse

    C. A physical therapist

    D. The nurse manager

    E. All of the above

    F. Only A, B, and D are needed

13. As a CNL in the ICU, you have observed several prolonged and fragmented processes of starting an intravenous line in a critically ill patient. All of the following considerations are necessary in identifying **a theme** for your improvement process except:

    A. A thorough review of the clinical unit

    B. The manager's mandate for change

    C. The alignment with the organization's strategic priorities

    D. Input from the patient's family

14. The hospital is looking to utilize cardiac monitor watchers. Your analysis includes all of the following except:

    A. A review of an online ECG monitoring education program

    B. Identifying a clinical issue with a focus on a specific population

    C. Conducting a trend analysis of outcome data

    D. Analyzing barriers and facilitators with the organization

15. Several near misses were identified by ICU nurses who had mistaken invasive lines for intravenous ports for medication administration. You have completed an analysis of the issue. Your recommendations include:

    A. A visual signal on all ports not intended for intravenous drugs

    B. A double-check system for medication administration

    C. To facilitate a critical incident reporting structure that fosters a "without blame" unit culture

    D. All of the above

    E. Only C

16. Data reported by the ICU quality committee reflect challenges in the management of the septic patient. As a CNL in the ICU, all of the following are first steps in evaluating the delivery of client care except:

    A. Knowledge of sepsis guidelines

    B. Critical care clinicians staffing ratios

    C. Use of clinical decision support systems

    D. Differentiating sepsis from systemic inflammatory response syndrome (SIRS)

17. A fellow staff nurse is struggling to understand the use of a clinical decision support system (CDSS) in the management of her septic patient. Your initial teaching strategy includes:

    A. Sharing the latest clinical research

    B. An understanding of expected and actual outcomes

    C. Defining the purpose of CDSS

    D. Exploring challenges, risks, and benefits

18. You are using failure mode and effect analysis (FMEA) to anticipate the risk of medication errors in the ICU related to invasive lines. You begin your FMEA analysis with:

    A. The effects of each failure

    B. The potential cause of each failure

    C. Process mapping

    D. Specific defects and delays in the medication administration process

19. Your colleagues have identified challenges in the process of inserting an intravenous line. To gain a better understanding of what this process entails, you:

    A. Directly observe the intravenous line insertion process and time each step of the process

    B. Create a workflow diagram tracing the path of the nurse during the line insertion process

    C. Engage the IV team to reeducate the nurses

    D. All of the above

    E. A and B

20. The result of a workflow diagram of a clinician illustrates an excessive amount of walking to obtain supplies. Reducing the waste of motion adds value-added time that ultimately benefits:

    A. The patient

    B. The clinician

    C. Documentation

    D. None of the above

21. Your team is looking at the delays in the discharge process. Your cause and effect diagram includes:
    A. A run chart
    B. A Gantt chart
    C. A fishbone diagram
    D. A high-level flowchart

22. You are leading a palliative care team in the ICU. Ethical competence is best defined as:
    A. The ability to recognize potential and actual ethical issues arising from clinical practice
    B. The collaboration with a multicultural workforce
    C. The understanding of the physical, emotional, and spiritual heath parameters of the ICU patient
    D. The skill set to define, design, and implement culturally competent health care providers

23. Opportunities that reflect human diversity include:
    A. Promoting effective communication for injured veterans
    B. Stressing the importance of family health history
    C. Standardizing the discharge process
    D. Decreasing the admission lead time to the pediatric unit

24. Survey results of the nursing staff reflect poor perceptions and a discomfort with addressing spiritual issues with patients. The ultimate success of focused staff education can be measured by:
    A. Trending quarterly patient satisfaction scores pertaining to spiritual care during hospitalization
    B. A follow-up survey of the staff after the education to solicit feedback
    C. An open discussion of how the nurse would address spiritual care in a given scenario
    D. Feedback shared during discharge phone calls

25. Sustaining process improvement requires the use of appropriate learning principles and strategies. The CNL function that best utilizes this competency is:
    A. Advocate
    B. Educator
    C. Clinician
    D. Information manager

26. How can the CNL make the greatest impact on the health care organization?
    A. By representing the microsystem
    B. By representing the mesosystem
    C. By representing the patient and family
    D. By representing the nursing profession

27. By leading which unit initiative can the CNL directly impact the financial health of the entire institution?

    A. Reducing readmissions

    B. Recruitment of new nursing staff

    C. Improving documentation compliance

    D. Encouraging staff to report safety events and near misses

28. The concept that an organization is in a continued state of change describes which organizational theory:

    A. Systems theory

    B. Classical theory

    C. Contingency theory

    D. Chaos theory

29. The new hospital CNO works hard to cultivate a shared vision of leaders and followers motivating each other toward their highest potential. This is an example of which type of leadership:

    A. Transformational leadership

    B. Transactional leadership

    C. Situational leadership

    D. Hierarchical leadership

30. Before beginning data collection, what is the primary key factor to determine?

    A. Personnel to collect data

    B. A secure database for holding data

    C. Operational definitions of data

    D. A user-friendly collection method

31. You are the CNL on a 25-bed cardiac unit. You are completing afternoon rounds with the patients. Upon entering Mr. K's room you notice that his son has brought him fried chicken, soda, and fries. How should you address this?

    A. Don't say anything to the patient or family and tell the interdisciplinary team at morning rounds

    B. Provide education to the patient and family about consuming a heart healthy diet

    C. Place a consult in the computer for the nutritionist to assess the patient

    D. Remind the patient why he is in the hospital and remove the food

32. As the CNL on a cardiothoracic step-down unit, what is the one recommendation you would make to decrease the chance of readmission of your patient population?

    A. Visiting nursing for all patients

    B. All follow-up appointments scheduled prior to patient discharge

    C. Pharmacy to visit with each patient prior to discharge home to review medications

    D. All patients should be enrolled in a cardiac rehabilitation program

33. You know teaching was effective to a cardiac patient and his wife with the following statement:

    A. "I can still have a burger and fries one to two times a week"

    B. "It is okay for my wife to bring in a pizza while I'm here; after all the hospital food is not that good"

    C. "I should limit my salt intake and increase fiber in my diet"

    D. "If my husband wants fried shrimp, it's okay because it is seafood"

34. You are the CNL on a geriatric unit. When walking down the hall, you notice a high-risk fall patient attempting to get out of bed alone. After assisting the patient and ensuring safety, what should you do?

    A. Report the incident to nursing management

    B. Identify the patient's nurse and nursing assistant and confront them with the incident

    C. Develop a new fall prevention policy and post it in the unit conference room for all staff to view

    D. Obtain the fall statistics and present them at the next unit staff meeting and develop a team to look at revising a fall prevention committee

35. As the CNL on a medical/surgical unit, you have noticed a trend over the last 3 months with patients having high blood glucose before lunch and dinner. What is the best way to address this problem?

    A. Investigate whether the blood glucose monitors on the unit are accurate

    B. Provide an educational in-service about diabetes to the staff

    C. Ensure all patients with diabetes receive a consultation with the nutritionist

    D. Determine what other changes in processes have occurred on the unit in the past 3 months that could influence this trend

36. After careful review of unit processes, you have determined that the self meal order program was introduced 3 months ago. With this program, patients have the ability to order meals when they are ready to eat rather than eating at predetermined times set by the hospital. This change has altered the timing of medications previously given with meals. What does the CNL do to improve the process?

    A. Develop an interdisciplinary team, including unit staff, nutritionist, diabetic educator, and meal service team members to investigate the self meal order program

    B. Have the nurse or nursing assistant order meals with patients; this way the nurse knows what time the patient orders meals

    C. When explaining the self meal order program to patients, instruct patients to notify staff when they order meals

    D. Have the meal service notify the unit secretary when meal orders are placed by patients

37. After completing unit audits, you have noticed the nurses are not completing AIR cycles documentation with pain management (AIR: assessment, intervention, reassessment). What should be done to improve documentation?

    A. Tell the unit management which staff are documenting inappropriately

    B. Reeducate staff on the hospital documentation policy

    C. Remind staff of pain documentation during staff meetings and charge report

    D. Provide staff with a self-audit sheet as a way to review their own documentation during their shifts

38. You are listening to report with a novice nurse. As part of mentoring new staff and supporting clinical decision making, you ask the new nurse which patient she would like to assess first. Which patient should this nurse assess first?

    A. 46-year-old receiving IV antibiotic therapy

    B. 60-year-old s/p liver biopsy

    C. 56-year-old with pneumonia

    D. 72-year-old hip replacement impatiently waiting for discharge

39. To help patients maintain healthy skin while in the hospital, all of the following should be considered *except*:

    A. Provide patient with Q2h positioning/turning if patient is unable to self-position

    B. Ensure adequate protein intake

    C. Use bed surfaces known to prevent skin complications

    D. Allow patient to refuse bathing for days if uninterested, as the patient has the right to refuse care

40. A nurse on the unit comes to you and says that every shift he works day or night he finds at least one of his patients without an identification band in place. He is very concerned about patient safety and feels a harmful mistake could occur in the near future if the practice on the unit is not improved. What do you do as the CNL?

    A. Perform daily audits on all the patients and report results to management

    B. Have the unit secretary make new identification bands for all the patients daily so the charge nurse can place new bands on the patients daily

    C. Research a new style of patient identification bands since the current product does not stay on the patient properly

    D. Provide support to the nurse on the unit who determines the problem and help him identify areas in the process to improve patient identification

41. Over the past few weeks, nurses on the 30-bed medical unit have been complaining the MD orders related to oxygen do not match what the patient is receiving. Often the patient has more than one oxygen order at the same time. This leads to confusion for nursing and respiratory care staff and could harm the patient. How can the CNL improve the practice?

    A. Using the informatics team as support, create a hard stop in the computer that does not allow the physician to activate a new oxygen order without discontinuing the previous order

    B. Tell the nurses they need to remind the doctors to keep orders up to date and have the nurses review orders at rounds with the team

    C. Meet with the unit hospitalist to make a plan to address the problem

    D. Do nothing since CNLs cannot write patient care orders

42. The hospital has a goal for patient transfers from ICU to be completed by 12 noon. Your unit has a very low percentage for meeting this hospital goal. How can you best address this problem as the CNL?

    A. Tell the charge nurse to discharge patients in the morning

    B. Ask the manager to staff an extra nurse on day shift to be the discharge nurse

    C. Use process mapping to determine all the possible factors that contribute to patient discharge and what barriers there are to discharge

    D. Don't worry about the number; your unit meets the other hospital goals, so it is okay to miss one

43. You are the CNL at an outpatient care clinic providing care to families in the area. You have noticed it is difficult to get families to bring their children in for their immunizations, and children are often off schedule. How can the clinic best address this issue to meet the needs of their patient populations?

    A. Educate families on immunizations, their purpose, and their children's schedule

    B. Provide reminder phone calls to families the day before a scheduled appointment

    C. If possible, offer extended clinic hours 1 to 2 nights a week, so parents can come in after work

    D. Use the clinic data to determine why families are not coming to appointments

44. You are the CNL in the day surgery center and have found that many patients come to the center unprepared on the morning of surgery. This delays surgery start times and backs up the operating room schedule for the day. The whole surgery team is frustrated. How can the process be fixed?

    A. Change the first surgery start time and delay it by 20 minutes

    B. Institute presurgery phone calls 2 to 3 days prior to a patient's scheduled appointment

    C. Stagger surgery start times more throughout the day

    D. Reschedule patients who come to the center unprepared

45. Per the epidemiology report, your unit's hand hygiene scores have steadily decreased over the past 3 months. When reporting these metrics at a staff meeting, most of the staff replies saying, "It's the doctors fault, we always wash our hands." How do you work to change the culture of the unit?

    A. Have secret shoppers monitor the staff and hand out tickets to hand hygiene offenders

    B. Collect hand hygiene metrics related to the unit staff only and use these data to educate staff

    C. Have a hand hygiene campaign to reinvigorate staff

    D. Investigate the barriers to hand hygiene and collaborate with staff to reduce these barriers

46. A new nurse on the medical/surgical unit approaches you with concerns about one of her patients. She states the patient has not turned on the lights or television all day and did not order breakfast or lunch. She had to ask the patient what meal they wanted and place the order. This nurse states she is concerned about the change in the patient's behavior. Looking at the patient's chart, you realize this patient is Jewish and it is Saturday. What is your best response to the nurse?

    A. "The patient is sick and needs extra support today"

    B. "The patient needs to be seen by the psychology team for an evaluation"

    C. "The patient may be following their religious practices and we need to support this"

    D. "Begin being in the hospital"

47. When trying to implement a change in the outpatient family clinic, which group of staff should the CNL focus on more?

    A. Late majority

    B. Early majority

    C. Laggards

    D. Innovators

48. As the CNL on a medical unit, which of the following interventions would you support to reduce the readmission rate on your unit?

    A. Keep patients one extra day to ensure they are prepared for discharge home

    B. Arrange for all patients to have at least 1 week of visiting nursing postdischarge

    C. Review discharge instructions with the patient and one family member

    D. Begin discharge planning and teaching on the day of admission

49. You are the CNL on a 32-bed medical–surgical unit. When you walk into the unit, you observe a novice nurse looking extremely busy and stressed. How can you best support her transition on the unit?

    A. Ask the charge nurse to decrease her patient assignment

    B. Give some of her morning medications

    C. Pull the nurse off the unit during her shift

    D. Meet with this nurse after the shift to discuss organization

50. Which type of evidence would you prefer to review and share with a team when trying to support whether an evidence-based intervention should be implemented on your unit?

    A. Meta-analysis

    B. Quasi-experimental

    C. Experimental

    D. Qualitative

51. Which group presents the highest challenge in attaining buy-in for a new innovation?

    A. Early innovators

    B. Early adopters

    C. Late majority

    D. Laggards

52. There has been disagreement regarding the suggested adoption of a patient transfer blackout period during change of shift. Staff on the inpatient units favor a 30-minute blackout period, while emergency department staff favor no blackout period. A team of stakeholders from all areas recently agreed on a universal blackout period of 15 minutes during shift change. What type of solution does this represent?

    A. Compromise

    B. Collaboration

    C. Accommodation

    D. Confrontation

53. The CNL can effectively design fiscally efficient patient care using which of the following strategies:

    A. Division of tasks and responsibilities among all team members

    B. Delegation of responsibilities according to job roles

    C. Seeking team members' input regarding their strengths and desired responsibilities

    D. Using input from the manager for job assignments

54. To demonstrate active listening, the CNL would exhibit which behavior:

    A. Avoid making any facial expressions

    B. Preserve at least 3 feet between the parties

    C. Lean slightly forward

    D. Fold hands in the lap

55. To confirm a scope of practice question, the CNL should consult which administrative body guidelines:

    A. The Joint Commission

    B. Centers for Medicare and Medicaid Services

    C. Hospital Policy and Procedure Manual

    D. State Nursing Practice Act

56. Team coordination skills can help avoid all but

    A. Undefined team member roles

    B. Poor membership involvement

    C. Member conflict

    D. Confusion regarding next steps

57. An important element of an effective team meeting is the creation of minutes to be distributed after the meeting. Who is the most appropriate team member to create the minutes?

    A. The meeting facilitator

    B. Any group member

C. A preidentified team member

D. The meeting scheduler

58. Which of the following may be a beneficial tool for an interdisciplinary team to use to focus many ideas for improvement of patient satisfaction scores?

A. Root cause analysis

B. Multivoting

C. Development of a subcommittee

D. None of the above; the group should work on all the ideas generated by the group

59. Who can function as an important ally to the CNL in engaging frontline staff in a major initiative?

A. Content expert

B. Unit champion

C. Initiative sponsor

D. Senior leadership

60. A team approach utilizing the integration of many different roles working toward common patient and family goals describes the objective of which type of team:

A. Multidisciplinary team

B. Interdisciplinary team

C. Patient advocacy team

D. Care coordination team

61. Individual consults by many different health disciplines represent which type of approach:

A. Multidisciplinary

B. Interdisciplinary

C. Team

D. Intradisciplinary

62. In order to generate ideas aimed at designing an implementation plan, a team reviews the topic and members verbalize solution ideas in a random fashion. This is an example of which of the following strategies:

A. Multivoting

B. Process mapping

C. Brainstorming

D. Nominal group technique

63. Your unit has worked hard to maintain a very low fall rate. There has now been a sharp increase over the past 2 months. In looking at control chart data related to falls, you see that all of these falls occur on the night shift. What is the most likely reason for this shift?

A. A common cause

B. A special cause

C. A coincidence

D. A trend

64. From which database would the CNL collect the most useful nursing-sensitive indicator metrics?

   A. NDNQI

   B. Hospital Compare

   C. TJC

   D. NQF

65. What is the appropriate ending point of a root cause analysis (RCA)?

   A. When several possible reasons for the error have been identified

   B. When staff have identified what they think is the reason for the error

   C. When the list of causes is exhausted to no more possible causes

   D. The CNL can identify reasons for occurrence

66. When is an RCA performed?

   A. Prior to the initiation of a new treatment to anticipate possible problems

   B. During a process to evaluate ongoing problems

   C. As part of data analysis to understand why an intervention led to poor results

   D. After a serious safety event has occurred

67. Your unit has recently been relocated to the new hospital wing. This area is more spacious and modern than the unit's previous environment. Patient satisfaction scores in the area of "physical environment of care" have improved significantly. The added distance that staff must walk to answer call lights has resulted in decreased patient satisfaction scores in the area of "Call bell answered immediately." Based on this, the hospital budget was realigned to build an additional nurses station at the midpoint of the unit. What is the relationship between these two measures?

   A. Confounding measures

   B. Balancing measures

   C. Opposing measures

   D. Concurrent measures

68. Your geriatric unit shows the highest average restraint episode duration in the hospital. You have been asked to lead an improvement project to reduce duration. What would be your first step?

   A. Obtain national restraint episode duration benchmark data

   B. Conduct a full assessment of your unit, including all restraint-related data and processes

   C. Conduct a literature search to obtain current best practices for geriatric patients in restraints

   D. Speak with staff and leadership of other units with lower restraint episode durations

69. What is the purpose of a fishbone diagram?

    A. To identify the cause and effect of multiple factors that lead to a result

    B. To identify the root cause of a serious safety event

    C. To aid in the development of an improvement project timeline

    D. To create the goals and objectives of an improvement project

70. Nurses on your unit have complained that equipment kept on the unit is not readily available. They have indicated that it often takes a considerable amount of time to locate. You realize that this is a waste of valuable human work resources. An effective process to utilize in solving this problem is the _____ principle.

    A. 5P

    B. SIPOC

    C. FMEA

    D. 5S

71. A process improvement project charter or establishment of specific aims can help a project group to avoid which difficulty:

    A. Scope creep

    B. Meeting time confusion

    C. Budget constraints

    D. Team communication problems

72. You have been charged with examining the heart failure 30-day readmission rate of your unit. In doing so, it is important for you to examine data from what other sources:

    A. National and state readmission rates

    B. National benchmarks

    C. Readmissions to other units in your hospital

    D. All of the above

73. One of the nurses on your unit was involved in a medication error. She revealed the error to both you and the nurse manager and documented the error in the online safety event reporting system. You meet with her and begin the process of identifying causes that led to this event, so the risk for future medication errors can be minimized. As evidenced by these actions, what is the culture of your hospital?

    A. A laissez-faire culture

    B. A just culture

    C. A punitive culture

    D. A structural culture

74. You are working with a team to reduce patient waiting time for transport to diagnostic imaging. An effective goal would be to:

    A. Decrease waiting time during the evening shift

    B. Increase monthly patient satisfaction

C. Improve communication between the ED and the DI departments

D. Decrease the waiting time for diagnostic imaging by 5%

75. When conducting a literature review, the publication that would provide a comprehensive summary of research on that topic would be:

A. Nonexperimental

B. Experimental

C. Case study

D. Meta-analysis

76. When incorporating evidence-based practice interventions into your health care setting, it would be best to:

A. Do what everyone else is doing

B. Do what you think would work in your setting

C. Choose the interventions you think would work for your setting and perform a rapid cycle test to evaluate the impact

D. Do everything the literature suggests to improve your chances of a good outcome

77. All of the following are steps of evidence-based practice except:

A. Integrating evidence with clinical expertise, patient preferences, and values when making a decision or change

B. Asking the question in a PICO format

C. Obtaining informed consent from patients involved in the practice change

D. Critically appraising the evidence

78. You are trying to encourage nurses on your unit to become more active in utilizing research in practice and to learn more about evidence-based practice. What would be a good activity to promote your idea?

A. Leave a few nursing journals on the unit

B. Make a point of discussing research articles you have read with nurses on the unit

C. Form a journal club on the unit

D. E-mail the nurses articles to read

79. What type of study would not be included in evidence-based practice if the nurses were looking for quantitative research?

A. Meta-analysis

B. Experimental

C. Quasi-experimental

D. Phenomenological

80. In assessing your organization for evidence-based practice environmental readiness, you would evaluate all of the following except:

A. Do advance practice nurse and educators model evidence-based practice?

B. Are the nurses expressing an interest in evidence-based practice?

    C. Are the librarians available to assist nurses with evidence-based practice research?

    D. Are computers readily accessible to staff?

81. Strategies for advancing evidence-based practice in health care settings include:

    A. Skill-building workshops

    B. Evidence-based practice poster presentations

    C. Evidence-based practice rounds

    D. All of the above

82. You are considering using a new type of Foley catheter in your setting when the sales representative mentions a study that the manufacturer conducted that showed a reduction of catheter-associated infections with the use of the new device. Which type of study would be most convincing of this new product's potential value:

    A. Case study

    B. Randomized controlled trial

    C. Expert opinion

    D. Nonrandomized controlled trial

83. In an effort to reduce central line infections, you have done some research and found evidence-based guidelines that you would like to implement at your organization. Your next step would be to:

    A. Gather data regarding central line infection rates at your institution

    B. Convene a team meeting to discuss the problem and impact of central line infections

    C. Run a PDSA of the new guidelines

    D. Share what you have found with the manager

84. You have evaluated the fall rate for the previous 12 months on the medical–surgical unit where you work as a CNL. You find that your fall rate is above the national benchmark. Your next step is to:

    A. Implement a new fall prevention tool

    B. Review the literature

    C. Review current hospital policy and find out what fall prevention strategies are currently being used on the unit

    D. Assemble a team from the unit to brainstorm ideas to reduce the fall rate

85. You have reviewed the most recent pressure ulcer prevalence data for your unit. Although your unit's pressure ulcer rates are below national benchmarks, they have been steadily climbing over the past year. Your next step should be to:

    A. Make sure you assess all patients' skin daily

    B. Schedule brief in-services for the staff on the unit to review the pressure ulcer prevention policy and strategies

    C. Evaluate the pressure ulcer prevention policy

    D. Assess the bed surface on your unit

86. The manager of the medical unit where you work has just shared some data with you. She is concerned because the 30-day readmission rate for COPD patients is 15%. Your next step should be to:

    A. Schedule a meeting with the staff to discuss the problem

    B. Compare your hospital's 30-day readmission rate with other like hospitals on the CMS website

    C. Perform a literature review in preparation for making changes to the current COPD pathway at your hospital

    D. Monitor the data over the next 6 months to see if there really is a problem

87. You have done some research and found a new fall prevention tool that you would like to trial on your unit. The tool was recently developed and tested at a large city hospital with a population of open heart patients. You are not sure that this tool can be effectively implemented in your small community hospital. You are questioning the tool's:

    A. Relative risk

    B. External validity

    C. Transportability

    D. Causal association

88. A patient who has been diagnosed with colon cancer remarks that since his diagnosis, many people he knows have mentioned someone they know who has colon cancer. Most of these people live nearby. The patient asks you if colon cancer rates in the area have been increasing recently. The patient is asking about what type of measure:

    A. Incidence

    B. Prevalence

    C. Mortality

    D. Correlation

89. Your hospital has just completed a study comparing outcomes in rehospitalization rates for CHF patients who either received predischarge teaching from an APRN with those who received predischarge teaching from an RN. In the analysis of data, what resulting p-value would indicate that the intervention had a significant result?

    A. $<.05$

    B. <0.8

    C. $<.10$

    D. $<.22$

90. You are trying to reduce admission time to your unit from the emergency department. You have completed several PDSA cycles and have reduced the time by 21 minutes. But in the most recent PDSA, the time actually increased by 6 minutes. What stage of the PDSA cycle should the team go to in order to plan the next steps?

    A. Act

    B. Plan

C. Do

D. Study

91. A patient admitted to the hospital in hypertensive crisis is now receiving care at what level of prevention:

    A. Primary

    B. Secondary

    C. Tertiary

    D. None of these

92. Vaccinations are considered what level of prevention:

    A. Primary

    B. Secondary

    C. Tertiary

    D. None of these

93. Patient satisfaction scores on your unit have declined over the last quarter. There are several new nurses on the unit. You suspect that the novice nurses may be contributing to this decline in satisfaction scores. What would be a good strategy to address the issue?

    A. Schedule a group education session with the new nurses to discuss patient satisfaction

    B. Have the novice nurse shadow an experienced nurse for the day

    C. While doing patient rounds, apologize for the number of new nurses on the unit

    D. Hang signs around the unit reminding staff that patient satisfaction is the goal

94. In your role as a CNL, you have implemented some practice changes on your unit that have resulted in an overall reduced LOS for the pneumonia patients. The cost savings will be reflected in which budget:

    A. Operating budget

    B. Capital budget

    C. Cash-flow budget

    D. Long-term budget

95. The manager on the unit where you work really encourages the staff to learn and grow professionally as individuals and as a group. Several of the staff have earned advanced degrees and moved onto other roles in the hospital. Her goals always seem to be aligned with the organization's vision. This is what type of leadership style:

    A. Charismatic leadership

    B. Relational leadership

    C. Transformational leadership

    D. Transactional leadership

96. The type of care delivery system where the nurse assumes 24-hour responsibility for patient care from admission through discharge is known as:

    A. Primary nursing

    B. Functional nursing

    C. Case management

    D. Total patient care

97. Medicaid covers which population:

    A. Employed

    B. Underinsured

    C. Unemployed

    D. Poor and disabled

98. Currently Medicare is moving from a fee-for-service model to a:

    A. Managed care model

    B. Pay-for-performance model

    C. Private insurance model

    D. Advantage care model

99. Which most demonstrates advocacy toward a patient?

    A. Led interdisciplinary rounds on a group of patients

    B. Consulted a diabetic instructor for a patient who was found to have an HgB A1C of 13.1

    C. Met with the trauma team of physicians to update patient plans of care

    D. Conducted an in-service with the nursing staff on how to reduce falls for the unit

100. To be culturally competent as a clinical nurse leader is best found to be an example of which form of nursing leadership?

    A. Lateral integration of care services

    B. Horizontal leadership

    C. Advocacy

    D. Vertical leadership

101. Which clinical nurse leader role from the White Paper best describes advocacy?

    A. Delegating and managing the care team

    B. Using appropriate teaching strategies when teaching clients

    C. Making sure that patients and families are well informed

    D. Using information to achieve the best outcomes for patients

102. Which of the following is a demonstration of how the CNL can be an effective use of self through routine presence?

    A. Develops a therapeutic alliance

    B. Uses the most up-to-date technology

    C. Monitors the environment

    D. Provides a comprehensive health assessment

103. In what way can the CNL serve as an advocate for the patient through other nurses?

    A. Delegate to other members of the profession

    B. Serve as an advocate for the profession of nursing

    C. Advocate for the staff to have better hours

    D. Research best practice methods for your unit

104. Which method of payment accounts for only 5% of the U.S. population?

    A. Out-of-pocket payments

    B. Employment-based private insurance

    C. Government financing

    D. Individual private insurance

105. What is considered to be the highest form of knowledge worker?

    A. Data gatherer

    B. Knowledge builder

    C. Knowledge user

    D. Information user

106. Which level depicts a nurse with basic computer technology skills?

    A. Informatics innovator

    B. Experienced nurse

    C. Beginning nurse

    D. Informatics nurse specialist

107. Which is *not* considered an activity of daily living necessary for coverage by insurance?

    A. Bathing

    B. Dressing

    C. Taking medications

    D. Going to the park

108. Which group represents the single largest health profession in the United States?

    A. Registered nurses

    B. Physicians

    C. Nursing assistants

    D. Clinical case managers

109. B.F. is a 52-year-old female recently placed with palliative care. She is transferred to another unit with a specific palliative care section. How is this demonstrative of advocacy?

    A. Works between the patients and the health care team to deliver care

    B. Ensures that the system meets the needs of the population

    C. Advocates for the professional nurse

    D. Applies ethics toward patient care

110. All of the following are found to be an effective use of self except?

    A. Managing group processes

    B. Communicating with other disciplines

    C. Dictating to other staff

    D. Negotiating

111. While admitting a patient to the unit after a car accident, the patient informs you that she has been off her psych meds Seroquel and Celexa due to the cost and no longer has a doctor. As an advocate you would talk with the physician in hopes of obtaining what two consults?

    A. Medicine and clinical case manager

    B. Psychiatry and social worker

    C. Clinical case manager and social worker

    D. Medicine and psychiatry

112. The CNL is performing rounds with the physician team on a patient that has a chest tube placed for a collapsed lung. Which is a priority in telling the medical team first?

    A. The patient has continued pain where the chest tube was placed

    B. There is no diet ordered for this patient

    C. The patient's incentive spirometer results decreased from 1,500 to 750

    D. The patient complains of a sore throat

113. Which of these actions can a clinical nurse leader take to help protect a patient admitted for suicide?

    A. Call to have a screen placed on the window

    B. Call dietary to have only plastic utensils delivered on meal trays

    C. Move the patient close to the nursing desk for more frequent monitoring

    D. Order a psych consult

114. A patient is admitted to the unit postoperative fixation of the femur. What is a priority for the clinical nurse leader?

    A. Make sure a diet is ordered post-op

    B. Make sure the physician addressed or filled out the venous thrombosis embolism or VTE sheet with type and time of anticoagulation

    C. Make sure the family in the waiting room knows where the patient is

    D. Place the phone near the patient

115. C.W. is a 92-year-old male who is a do-not-resuscitate (DNR). There is no family to visit this patient, and the patient's status has declined over the past 24 hours. The patient's breathing is labored and the physician tells the staff there is nothing else to do. What is an effective use of the CNL?

    A. Spend time talking with staff on their views of the dying process

    B. Call bed management and let them know there will be a bed available soon for a postoperative patient

    C. Consult pastoral care to come with the patient

    D. Call dietary and tell them to stop bringing the patient food

116. A Korean patient is admitted who speaks little English. An example of culturally competent care is:

    A. Finding a nurse who speaks some Korean

    B. Transferring that patient to a floor that has a Korean-speaking secretary

    C. Calling the patient's family to see if they speak any English

    D. Obtaining a Korean translator

117. What part of the interdisciplinary team is most important postoperative day 1 from a knee replacement?

    A. Physical therapy

    B. Speech therapy

    C. Dietary

    D. Financial counselor

118. M.L. is a 42-year-old female admitted for domestic violence and being shot by her husband. Which is a priority at this time?

    A. Inform the social worker of the situation

    B. Place the patient under an alias name with her permission

    C. Inform the police

    D. Call the domestic violence nurse

119. An example of true advocacy is:

    A. Telling dietary staff if the patient has any concerns with her food

    B. Calling a patient's family to give them updates on a patient's health

    C. Establishing goals to promote patient health

    D. Performing handoff communication at change of shift

120. As a member of the interdisciplinary team, the CNL is effective in all the following except:

    A. Maintaining and updating the plan of care

    B. Collaborating with other members of the team for the care delivery

    C. Delegating to other staff

    D. Taking charge of all patient care

121. While admitting a patient for COPD, a nurse notices the patient has had two other admissions this month for the same diagnosis and is homeless. A key part of this admission is:

    A. Consult a social worker on admission

    B. Notify the physician

    C. Consult a clinical case manager upon discharge

    D. Consult financial counseling

122. D.M. is admitted for a hip fracture, a fall from standing. As a clinical nurse leader, you would know such a fracture obtained this way is best found from what?

    A. Osteomyelitis

    B. Osteoporosis

    C. Anemia

    D. Rheumatoid arthritis

123. B.L. is a 91-year-old male who was transferred to a skilled nursing facility from an acute care hospital. Upon transfer, the patient's Lasix for CHF was not transferred with the patient. Once the medication error is found and re-started, it is the CNL's job to:

    A. Notify the hospital of the error

    B. Notify the skilled nursing facility of the error

    C. Go back through all pathways and find where the error in this transfer process occurred

    D. Notify the family

124. A new graduate RN who recently got out of orientation approaches you, the clinical nurse leader (CNL). One of her patient's physicians wrote an order to place an NG tube. The RN has not done this since nursing school and asks for your help. How do you respond?

    A. Tell her to ask the charge nurse, as this is not one of your CNL roles and you really do not have time at the moment

    B. Direct her to get the policy and procedure guidelines, review it, assemble the needed supplies, and then you will review it with her and assist her with placing the NG tube

    C. Direct her to review the policy and procedure guidelines, assemble the needed supplies, and ask an available LPN to assist her with placing it

    D. Review the order, gather the needed supplies, and have her watch you place the NG tube, as she has not done it before as an RN

125. As you, the CNL, are reviewing one of your patient's charts, you notice that he recently tested positive for methicillin-resistant *Staphylococcus aureus* (MRSA) in his open wound. He has been in the hospital for 2 days, and as far as you can tell, this result has not been addressed. You bring the result to the attention of the primary nurse, who says that the night shift nurse told her about that, but no one has had a chance to "deal with it" since each nurse has six or seven patients. How do you respond?

    A. Tell the nurse you understand how busy she is, and to please make it a priority to "deal with" as soon as possible for patient safety

    B. Tell the nurse you understand how busy she is, and offer to call the physician yourself as well as place the patient on contact precautions

    C. Ensure the nurse knows why this is a priority, especially since she does have so many other patients, and help her to make time to notify the physician as well as immediately place the patient on contact precautions

D. Notify the charge nurse so that he may either take the needed steps himself or delegate it to another available nurse

126. You are the CNL on a busy high-risk antepartum unit. One of the nurses comes to you because she is "sick of dealing with a noncompliant patient." The nurse tells you the patient is refusing all of her treatments, including fetal monitoring, vital signs, and insulin administration, and she cannot bear to take care of the patient who does not even care about her baby. What do you do?

A. Tell the nurse you understand how she feels, but as the nurse, she is going to have to deal with it, at least until the end of her shift. All patients deserve excellent nursing care, even difficult, noncompliant patients

B. Ask the nurse what has happened between her and the patient, as she was not acting like that previously

C. Take the issue to the charge nurse and have the nurse's assignment changed so that another nurse may take care of this patient

D. Go into the patient's room and ask her if you may talk. Sit down with the patient and try to understand what is going on and why she is refusing all of her treatments

127. One of your patients, a widow, is reaching end of life. The physician has adamantly suggested to the patient's family to plan for death and to make the decision to remove life support, as he feels it is futile at this point and most likely causing more agony to the patient. The patient has three children, and they cannot agree on a decision. The oldest daughter feels that they should abide by the doctor, as he knows best. The middle child does not agree with "killing" his mother. The youngest child just wants to be with her mother and cannot make a decision. You decide the best thing to do now is hold a patient-care conference. Whom do you invite?

A. The family, the team of physicians, the primary nurse, the case manager, the chaplain, an ethics committee member, and the social worker

B. The family, the team of physicians, the primary nurse, the nurse manager, the chaplain, the respiratory therapist, and the nutritionist

C. The team of physicians, the primary nurse, the nurse manager, the case manager, the chaplain, an ethics committee member, and the social worker

D. The team of physicians, the primary nurse, the chaplain, the respiratory therapist, and the nutritionist

128. Nurse Alice, whom you work with on a busy antepartum unit, comes to you one Monday morning because she does not agree with one of her patient's medical management. The patient, who is $35\frac{5}{7}$ weeks' gestation, has been NPO (nothing by mouth) since Friday at midnight. She was supposed to have a repeat cesarean section Friday morning for mild preeclampsia and has demonstrated positive lung maturity via an amniocentesis. However, the labor and delivery unit is extremely busy and short staffed due to an outbreak of influenza. The patient is getting upset because she was told she was going

to have her baby on Friday and is "sick of being pregnant and is starving." Alice says she talked to the physician on Sunday about it and was told that the patient just needs to be patient. You, the CNL, take these next steps:

A. Tell Alice you understand how she feels, but since she already spoke with the physician, the team needs to work together and respect the physician's order. You talk with the patient and explain why she needs to continue to be NPO, and hopefully it will not be much longer

B. Call the labor and delivery charge nurse to discuss this patient and see when she will be able to get delivered. You are told it will be this evening at the earliest, so you call the physician and get a diet ordered for this morning, and return to NPO status after lunch with IV fluids to start when NPO. You share this plan with Alice and the patient

C. Call the labor and delivery charge nurse and demand that this patient be delivered this morning, as she is preeclamptic and has been waiting since Friday

D. Find out that the patient most likely will not be delivered today, and if so it will be late tonight. You allow the patient to eat breakfast and a light, early lunch, returning to NPO afterward. Alice and the patient agree with and are happy about this plan of care

129. You are the CNL on a busy medical–surgical unit. One of your patients, Mr. Thompson, a Type 2 diabetic, has been on your unit for 5 days following a right foot amputation due to necrosis. He has been on IV antibiotics and has now been afebrile for 24 hours. Mr. Thompson, 67 years old, lives alone, but his son lives two miles away and says he will be able to check on his dad at least daily once he is discharged home. In preparation for discharge, you realize Mr. Thompson will need someone to assist him with his dressing changes and to check his vital signs for several days. You think he will also need outpatient physical therapy. You discuss with the physician your thoughts on discharging Mr. Thompson home with home health. The physician agrees with your plan of care, so you consult the case manager to set up home health and outpatient physical therapy. You also consult with the physical therapist for recommendations on home needs. You assist with making follow-up appointments for Mr. Thompson. Mr. Thompson is able to be discharged home the next day. This is an example of which CNL role?

A. Lateral integration of care

B. Risk anticipation

C. Management and use of client-care and information technology

D. Clinical decision making

130. Because you are the CNL on a postsurgical unit, staff are regularly bringing you new ideas and questions about current treatment regimens. Today two nurses come to you with conflicting ideas. One nurse, Rachel, says that she will not allow her patients to have anything PO except for clear liquids postsurgery until they are passing flatus. She says that she has worked on this unit for 20 years and that the more experienced doctors support this thought.

Tom, a newer nurse of 2 years, says he was taught that patients may eat and drink whatever they want post-op as long as they have positive bowel sounds and are not nauseous. They want to know "who is right." In response, you:

A. Tell them they are both right, depending on the patient, and it is up to the physician's orders

B. Tell them that is a great question, and instruct them to both do research on the topic, bring it back to you, and you will help them take their information forward for a potential practice change

C. Thank them for bringing up such an important question, and tell them you do not know the answer. Guide them to discuss this with the physicians

D. Assist them in researching this topic in research and evidence-based articles, and evaluate the information. Bring your findings to the unit staff and physicians and come to an agreement on the best practice

131. You are the CNL on a busy medical unit. You get a new patient, Mrs. Garcia, admitted through the emergency department (ED) for abdominal pain. Mrs. Garcia is a 37-year-old Spanish-speaking woman. She has her 12-year-old son with her, who has been translating for the medical staff in the ED. Mrs. Garcia is clearly in a lot of pain, but you cannot give her any pain medications until she is admitted into the system. Your next steps are to:

A. Allow the son to translate enough to get Mrs. Garcia admitted so that you may give her some pain medications and then get an interpreter to complete her admission history

B. Ask Mrs. Garcia, through her son, if it is okay with her to use her son as the interpreter. You explain to her this will expedite her pain relief and she agrees

C. Request an interpreter to come as soon as possible and tell Mrs. Garcia through her son that you will make her comfortable as soon as possible. Notify the primary RN who will be caring for her

D. Explain to Mrs. Garcia that you are unable to give her medicine until she is admitted and that you need an interpreter to admit her. You will give her medicine as soon as possible. You stay with Mrs. Garcia until the interpreter gets there, and try to help relieve her pain with other nonpharmaceutical therapies

132. You, the CNL, work on an infectious disease unit in the hospital. Your patients tend to have long lengths of stays, sometimes weeks to months. During your 5Ps assessment, you discovered that the nursing staff is not satisfied with hand-off communication. They feel like important information is often left out of report. As a leader of this team, the most appropriate next step would be to:

A. Create a new process based on evidence and implement it

B. Assess the current communication handoff process

C. Ask the nursing staff what they think would be the best way to give report

D. Bring this issue up at the next staff meeting

133. You, the CNL, are putting an interdisciplinary group together to make improvements to your high falls rate. You are seeking members to be on this

team. Carly, an RN, volunteers to be on this team. You and Carly have had many differences in the past and because of personality conflicts have not been able to work well together historically. What should you do?

A. Thank Carly for volunteering, but politely tell her you will not be needing her for this particular team

B. Allow Carly to be part of the team—your personal issues should not affect this group's progress

C. Invite Carly to be part of the team, but do not give her any major responsibilities

D. Tell Carly that you think it is best if the two of you just avoid each other

134. One morning as you, the CNL, are walking into the nurses' lounge, you hear a lot of talk about a nurse who has called out sick that day. The nurses are griping about how this nurse *always* calls out, especially on Fridays. The best response is to:

A. Sympathize with your team, saying you have no idea how she does not get in trouble or fired. This kind of behavior should not be tolerated

B. Tell the nurses to stop talking about one of their teammates, especially in front of a new employee

C. Listen to what the nurses are saying, and notify the manager to address it

D. Listen to what the nurses have to say, and then address that it is not our business to discuss someone else's personal life. That nurse's sick days and disciplinary action are up to that nurse and the manager. Ensure they have adequate staffing to make up for the sick call/help to adjust assignments

135. You are the CNL on a postpartum unit. You have noticed that lately you have had an increased number of patients readmitted with wound infections. You know that the most appropriate next step is to:

A. Perform a failure mode and effects analysis

B. Ask the doctors why their patients are getting so many infections lately

C. Perform a root cause analysis

D. Consult the wound-ostomy care nurses

136. As the CNL on a medical–surgical unit, you are asked to participate in a root cause analysis of a group of sentinel events that have occurred recently throughout the hospital. Your team determines that a lack of effective communication in emergent situations is the root problem. Now what?

A. Lead the team in researching evidence-based practice improvements to implement a better way of communicating during emergencies

B. Submit your findings to the administration that assigned you this task

C. Share the findings with the units that had these sentinel events and instruct them to come up with better, research-based communication techniques

D. Take the findings directly to the individuals involved in the sentinel events and show them what they need to improve to prevent these adverse outcomes

137. A medical equipment representative approaches you to incorporate his new product into your unit supplies. He tells you that this new device has been proven to be the best device in its arena to prevent DVTs. Preventing DVTs is one of your goals as the CNL on this medical–surgical unit. The price is only slightly higher than the current equipment you use now, but he says the research shows you will save money in the long run by preventing more DVTs. How do you go about getting this new device?

A. Since you do not have any purchasing power as the CNL, you direct him to the director of the purchasing department

B. You have the representative speak with your manager, since your manager must approve all items purchased for your unit

C. You thank him for the information, but pass on the offer since it costs more than the equipment you currently use, and as a CNL you are only looking for cost-effective ventures

D. You perform your own research on the device and compare it with the equipment you have now. If it proves to be as good as the representative says it is, you will take it forward to administration

138. What is the best way for the CNL to analyze systems and outcome datasets to anticipate individual client risk and improve quality care?

A. Perform a root cause analysis of all postoperative patients who have been readmitted to your unit within the last year

B. Perform a failure mode and effects analysis on all congestive heart failure patients on your unit within the last year

C. Implement the Systems Theory to evaluate individual risks to each patient population on your unit

D. Utilize the Complexity Theory to make the needed changes to the defective systems

139. You work in the emergency department at a major public hospital. You have noticed that you see the same diabetic patients regularly. They are indigents and do not have primary care physicians. They never check their blood sugars at home because they do not have a glucometer, so by the time they get to the emergency department their blood sugars are well into the 300s and 400s. Usually the plan of care involves treating the blood sugars, instructing them to follow up at the clinic, and giving them a snack for the road. What would be a positive change in the plan of care from the CNL perspective?

A. Set up a program to give free glucometers to these patients who do not have one and schedule the follow-up appointment for them before they leave the emergency department, sending them home with information

B. Admit the patients to the hospital so they can get instruction on diabetes care, including diet, exercise, insulin administration, and blood glucose monitoring

C. Instruct the patients on where to purchase an inexpensive glucometer, and instruct them on the importance of checking their blood sugar regularly and making and keeping follow-up appointments

D. Incorporate diet teaching into their visit. Stress the importance of a diabetes-friendly diet, and send them home with a packet of information and a healthy snack

140. Of the following choices, what is the best way that you, the CNL, could have an environmentally positive impact?

A. Incorporate the importance of the environment into your teaching with each of your patients

B. Institute a recycling program into your hospital

C. When teaching patients and families, make sure they know how to properly dispose of their medical waste

D. Have patients start calling their physicians instead of going to their appointments to save on gas and time

141. You are caring for Mrs. Jackson, a patient with congestive heart failure, on a cardiac unit. As you are looking through Mrs. Jackson's chart, you notice her last blood pressure was 188/110, following a blood pressure of 176/106. You see an order for labetalol 20 mg IV × 1 now written on her chart. What do you do now?

A. Find the primary nurse and make sure she has given the labetalol

B. Get an order for a second dose of the labetalol, as this first dose clearly has not been effective and Mrs. Jackson's blood pressure is rising

C. Verify Mrs. Jackson's allergies and the order and ensure the medication is on the unit ready to be given

D. Get the order discontinued and make sure it has not been given

142. You are caring for Sara, a 76-year-old grandmother recovering from heart failure. You know that she is ready to go home because:

A. Her ECG is normal, her pulse oximetry is normal, and she has a supportive family to help care for her at home

B. She tells you she is ready to go home

C. You observe her ambulating in the hallway, free from dyspnea

D. She is free from dyspnea and fatigue, she has a follow-up appointment set up for the following Monday morning, and her daughter said she can drive her to the appointment

143. As the CNL, you know that one of the first steps in building a team is to:

A. Build trust

B. Assign roles to each member

C. Designate a mission of the team

D. Determine meeting times and locations

144. You are working with your team to modify the unit's budget. You know that the best way to create a budget is:

A. Looking at the previous budget's variance

B. Requesting a large capital budget

    C. Being in line with your budget goal

    D. Utilizing a case mix

145. You know that regulatory agencies' purpose is to:

    A. Stress out hospital employees

    B. Decrease fragmentation and medical errors resulting in deaths

    C. Give the public a source of standards for health care facilities

    D. Make the public feel safe and give them guidelines to follow with lawsuits

146. A new health policy is being voted on in Congress. Your professional organization supports this policy and is recruiting nurses to go to Washington, DC, to help promote their view and to have a bigger voice. You do not support this policy. Your manager wants you to go as a leader and represent your unit. What should you do?

    A. You should go, as you need to stick together with your professional organization and yield to your manager

    B. Learn more about the policy and why your organization supports it

    C. You should politely decline, as you do not agree with the policy

    D. You should go, but rally against the policy since you do not agree with it. This is America and you are exercising your freedom of speech

147. You want to do some research for a potential policy change. All of the following are excellent resources, except:

    A. Centers for Disease Control

    B. Wikipedia

    C. American Diabetes Association

    D. WebMD

148. As a CNL, what is your number one priority?

    A. Cost-effectiveness of care

    B. Improving quality of care

    C. Patient safety

    D. Decreasing fragmentation of care

149. Leah, a CNL on an obstetrical high-risk unit, looked at the evidence regarding women taking folic acid during pregnancy. Because it shows evidence to prevent neural tube defects in the fetus, she recommends this be included on the order set for antepartum patients. This is an example of which of the following:

    A. Health promotion

    B. Health literacy

    C. Qualitative review

    D. Quantitative analysis

150. Sam is a homeless 59-year-old male admitted with CHF. He arrives alone and crying. His vitals are BP = 173/96, HR = 83, O2 = 86%, and temperature = 98.9°F. During your assessment, you notice multiple bruises and lacerations.

His clothes are torn and soiled. According to Maslow's Hierarchy of Needs, what should you do first?

A. Inquire about his bruises and lacerations

B. Call the social worker regarding shelter placement

C. Ask why he is crying

D. Apply oxygen

151. Which of the following would not correlate with a major goal of Healthy People 2010?

A. Providing free clinics for underprivileged children

B. Educating a 76-year-old on smoking cessation

C. Implementing a unit to place all positive HIV patients

D. Designing a nutritious meal plan for school systems

152. Tim is a 31-year-old admitted for pneumonia. During his hospitalization, you discovered he smokes cigarettes 1 ppd. You provided handouts on smoking cessation and gave him a helpline number. At discharge you made a follow-up appointment with his PCP for his pneumonia and smoking cessation. What did you forget to do?

A. Ask

B. Advise

C. Assist

D. Arrange

153. Marie's capstone project for her CNL immersion experience focused on wound infections and readmission rates. She conducted a literature review on the best way to provide education to surgical patients, reduce surgical infections, and prevent readmissions. On the basis of literature review and evidence-based practice, she developed a protocol for this patient population. What key principle did Marie use by incorporating this protocol?

A. Team coordination

B. Risk reduction and prevention management

C. Lateral integration of care

D. Information management

154. Tim, a CNL in the clinic setting, begins seeing a lot more Hispanic patients with high blood pressure and/or diabetes and many with a lack of knowledge on nutrition. They often say someone in their family has the same problems. He knows the best way to educate them is to:

A. Set aside extra time at each appointment to focus on education

B. Set up educational posters at a local Hispanic supermarket

C. Set up a health fair with bilingual educators at a local highly populated park in a Hispanic neighborhood

D. Make up handouts to be given to patients at their appointments to take home

155. Marcia, a CNL, reviews the diet with a newly diagnosed gestational diabetic. She inquires about the patient's previous diet and habits, and after spending much time with the patient and asking questions, she discovers the patient eats a lot of fast food. She says she rarely has time to cook and has four kids who are always on the go. What should Marcia do?

    A. Look up the nutritional information on the patient's favorite fast food places and pick out good food choices together with which she can be compliant

    B. Tell her it does not really matter what she eats because she only has gestational diabetes

    C. Tell her she cannot eat fast food and give her another list of what she can eat

    D. Consult the dietician again to review her meal plan

156. A 6-year-old boy named Braden is a patient in your microsystem. He is terrified of the shots he has to get twice a day for the next 3 weeks. It is the most therapeutic medication and route for his illness. He becomes hysterical every time the medication is due and has to be held down by two people while the nurse gives the injection. They will not have three people at home to do this. Working on discharge planning, what should you do?

    A. Plan on Braden being in the hospital for the next 3 weeks to receive his injections

    B. Obtain restraints for the parents to use at home in order to give the injection

    C. Talk with the physician to prescribe a pill instead

    D. Work with the child specialist and sit down with Braden to find out what scares him about the injections

157. A CNL on an orthopedic floor notices the legs on several of the walkers are not secure. She immediately calls medical equipment to replace the walkers on the floor and puts defective stickers on the current walkers. This is an example of:

    A. Health promotion

    B. Injury prevention

    C. Health care informatics

    D. Delegation

158. Jen is an obese patient admitted with COPD and CHTN. Part of her social history is that she smokes 2 ppd. Her CNL, Erika, makes a goal for her to decrease by one cigarette a day until there are no more by August 1. This goal will not work because:

    A. There is not a measurable outcome

    B. Jen should decrease by two cigarettes a day

    C. The patient has COPD

    D. Jen should help make the goal

159. Elizabeth performed a CNL capstone project on group shift report. First she conducted a literature review and then developed new guidelines based on the research in the literature review. She measured the amount of time the report took prior to and after the change. This is an example of what type of research?

    A. Evidence-based practice

    B. Randomized control trial

    C. Cohort

    D. Ethnography

160. All of the following are components of evidence-based practice and clinical decision making except:

    A. Clinical expertise

    B. Information about patient preferences and values

    C. Research utilization

    D. Evidence from research and theories

161. Pam, a CNL on a surgical unit, posted new evidence-based guidelines on preventing constipation in post-op patients. Pam notices an experienced nurse is not following these guidelines correctly. She realizes this nurse is demonstrating what behavior?

    A. Avoidance

    B. Angry there are more changes

    C. Lack of nursing competence

    D. Lack of knowledge

162. Angela, a CNL, reviews RCTs on care for preterm labor patients. She discovers bedrest has not been proven to prolong pregnancy for preterm labor patients. This is typically ordered for all preterm labor patients at her facility. She posts her findings for the staff to review and gives an in-service to the nurses. Angela goes to the physicians to get the orders changed for her group of patients. What should Angela have done before implementing this change?

    A. Look at case studies

    B. Meet with the interdisciplinary team to discuss protocols before initiating change

    C. Meet with the nurse manager to discuss the research

    D. Look at more qualitative studies to get more information

163. A patient care nurse, Kristin, comes to you about a new idea she has to provide better patient care. You agree this is a great idea. You should:

    A. Research the latest evidence on this topic

    B. Set up a meeting with the interdisciplinary team to discuss

    C. Start implementing the change

    D. Encourage Kristin to take on this project

164. Julie, a CNL, hears that another hospital does hourly rounding and thinks this is a great idea to reduce falls on her unit. She meets with her interdisciplinary team and they decide to try this on their unit. She informs the rest of the staff and makes a start date. What did Julie forget to do?

    A. Look at the latest evidence/literature review

    B. Ask her nurse manager

    C. Ask other units if they do hourly rounding

    D. Get data from the other hospital

165. According to the PICOT method to make a search for your clinical question, the "P" stands for:

    A. Processes

    B. Population

    C. Patterns

    D. Practice

166. Carey, a CNL, thinks utilizing volunteers in a microsystem will benefit the staff and the patients. She performs a literature review and does not find much literature evaluating volunteers being effective in a health care setting. She decides to go ahead and implement a volunteer program and collects data to see whether this is an effective change. Should Carey have implemented this?

    A. No, there was no evidence volunteers would be beneficial

    B. No, she should have waited until there were data on this topic

    C. Yes, if there is no literature on a topic, data should be collected to evaluate the change to see whether it is effective

    D. Yes, it is always good to try something new

167. You are trying to get literature on using music to relieve pain. One research article uses methods you forget how to interpret. You should:

    A. Not use this article

    B. Google the methods to try and figure it out

    C. Look at the conclusion and just use that information

    D. Ask a mentor to assist you, so you understand the data

168. What is the first essential key to implementing a change in a microsystem?

    A. A clear vision of what outcomes are to be accomplished

    B. A strategic plan

    C. Persistence on the change implementation to be successful

    D. Belief the change will be a success

169. Cassidy, a CNL at an outpatient setting, starts seeing an increase of Japanese patients. This is a culture she does not know much about and does not have very much educational materials to give to patients in this language. She goes online to valid websites and learns more about their culture and health care practices. She also discovers a site within her health care system that

translates information and has handouts in 12 different languages. Cassidy demonstrated knowledge of:

A. Team coordination

B. Injury reduction

C. Health care informatics

D. Health care policy

170. Many handouts are given to all the patients on admission to the hospital. The CNL notices many patients leave them or throw them away. She decides to make binders for all the rooms with laminated copies of the information and lets each patient know they can get a copy to take home if wanted. This CNL exhibited what concept?

A. Health care informatics

B. Fiscal responsibility

C. Team coordination

D. Health promotion

171. Chloe, a CNL, walks into a patient's room and notices she has labored respirations and is pale. She immediately takes her vitals and calls the patient care nurse. Her vitals are BP = 183/101, HR = 121, R = 28, T = 98.1, O_2 = 90%. What should Chloe do?

A. Call the doctor

B. Lay the patient down and recheck the VS in 30 minutes

C. Give labetalol 20 mg IVP

D. Instruct the patient care nurse to call the doctor

172. A 5Ps assessment was completed by each CNL in the hospital. As a CNL, you know this is an assessment of the:

A. Microsystem

B. Mesosystem

C. Macrosystem

D. Health care system

173. A patient asks the CNL about the regulations on abortion in North Carolina. What should the CNL do?

A. Tell the patient you cannot answer that because it is an ethical situation

B. Let the doctor know the patient is asking about abortion

C. Inform the patient care nurse

D. Look up the regulations in North Carolina and share them with the patient

174. A nurse approaches you and expresses her knowledge deficit regarding the difference between signs and symptoms of left- and right-sided heart failure. You explain the physiology between the two types of heart failure and identify which of the following as a primary symptom of right-sided heart failure?

A. Shortness of breath on exertion

B. Heart murmur and distended veins

    C. Peripheral edema

    D. Cool extremities and weak peripheral pulses

175. As a CNL you know that the most important nursing intervention to monitor a patient with CHF includes which of the following?

    A. Assessing the patient's knowledge of the disease

    B. Encouraging coughing and deep breathing

    C. Encouraging frequent ambulation

    D. Monitoring fluid intake and output

176. A nurse notifies you that her patient is complaining of chest pain. As you enter the room, the patient becomes unresponsive. Upon verification that a pulse is absent, the cardiac monitor reveals the patient is in ventricular fibrillation. The nurse begins CPR. As a CNL, you anticipate the need for which treatment next?

    A. Amiodarone (Cordarone)

    B. Labetolol (Normodyne)

    C. Defibrillation

    D. Cardiac catheterization

177. Your patient was recently diagnosed with non–small-cell cancer to the lung. Postradiation she reports to the nurse that she has a sore throat. The nurse approaches you indicating that he is unaware of what to do. You explain to the nurse that mucositis is a common side effect for patients receiving radiation treatment. What will you instruct the nurse to do next?

    A. Assess the patient's oral mucosa for swelling and redness with ulcerations

    B. Call the physician and obtain an order for an antiseptic mouthwash

    C. Instruct the patient to rinse her mouth before and after meals with a solution of salt and sodium bicarbonate

    D. Use a soft-bristled toothbrush to clean her teeth and tongue

178. You are providing discharge instructions to a young patient with sickle cell anemia. What statement made by the patient would concern you most for the potential of this patient readmitting to the hospital?

    A. "I am scared about my pain being kept under control"

    B. "I will need to find someone to take me to my hematology follow-up appointment"

    C. "My mother helps me manage my pain medicine"

    D. "I get tired throughout the day and often have to take naps"

179. As a CNL you are educating a patient with type 1 diabetes mellitus about the potential advantages of an insulin pump. The patient has been frequently readmitted with labile blood sugars although she has followed her prescribed insulin regimen of Lantus and Humalog. What is most important to emphasize on the benefits of an insulin pump?

    A. An insulin pump allows you to decrease the number of injections throughout the day

B. An insulin pump will provide intermittent doses of insulin in response to the patient's blood sugar

C. An insulin pump has the capability to read your blood sugars throughout the patient's waking hours

D. An insulin pump provides continuous doses of insulin around the clock as a basal rate that can be adjusted

180. You are caring for a patient who has suffered a cerebrovascular accident. The patient's daughter approaches you expressing that the patient has been frequently crying during her visits. What would be the best explanation to help the daughter cope with her mother's emotions?

A. "I will call the doctor and get medication ordered for depression"

B. "Emotional responses may be unpredictable after a stroke"

C. "Your mother is dealing with her hospitalization and diagnosis appropriately"

D. "Your mother may need an increased amount of family support during this difficult time"

181. A nurse has called you into a room with a patient who is newly admitted to your unit with a diagnosis of urinary tract infection. The patient is 86 years old, and his vital signs reveal a temperature of 97.8°C, respiratory rate of 24, heart rate of 115, and blood pressure of 75/48. The nurse has called the doctor and has received orders to bolus that patient with IVF that the patient is currently receiving. The patient is becoming increasingly confused. What is the *most appropriate* response to delegate to the nurse while you stay with the patient?

A. Recheck the vital signs in 15 minutes to ensure the blood pressure is rising

B. Call the patient's family to obtain a full medical history

C. Ask the nurse to call the physician and notify him of the need to evaluate the patient for a higher level of care

D. Give the patient a prn dose of Ativan to help with the patient's confusion

182. You are working in a unit that has recently seen an influx of patients with substance-related disorders. The nurses on the unit are complaining that frequently these patients are "drug seeking" and often signing out against medical advice in order to receive drugs elsewhere. What is an intervention that a CNL may implement to improve the treatment for this patient population?

A. Educate the staff on not labeling the patients as "drug seekers" because they often require higher doses of pain medications to achieve an acceptable level of comfort

B. Provide an in-service to the staff about patients' withdrawal symptoms

C. Follow each patient that comes in with a diagnosis of a substance-related disorder in order to identify trends in mistreatment

  D. Research on whether the hospital uses an evidence-based tool that may help with the assessment of patients for alcohol addiction and/or withdrawal

183. You are reviewing a patient's morning laboratory values. The patient's hemoglobin has dropped from 12.5 to 7.3. The nurse has called the physician and received orders for two units of packed red blood cells to be transfused. The patient was admitted for diabetic ketoacidosis. What is the next step you should perform?

  A. Research whether the patient has ever had a history of any anemia or gastrointestinal bleeding

  B. Assess the patient for any signs and/or symptoms of bleeding

  C. Call the physician and inform him to redraw the labs

  D. Review the rest of the patient's laboratory values

184. You are helping a new nurse with the admission of a patient with the diagnosis of COPD exacerbation. You explain the differences between the two types of COPD. Together you review the findings that you would expect to assess on a patient with chronic bronchitis versus emphysema. Which of the following would not be an expected finding on a patient with chronic bronchitis?

  A. Wheezing and bronchi upon lung field auscultation

  B. Dry cough with little sputum production

  C. Cyanotic

  D. Hypercapnia and respiratory acidosis

185. Which of the following is an example of knowledge management?

  A. Forming a multidisciplinary team to evaluate your patient's plan of care

  B. Provide counseling for patients and families on smoking cessation

  C. Presenting to your unit's staff a comparison of your institution and unit fall rates against national benchmarks

  D. Participating in a community event that focuses on cholesterol screening

186. Your unit has recently been participating in a study to evaluate the use of new, more affordable gloves. You have noticed that many of the nurses are complaining that the gloves are cheap and tearing easily. You present this to your unit manager and discuss the risk of infection. What is this an example of?

  A. Patient advocacy

  B. Evidence-based practice

  C. Team coordination

  D. Knowledge management

187. Your unit has recently had an increase in fall rates. When you compare what other units in your department are doing, you identify that each unit is using a different fall risk assessment tool. You research each tool and identify which one has the strongest evidence-based research in preventing patient falls. This tool is later standardized throughout the hospital. What is this an example of?

    A. Applying tools for risk analysis

    B. Patient advocacy

    C. Gathering, analyzing, and synthesizing data related to risk reduction and patient safety

    D. Demonstrating accountability for the delivery of high-quality care

188. As the CNL, you have identified that postsurgical pneumonia has been a frequent occurrence within your unit. Your manager approaches you and identifies that each occurrence of postsurgical pneumonia costs the unit $5,000. You develop a respiratory program that includes frequent incentive spirometer use, ambulation at least three times a day, if warranted, and frequent mouth care. You are able to reduce the unit's occurrences of postsurgical pneumonia by 75%. What is this an example of?

    A. Conceptual analysis and implementation of the CNL role

    B. Knowledge management

    C. Effective use of self

    D. Horizontal leadership

189. You have noticed that on your unit many elderly patients are unable to return home with their family members due to loss/decrease of their functional abilities. You research and implement a tool that scores a patient's functional ability when they enter the hospital and once upon discharge. You use these data to share with staff and create ideas to improve maintenance of an elderly patient's functional ability. What is this an example of?

    A. Interpreting and using quantitative data

    B. Interpreting and using qualitative data

    C. Risk analysis

    D. Using evidence to identify and modify interventions to meet specific client needs

190. You are providing discharge education to a patient who was diagnosed with Parkinson's disease. The patient is being discharged with a home health nurse and physical therapist. Which of the following statements made by the patient's wife identifies a need for more education?

    A. "I am afraid my husband will fall"

    B. "I am uncertain that I will be able to provide the right care for my husband"

    C. "My husband enjoys watching TV for long periods of time"

    D. "I may ask my daughter to stay with us for the next couple of weeks"

191. You are discharging a young patient diagnosed with a urinary tract infection. To help prevent future urinary tract infections, you instruct the patient to do the following:

    A. Urinate forcefully to clear bacteria from the tract

    B. Urinate before sexual intercourse to limit transmission

    C. Wear cotton underwear to prevent moisture

    D. Pat dry after urinating to prevent infection

192. Which of the following is an example of transcultural nursing?

    A. Maintaining eye contact with an Asian family

    B. Reporting to the physician that you are unsure your American Indian patient understands his plan of care because he stares at the floor when you talk to him

    C. A male nurse giving his Hispanic female patient a hug

    D. Alerting the physician to write for a pork-free diet for your Islamic patient

193. You are caring for a patient with CHF. He has just completed a transfusion of 2u of PRBCs. Upon entering the room, he complains of shortness of breath. His O_2 saturations are 85% on 2 L and he is breathing 28 respirations a minute. What drug do you anticipate administering?

    A. Nitroglycerin SL

    B. Lasix IV

    C. Albuterol HHN

    D. Prednisone PO

194. Your manager has approached you regarding her need to decrease the unit's budget. Which of the following would have the greatest impact on decreasing the unit's budget?

    A. Exploring why staff is not leaving on time and creating overtime

    B. Eliminating unused supplies on the unit

    C. Increasing nurse to patient ratio

    D. Deciding not to update the unit's computers

195. Which accrediting body is an independent, nonprofit organization that works outside of government to provide unbiased and authoritative advice to decision makers and the public?

    A. Centers for Medicare and Medicaid Services (CMS)

    B. Institute of Medicine (IOM)

    C. Institute for Safe Medication Practices (ISMP)

    D. Division of Health Service Regulation (DHSR)

196. Which of the following is not part of the PDSA change model?

    A. Plan

    B. Assess

    C. Do

    D. Study

197. You have recently encountered many people in your community who have been sick from drinking park water. As a CNL, which of the following actions would have the greatest impact for your community?

    A. Inform your local news station

    B. Participate in a petition to send to legislators

    C. Research whether this has become a national problem

D. Do nothing

198. Which accreditation body is responsible for overseeing medical, mental health, and adult care facilities; emergency medical services; and local jails?

    A. Institute of Medicine (IOM)

    B. The Joint Commission (TJC)

    C. Division of Health Service Regulation (DHSR)

    D. Centers for Medicare and Medicaid Services (CMS)

199. A 65-year-old man with a history of chest palpitations was seen by his cardiologist for new onset palpitations and put on a beta blocker and told to return for a follow-up in 1 week after taking a stress test. The beta blocker's action includes:

    A. Increasing the consistency of the heart rate

    B. Decreasing the ability of the heart muscle to contract

    C. Decreasing the chance of dysrythmia

    D. Increasing contractility and decreasing heart rate

200. When assessing a patient for a diagnosis of pneumonia, it is more difficult to make a proper diagnosis in the absence of the following symptom:

    A. Cough

    B. Cyanosis

    C. Tachycardia

    D. Bradycardia

201. In order to complete a thorough assessment of a 55-year-old male beginning an exercise program, the CNL should include the following in the instructions:

    A. Begin an exercise program of a minimum of 60 minutes of vigorous exercise each day

    B. Keep a daily written log of exercise and include the type of exercise, time of exercise, and the intensity of the exercise

    C. Avoid drinking more than 8 oz of water per day when exercising

    D. Side effects are common when beginning exercising and should be ignored

202. An 88-year-old lady suffers a stroke in the nursing home and develops pneumonia and is transferred to the hospital. She continues to decline, is having trouble breathing, and becomes unconscious with little hope of recovery or quality of life. She has no family and no health care proxy, living will, or directions about whether she wants to be intubated or not. The physician wants to intubate the patient. The staff nurse strongly believes the patient would not want to be intubated, as she had cared for the lady before she became unconscious. What is the BEST thing for the CNL to do first:

    A. Take a vote among the staff nurses

    B. Call for an ethics consultation

C. Ask the social worker to make a recommendation or decision

D. Do a literature review on quality of life of elderly patients with pneumonia

Case Study 1

You are a CNL in a critical care unit. You have recently been asked to join a task force to address specific clinical outcomes. The first priority of the group is to address critically ill patients intubated for more than 24 hours who are at high risk of developing ventilator-associated pneumonia (VAP). Other risk factors for VAP include decreased level of consciousness, supine positioning with a head of bed less than 30°, gastric distension, trauma, and a COPD diagnosis.

1. Ventilator-associated pneumonia (VAP) in mechanically ventilated patients is a complication that can be prevented. Your ICU has an opportunity to improve. Choose the best response that illustrates the incidence of VAP in your unit.

   A. Trend analysis of ICU-acquired pneumonia for the last fiscal year

   B. Average length of stay in the ICU

   C. The latest research

   D. All of the above

2. Reviewing and evaluating the current patient care guidelines and protocols for all intubated patients demonstrates which CNL role function:

   A. Member of the profession

   B. Team manager

   C. Advocate

   D. Systems analyst

3. Understanding of the ICU as a clinical microsystem includes an exploration of its:

   A. Processes, patients, and paperwork

   B. Paperwork, purpose, and professionals

   C. Professionals, patterns, and paperwork

   D. Purpose, patients, processes, patterns, and professionals

4. Process mapping is a method of creating a diagram showing the steps and the flow of the intubated patient's care process. Flowcharting:

   A. Identifies unwanted variation, rework, and waste

   B. Engages the interdisciplinary team

   C. Replaces words with a picture

   D. All of the above

5. The standard of care for all intubated patients now includes a 30° head of bed position and oral care with chlorhexidine every 4 hours. After two quarters of practice, the incidence of VAP can be best trended using:

A. Root cause analysis

B. An audit by the nurse manager

C. A run chart

D. A pie chart

Case Study 2

Jenny, an 18-year-old, was admitted through the ED to your general medical unit during the night. Her admitting diagnosis is asthma exacerbation. Six months ago she was transferred from receiving care at the hospital pediatric clinic to the adult women's health clinic. This is her second admission in 3 months.

1. What are important components of your initial nursing assessment?

   A. Her ED course of treatment, medication history, living situation

   B. Her medication history, lab work, living situation

   C. Medications, labs, family, clinic appointment history, smoking history

   D. Her ED course of treatment, present vital signs, medication history, living situation, social history, smoking status

2. Jenny's clinic history shows a history of appointment noncompliance and failure to fill her prescriptions. When Jenny does take her medication, she tells you that she uses a steroidal inhaler once or twice a day if she feels she needs it. She does not take a rescue inhaler (bronchodilator) unless she has very bad wheezing because she complains it makes her "jittery." You recognize that:

   A. This is the correct sequence for her medications

   B. She is taking both medications incorrectly. She needs medication administration instructions

   C. You need to assess Jenny's knowledge regarding the mechanism of actions and administration of her medications prior to any further action

   D. You should ask the physician to prescribe other medications

3. Jenny lives with her mother and two younger siblings. She is a nonsmoker, but her mother smokes one to two cigarettes per day. Jenny's mom states she only smokes outside the house. There are also two cats in the home. You feel it is important to:

   A. Tell Jenny's mother that it is irresponsible to smoke in the house, as it may make Jenny's symptoms worse, and provide informational pamphlets about smoking cessation programs

   B. Suggest that the cats be removed from the home and offer to facilitate communication with pet adoption agencies

   C. Speak with Jenny and her mother together and explain the role that allergens, such as smoke and cat hair, may have in exacerbating asthmatic symptoms

   D. Inform the family to keep cats and smoke outside of the house

4. Beginning with your first visit, you begin to prepare Jenny for discharge. You feel that her needs would be best served by conducting an interdisciplinary meeting to discuss her discharge plan and future care. You invite the following people to this meeting:

   A. Pulmonologist, social worker, dietician

   B. Pulmonologist, PMD, former pediatrician, Jenny, Jenny's mother, school nurse

   C. Pulmonologist, PMD, Jenny, dietician

   D. PMD, Jenny, Jenny's mother, social worker

5. As a CNL, you know that a key part of Jenny's ongoing care after discharge that would help improve her outcome is:

   A. A medication reconciliation record

   B. An asthma plan

   C. A peak flow diary

   D. Discharge instructions

6. Prior to discharge, the CNL should pay particular attention to:

   A. Vaccination status

   B. Diet plan

   C. Exercise plan

   D. Labwork

Case Study 3

You are a CNL on a medical–surgical unit in a community hospital. A few of the nurses from the unit come to you because they are concerned about a recent increase in falls on the unit. They tell you that they believe that the increase is due to insufficient staffing on the unit. They would like you to help them investigate this topic.

1. What should be your first step?

   A. Compare your unit's fall rate to similar like-sized hospitals nationwide

   B. Look at your current rates for this unit and see if there has been an increase in the fall rate over the last year, as the nurses suspect

   C. Compare your fall rates to other units in the hospital to see if they are higher or lower

   D. Look at staffing ratios over the last year to see if they have changed

You find that the fall rate on your unit has in fact been increasing over the past 6 months. More troubling is that the number of patient injuries due to falls has also increased. You decide to form a unit-based subcommittee to look into the issue further.

2. Who should be the initial members on the committee? (Check all that apply)

   A. Physical therapist

   B. Nurses

   C. Housekeeper

   D. Nurse manager

   E. Nurses' aides

   F. Secretary

   G. Physicians

   H. Coordinator of patient safety

   I. Risk manager

3. What information should the committee evaluate in the initial phase of this project? (Choose all that apply)

   A. What types of injuries the patients are sustaining when they fall

   B. The current fall policy

   C. Chart audits of documentation related to falls and safety assessments

   D. The current fall prevention tool

   E. Current research on the topic

   F. Staffing ratios on the unit

   G. Current fall prevention strategies on the unit

You find that staffing ratios have not changed on the unit. There have been several days when the unit has been short staffed, owing to staff resignations, but there has not been a higher fall rate on those days as compared with days when the unit is well staffed. New staff have been hired for the unit and will be starting over the next few weeks.

There is a fall prevention policy in place and a fall prevention tool that is to be filled out each shift by the nursing staff. The problem seems to be lack of documentation and consistent implementation of fall prevention strategies by the nursing staff.

4. What would be the best way to find out what the barriers are for the nursing staff with documentation and implementation of fall prevention strategies?

   A. Create a written survey and ask all of the nurses and nurses' aides on the unit to complete it

   B. Brainstorm with the other members of the committee on ways to improve documentation among the staff

   C. Get a group of nurses and nurses' aides together, representing each shift and go through the fall prevention tool with them item by item to find out where the barriers are

   D. Go around the unit and question the staff who have had a patient fall over the past 6 months about what they think led to the fall

After meeting with a group of nurses and nurses' aides, you learn that the responsibilities for each group were not clear, and that led to fall prevention strategies not being consistently implemented on patients who were identified as being at risk for falling.

5. What should the subcommittee's next step be?

   A. Make sure that the nurses understand that they are solely responsible for fall prevention on the unit

   B. Look for a new fall prevention tool to implement and revise the current policy. Then provide education for the staff regarding the new tool

   C. See if they are having the same problem on other units in the hospital

   D. Develop an educational tool based on the current fall prevention policy and tool. Provide education to all of the staff, so they understand their own and each other's role in fall prevention

Case Study 4

You are a CNL on an oncology unit. A nurse comes to you to share concerns about Mrs. Lopez, an 84-year-old patient admitted for shortness of breath. The patient was diagnosed 6 months ago with small cell lung cancer treated with chemotherapy and radiation therapy. On admission to the hospital, the patient had evidence of significant metastatic disease. The patient is being treated with morphine and oxygen, but remains significantly short of breath. The physician meets with the patient and family to share the plan for radiation treatment in an attempt to reduce the size of the current tumors. When the physician and family leave, the patient shares that she no longer wants aggressive treatments, but prefers to be comfortable and would like to go home, if possible.

1. Which of the following is an appropriate intervention for the nurse to suggest to the concerned nurse to do first?

   A. Report the patient's wishes to the physician

   B. Take the family aside and tell them what the patient shared

   C. Call an immediate family meeting with all members of the patient's health care team to discuss the matter

   D. Ask the patient if she would like to see the palliative care nurse and discuss options regarding her wishes for care

2. Mrs. Lopez shares with her physician and family that she does not plan to have the suggested radiation and would like a plan for a safe discharge with the support of hospice. All involved are supportive of this plan except for one daughter, who is very opposed to withdrawing treatment. Mrs. Lopez is concerned that the conflict among her children will impact her wishes when she can no longer make her own decisions. The best recommendation to Mrs. Lopez would include:

   A. Have the physician speak to all of Mrs. Lopez's children to explain the prognosis

   B. Contact the Pastoral Care department to speak to the daughter who is resisting the current plan

   C. Support the necessary steps to help Mrs. Lopez create an advanced directive

   D. Support the necessary steps to develop the patient's do-not-resuscitate orders for her hospital stay

3. The events of the past 48 hours have been very stressful on Mrs. Lopez and her family. The CNL recognizes this emotional distress and offers to have a certified therapeutic touch volunteer come and visit the patient. This action is best described as:

A. Inappropriate, given the patient's circumstances

B. Appropriate to the holistic needs of the patient

C. A standard practice for hospitalized patients

D. An example of a quality improvement initiative focused on increasing patient satisfaction for the long-term purpose of increased financial reimbursement

4. On day 4 of the admission, Mrs. Lopez is ready for discharge home with home care services and hospice care. The discharge process represents what opportunities regarding assuring a safe transfer of care in all of the following?

A. Risk anticipation—through medication reconciliation and education, because Mrs. Lopez is being discharged on a high-risk medication (morphine)

B. Knowledge management—as information about Mrs. Lopez is communicated to her hospice nurse in a written plan as well as oral communication

C. Advocacy—as the nurse should ensure that a copy of any advance directive is provided to the homecare agency and confirmed through verbal communication

D. Tertiary health promotion through the continuation of physical therapy to maximize physical mobility and minimize preventable complication of her condition

E. All of the above

Case Study 5

Walter is a 63-year-old African American who was readmitted to the telemetry unit of your hospital after being home for just 8 days. He has previously been diagnosed with stage 2 left heart failure secondary to a septal myocardial infarction (MI) that occurred 2 years ago. He has a 40-pack smoking history but quit at the time of the MI. Walter has had to retire from his job as a postal service employee and lives with his wife who continues to work full time. On this admission, Walter had the following data collected in the Emergency Department:

Blood pressure: 150/90	Respiratory rate: 28
Heart rate: 124 bpm	BMI: 29
Arterial blood gas:	
pH	7.48
PaO_2	78%
$PaCO_2$	28 mmHg
HCO_3	24 mEq/L
Sao_2	88%

1. Based on the results of the ABG, your preliminary classification of the patient would be:
   A. Respiratory acidosis
   B. Respiratory alkalosis
   C. Metabolic acidosis
   D. Metabolic alkalosis

2. Walter is preparing for discharge on day 3 of hospitalization. The CNL chooses the following next step in discharge preparation:
   A. A discussion with Walter's wife regarding their home situation
   B. A team meeting with those involved in Walter's care with inclusion of the outpatient team members
   C. A session of patient education focused on teach-back techniques to assure knowledge
   D. A conversation with Walter regarding what factors he felt contributed to his readmission

3. Based on priorities of care for those with heart failure, which intervention should the CNL ensure is part of Walter's discharge plan?
   A. Scheduling of a follow-up appointment with the primary care provider within 7 days
   B. Smoking cessation
   C. Cardiac rehabilitation
   D. Visiting nurse services

4. In preparation for discharge, the CNL ensures that the patient understands the medication plan for home and provides a written plan to the patient. The patient is being discharged on metoprolol. The CNL understands this drug is used for which of the following purposes:
   A. To reduce myocardial oxygen consumption
   B. To reduce platelet aggregation and risk of coronary occlusion
   C. To reduce cardiac workload and oxygen demands of the heart
   D. To reduce plasma aldosterone concentrations

Case Study 6

You are receiving a 24-year-old patient from the intensive care unit (ICU). The patient has been in ICU for 1 week. He was admitted due to a motor vehicle accident in which he had to have surgical repair of his femur and right hip. His medical history is significant for smoking (cigarettes) and occasionally drinking alcohol. Vital signs are stable and the patient is alert and oriented × 4. When you are reviewing his plan of care, he indicates that he has not been out of bed although he has been cleared by the surgical trauma physician.

1. Which of the following complications would you be most concerned about following this patient's surgery?

   A. Sepsis

   B. Bowel obstruction

   C. Acute respiratory failure

   D. DVT

2. The patient states that he does not understand why he would be at risk for pulmonary complications. You explain to the patient that pulmonary complications such as infection, aspiration, bronchospasm, respiratory failure, pleural effusion, and atelectasis are common after surgery. You indicate that all of the following are risk factors for developing postoperative pulmonary complications *except*:

   A. Hemoglobin level <10 g/dL

   B. Emergency procedure

   C. Respiratory infection during the previous year

   D. Older age

3. The patient acknowledges the importance of mobility to prevent these complications. What would be the next most important intervention to help further reduce that patient's chances for developing pulmonary complications?

   A. Smoking cessation education

   B. Appropriate pain management

   C. Nutrition

   D. Chest physical therapy

4. Your patient begins to complain of leg pain. When you assess his leg, he points to his thigh. His pulses are +1, where previously they have been +3. You notify the physician and he orders a Doppler ultrasound, which is positive for a DVT. What other complications are you most concerned about this patient developing?

   A. Pulmonary embolus

   B. Loss of blood flow to the patient's extremity

   C. Edema

   D. Immobility

5. Your patient suffers a pulmonary embolus, which leads to his requiring mechanical ventilation. The patient returns to ICU. As a clinical nurse leader, what would be the most appropriate intervention after caring for this patient?

   A. Perform a root cause analysis

   B. Forming a multidisciplinary team to review the patient's plan of care and gather whether anything could have been done to prevent this from occurring

   C. Review the case with your nurse manager

D. Review evidence-based practice and research on caring for and preventing pulmonary complications postoperatively

Case Study 7

You are the CNL on an obstetrical unit. You receive a patient, Sharon T, from the doctor's office, admitted with mild preeclampsia at 28 weeks' gestation.

1. Over the next 24 hours, you should review all of the following except:

A. Pregnancy history, allergies, medical history

B. Birth plan, sleep history, hobbies, exercise routine

C. Alcohol, drug, and tobacco use; social history; diet

D. Medications prior to admission, immunization status

2. As the CNL, what are some appropriate interventions that you can perform?

A. Consult the physical therapist

B. Give the patient an application for Medicare

C. Consult the social worker and case manager

D. Write an order to keep all staff out of her room between 2300 and 0600

Sharon is very grateful for your interventions and feels much better about her situation. She has now been on your unit for 2 ½ weeks and has developed gestational diabetes and severe preeclampsia. The doctors have told her that she will have to remain in the hospital on bedrest with bathroom privileges for the duration of her pregnancy. Sharon is not happy about this, but knows it is the best thing for her and her baby and is compliant.

3. As the CNL who is managing her plan of care, you will be sure to include in her plan of care all of the following except:

A. Daily rounding with her care team, and weekly interdisciplinary team meetings

B. Instructions on how to self-administer insulin, and daily walks outside

C. Physical therapy consult, visits with her family

D. Utilization of antithromboembolism pump/antithromboembolism therapy

Two weeks later, Sharon's vital signs and labs start going downhill and she is having subjective symptoms of preeclampsia. She is 32 ½ weeks pregnant, and the doctors have decided that it is time to move toward delivery. As it is not urgent at this time, they will allow Sharon to attempt a vaginal delivery.

4. As the CNL, what should you make sure happens prior to delivery?

A. Steroid administration

B. Blood glucose control

C. Neonatologist consult

D. Sharon's birth plan of no medications be upheld

The next day you go to check on Sharon. She had a successful vaginal delivery of a baby girl at 0249. The baby went to the NICU. Sharon is still in labor and delivery on magnesium sulfate. She will be transferred once her acuity level decreases enough not to have one-on-one nursing care. Her vital signs are stable, but her blood pressure is still elevated. Her labs are beginning to trend back to normal. Sharon thanks you for all your care.

5. What would your next priority be?

    A. Begin discharge teaching

    B. Have the transport team take Sharon to the NICU to see her baby

    C. Consult the social worker

    D. Consult child life

Case Study 8

Erika is a Caucasian 72-year-old female being admitted by her primary care physician for uncontrolled DM Type II.

1. What other information do you need right now upon admission?

    A. FSBG

    B. Mental status

    C. Does she live alone?

    D. Does she have a glucometer?

Her FSBG is 327 on admission. The primary care nurse gives her insulin on the basis of the physician's orders. You introduce yourself to Erika and start gathering information. You ask the patient whether she is taking her medication at home. Erika tells you, "I take my medicine all the time. I have no idea why my blood sugar is so high! It's never even close to that at home!"

2. What do you want to know next while gathering information?

    A. Does she have a glucometer?

    B. Falls risk score

    C. HgbA1c

    D. Mental status

3. From this HgbA1c, you know:

    A. It is normal

    B. It is high

    C. Erika is taking her medication

    D. It is inconclusive

4. What should you do next?

    A. Get a dietician consult to review her knowledge about diabetic diets and develop a meal plan

    B. Call her son, whom she lives with, to develop a POC

C. Call her PCP and see if she is compliant with her appointments and medication regimen

D. Tell her she cannot eat any potatoes, rice, or refined sugars at all

After the diabetes educator and dietician have seen the patient, you discover the patient did not have very much money and was having trouble buying the right foods. She was also having severe diarrhea from the metformin and was very embarrassed after she had a few accidents in public. You contact the social worker to come help the patient work on getting the right foods and you make a list of healthy foods that are not very expensive to help the patient make better food choices.

5. What else should you do?

A. Call her son to go get her metformin from the pharmacy

B. Tell the patient the metformin is important and to just wear some Depends

C. Discontinue the metformin and start glyburide

D. Call her PCP to discuss her side effect from taking the metformin and to develop a POC

APPENDIX D

Answers and Rationale

Kimberlee-Ann Bridges, MSN, RN, CNL
Care Coordinator
Western Health Network
Danbury, CT

Leah Ledford, MSN, RN, CNL, SANE
Clinical Nurse Leader
Charlotte, NC
Carolinas Medical Center

Marie D. Litzelman, MSN, RN, CMSRN, CNL
Clinical Nurse Leader
Carolinas Medical Center
Charlotte, NC

Danielle Morton, MSN, RN, CNL
Pediatric Nurse Educator
Yale New Haven Hospital
New Haven, CT

Sara Pratt, MSN, RN, CNL
Clinical Nurse Leader
Carolinas Medical Center
Charlotte, NC

Katarzyna A. Qutermous, MSN, RN, CNL
Clinical Nurse Leader
Carolinas Medical Center
Charlotte, NC

Josephine Ritchie, MSN, RN, CNL
Performance Improvement Manager
Norwalk Hospital, Norwalk, CT

Mary-Jo Smith MSN, RN, CNL
Patient Services Manager
Yale-New Haven Children's Hospital
New Haven, CT

Correspondence to:

Cynthia R. King, PhD, NP, MSN, CNL, FAAN
11313 Coreopsis Road
Charlotte, NC 28213
Cell phone: 336-416-8668
Home: 704-900-8097 answering machine
E-mail: Kingc@queens.edu

Sally O'Toole Gerard, DNP, RN, CDE, CNL
Assistant Professor
CNL Track Coordinator
Fairfield University
Fairfield, CT
sgerard@fairfield.edu

1. Patient satisfaction scores in the emergency department (ED) have shown a downward trend over the past three quarters. As a clinical nurse leader (CNL) in the ED, your focus is to:
   A. Create a script for the triage nurse in welcoming the patient
   B. Assign a volunteer to welcome patients to the hospital
   C. **Compare desired outcomes with national and state standards**
   D. Write a letter of apology to each dissatisfied patient

C: Client care outcomes are a measure of quality practice. CNLs must know how to compare desired outcomes that will improve safety, effectiveness, timeliness, efficiency, quality, and the degree to which they are client centered.

2. Which of the following actions illustrates the CNL professional value of altruism?
   A. Leading an interdisciplinary team looking at the remote cardiac monitoring process
   B. **Sponsoring a meeting with the monitor technicians to understand their barriers in the cardiac monitoring process**
   C. Flow mapping the admission process of the remote cardiac-monitored patient
   D. Editing the policy for the remote cardiac monitoring process

B: Altruism is a concern for the welfare and well-being of others. In professional practice, altruism is reflected by the CNL's concern for the welfare of clients, other nurses, and other health care providers.

3. You are a CNL on the telemetry unit and orienting a newly graduated nurse. Critical thinking is best demonstrated when:
   A. **The CNL discusses with the physician the rationale for discontinuing cardiac monitoring in the hospice patient**
   B. Drawing the scheduled cardiac enzymes every 8 hours
   C. Reviewing the patient care guidelines and protocols related to hourly rounding
   D. The CNL balances both the charge role and the preceptor role simultaneously

A: Critical thinking underlies independent and interdependent decision making. Critical thinking includes questioning, analysis, synthesis, interpretation, inference, inductive and deductive reasoning, intuition, application, and creativity.

4. You are a CNL selected to lead a team focused on implementing a multidisciplinary clinical pathway for acute ischemic stroke and transient ischemic attack. The risk assessment tool that you have adopted identifies all of the following as independent stroke risk factors except:
   A. Age
   B. Systolic blood pressure
   C. **Liver dysfunction**

    D. Current smoking

    E. Diabetes mellitus

C: Independent stroke predictors include age, systolic blood pressure, hypertension, diabetes mellitus, current smoking, established cardiovascular disease (any one of myocardial infarction, angina or coronary insufficiency, congestive heart failure, or intermittent claudication), atrial fibrillation, and left ventricular hypertrophy on ECG.

5. A lack of compliance with deep vein thrombosis (DVT) prophylaxis has been identified in retrospective chart reviews of all ischemic stroke patients in your organization. As a CNL on the neurological unit, your primary goal will include:

    A. Challenging the guidelines on primary prevention of ischemic stroke written by the American Stroke Association

    B. **Gaining an understanding of how DVT prophylaxis is initiated on each stroke patient on your unit**

    C. Developing an organization-wide educational program on DVT prophylaxis

    D. Developing a unit-based team of nursing personnel to investigate the problem

B: White Paper: One competency is that of a systems analyst. A CNL participates in a system review and conducts a microsystem analysis, identifying a clinical issue with a focus on a particular population.

6. You are working on improving the patient discharge process. Which of these targets would best reflect clinical microsystem outcomes?

    A. Hospital length of stay

    B. Time of discharge order for all medical patients to the actual time the patient left

    C. **Number of discharge orders on your unit entered before 11 a.m.**

    D. Total number of discharged patients leaving by 11 a.m.

C: A CNL as an outcomes manager uses data to change practice and to improve outcomes. Selecting the most appropriate goals and targets will provide meaningful information.

7. Electronic nursing documentation has recently been instituted in your organization. Select a response that best defines a clinical decision support:

    A. A reminder to save and sign your admission assessment

    B. A visual red alert when a patient's potassium is 6.8 mEq/L

    C. **A pop-up to initiate the discharge instruction sheet with every physician discharge order**

    D. An electronic nursing care plan

C: CDS is a computer-based program designed to assist clinicians in making clinical decisions by filtering and integrating vast amounts of information and providing suggestions for clinical intervention.

In 2008, the Centers for Medicaid and Medicare Services (CMS) collaboratively with the Centers for Disease Control and Prevention enacted a new payment provision related to eight hospital-acquired conditions. Hospital falls and traumas occurring during a hospital stay will not receive CMS reimbursement. Health promotion, risk reduction, and disease prevention are core competencies of the clinical nurse leader. As a CNL on the telemetry unit, you have recognized the importance of this issue.

8. Which level within a system does this issue affect?

   A. Microsystem

   B. Mesosystem

   C. Macrosystem

   D. **All of the above**

D: One concept of health care systems involves three levels of building together to make up complex organizations.

9. Clinical nurse leaders focus on projects within a clinical microsystem. A clinical microsystem can be best described as:

   A. A department-wide program focused on improving continuity of care and patient satisfaction

   B. Trending the postoperative care on all surgical units

   C. **The clinical and business processes of a single unit within an organization**

   D. All medical and surgical units guided by a chief nursing officer

C: The microsystem is described by the AACN White Paper as the practice level of the CNL.

10. All are part of the data necessary for a CNL to fully understand and assess his or her clinical unit except:

    A. **The organization financial statement**

    B. The target population and age distribution

    C. The percentage of full-time equivalents (FTEs)

    D. Rate of nosocomial infections

    E. Fall rates

A: A comprehensive assessment of the clinical unit is a foundation for the work of the CNL but does not include the financial statement of the organization. In comprehending the "big picture" of the organization, the CNL should have an understanding of the financial health of the institution.

11. The results of a quarterly report identify an increase in patient falls on the telemetry unit. Your first action will be to:

    A. Implement hourly rounding

    B. **Gain an understanding of patient care practices on the telemetry unit**

    C. Assign patient personal alarms to all patients at risk

    D. Revise the current fall risk documentation form

B: Assessment includes gathering information about the health status of the client and analyzing and synthesizing those making judgments about nursing interventions on the basis of findings, evaluation, and managing of individual care outcomes.

12. You have been asked to lead the telemetry fall prevention committee. Which combination of team members would best suit the initial phase of this group?

   A. A behavioral health APRN

   B. A staff nurse

   C. A physical therapist

   D. The nurse manager

   E. **All of the above**

   F. Only A, B, and D are needed

E: Health promotion and disease prevention knowledge includes methods to keep an illness or injury from occurring, diagnosis, and treating a disease in its early course. CNLs need to work with an interdisciplinary team to make ethical decisions, develop, and monitor comprehensive, holistic plans of care. There is a strong correlation between patient falls and delirium. Exercise programs focused on strength, functional performance, and balance training are effective steps in reducing inpatient falls.

13. As a CNL in the ICU, you have observed several prolonged and fragmented processes of starting an intravenous line in a critically ill patient. All of the following considerations are necessary in identifying *a theme* for your improvement process except:

   A. A thorough review of the clinical unit

   B. **The manager's mandate for change**

   C. The alignment with the organization's strategic priorities

   D. Input from the patient's family

B: Specific mandates for change would be considered as the team "drills down" for further information.

14. The hospital is looking to utilize cardiac monitor watchers. Your analysis includes all of the following except:

   A. **A review of an online ECG monitoring education program**

   B. Identifying a clinical issue with a focus on a specific population

   C. Conducting a trend analysis of outcome data

   D. Analyzing barriers and facilitators with the organization

A: Systems analysis and risk anticipation are the competencies of the CNL.

15. Several near misses were identified by ICU nurses who had mistaken invasive lines for intravenous ports for medication administration. You have completed an analysis of the issue. Your recommendations include:

   A. A visual signal on all ports not intended for intravenous drugs

   B. A double-check system for medication administration

C. To facilitate a critical incident reporting structure that fosters a "without blame" unit culture

D. **All of the above**

E. Only C

D: The CNL should support the staff to identify all opportunities for improving safety in this situation.

16. Data reported by the ICU quality committee reflect challenges in the management of the septic patient. As a CNL in the ICU, all of the following are first steps in evaluating the delivery of client care except:

A. Knowledge of sepsis guidelines

B. Critical care clinicians staffing ratios

C. Use of clinical decision support systems

D. **Differentiating sepsis from systemic inflammatory response syndrome (SIRS)**

D: Nursing leadership and advocacy reviews and evaluates care guidelines and protocols.

17. A fellow staff nurse is struggling to understand the use of a clinical decision support system (CDSS) in the management of her septic patient. Your initial teaching strategy includes:

A. Sharing the latest clinical research

B. An understanding of expected and actual outcomes

C. **Defining the purpose of CDSS**

D. Exploring challenges, risks, and benefits

C: CDSS supports a safe patient culture and should be designed to help providers.

18. You are using failure mode and effect analysis (FMEA) to anticipate the risk of medication errors in the ICU related to invasive lines. You begin your FMEA analysis with:

A. The effects of each failure

B. The potential cause of each failure

C. **Process mapping**

D. Specific defects and delays in the medication administration process

C: Utilizing tools for process improvement can provide new insights into routine practices.

19. Your colleagues have identified challenges in the process of inserting an intravenous line. To gain a better understanding of what this process entails, you:

A. Directly observe the intravenous line insertion process and time each step of the process

B. Create a workflow diagram tracing the path of the nurse during the line insertion process

C. Engage the IV team to reeducate the nurses

D. All of the above

E. **A and B**

E: Proper assessment of a clinical situation can expose issues of policy, compliance, or the need for education.

20. The result of a workflow diagram of a clinician illustrates an excessive amount of walking to obtain supplies. Reducing the waste of motion adds value-added time that ultimately benefits:

A. **The patient**

B. The clinician

C. Documentation

D. None of the above

A: Process improvement enhances patient safety and nursing time at the bedside for the patient and family.

21. Your team is looking at the delays in the discharge process. Your cause and effect diagram includes:

A. A run chart

B. A Gantt chart

C. **A fishbone diagram**

D. A high-level flowchart

C: A fishbone diagram is a useful tool to identify themes of clinical issues. Categories such as equipment, personnel, communication, and so on can be identified.

22. You are leading a palliative care team in the ICU. Ethical competence is best defined as:

A. **The ability to recognize potential and actual ethical issues arising from clinical practice**

B. The collaboration with a multicultural workforce

C. The understanding of the physical, emotional, and spiritual heath parameters of the ICU patient

D. The skill set to define, design, and implement culturally competent health care providers

A: The CNL's role in ethics is highlighted in AACN's White Paper.

23. Opportunities that reflect human diversity include:

A. **Promoting effective communication for injured veterans**

B. Stressing the importance of family health history

C. Standardizing the discharge process

D. Decreasing the admission lead time to the pediatric unit

A: Human diversity includes understanding the ways cultural, ethnic, socioeconomic, linguistic, religious, and lifestyle variations are expressed.

24. Survey results of the nursing staff reflect poor perceptions and a discomfort with addressing spiritual issues with patients. The ultimate success of focused staff education can be measured by:

    A. **Trending quarterly patient satisfaction scores pertaining to spiritual care during hospitalization**

    B. A follow-up survey of the staff after the education to solicit feedback

    C. An open discussion of how the nurse would address spiritual care in a given scenario

    D. Feedback shared during discharge phone calls

A: Application of knowledge that impacts patient outcomes is the most significant indicator.

25. Sustaining process improvement requires the use of appropriate learning principles and strategies. The CNL function that best utilizes this competency is:

    A. Advocate

    B. **Educator**

    C. Clinician

    D. Information manager

B: CNL competencies are described in the AACN White Paper.

26. How can the CNL make the greatest impact on the health care organization?

    A. **By representing the microsystem**

    B. By representing the mesosystem

    C. By representing the patient and family

    D. By representing the nursing profession

A: The CNL functions as the change agent at the microsystem level, engaging frontline staff in best practices to better patient outcomes.

27. By leading which unit initiative can the CNL directly impact the financial health of the entire institution?

    A. **Reducing readmissions**

    B. Recruitment of new nursing staff

    C. Improving documentation compliance

    D. Encouraging staff to report safety events and near misses

A: Medicare reimbursement rates include a penalty to those health care institutions with 30-day readmission rates that are higher than national benchmarks.

28. The concept that an organization is in a continued state of change describes which organizational theory:

    A. Systems theory

    B. Classical theory

    C. Contingency theory

    D. **Chaos theory**

D: The chaos theory is based on the principle that a system can maintain itself only if change is occurring somewhere in the organization all the time. Chaos and change are seen as means of survival.

29. The new hospital CNO works hard to cultivate a shared vision of leaders and followers motivating each other toward their highest potential. This is an example of which type of leadership:

 A. **Transformational leadership**

 B. Transactional leadership

 C. Situational leadership

 D. Hierarchical leadership

A: A transformational leader believes that leaders and followers motivate each other toward the end goal of developing followers into leaders. This is accomplished by leading and motivating by example.

30. Before beginning data collection, what is the primary key factor to determine?

 A. Personnel to collect data

 B. A secure database for holding data

 C. **Operational definitions of data**

 D. A user-friendly collection method

C: Operational definitions clearly define what is to be collected and avoid confusion for those collecting the data. Clear operational definitions also helps those who are interpreting the data. Failure to determine operational definitions may result in data that are inaccurate.

31. You are the CNL on a 25-bed cardiac unit. You are completing afternoon rounds with the patients. Upon entering Mr. K's room you notice that his son has brought him fried chicken, soda, and fries. How should you address this?

 A. Don't say anything to the patient or family and tell the interdisciplinary team at morning rounds

 B. **Provide education to the patient and family about consuming a heart-healthy diet**

 C. Place a consult in the computer for the nutritionist to assess the patient

 D. Remind the patient why he is in the hospital and remove the food

B: You are in the room currently and can provide real-time education to the patient and family. It is an opportunity to educate the patient/family on how to make heart-healthy choices. As a follow-up, you should place a consult for the nutritionist to follow up.

32. As the CNL on a cardiothoracic step-down unit, what is the one recommendation you would make to decrease the chance of readmission of your patient population?

 A. Visiting nursing for all patients

 B. All follow-up appointments scheduled prior to patient discharge

C. Pharmacy to visit with each patient prior to discharge home to review medications

D. **All patients should be enrolled in a cardiac rehabilitation program**

D: All patients should be enrolled in a cardiac rehabilitation program to assist the patient with making permanent lifestyle changes required to improve their health, well-being, and success after their illness. Because these programs provide ongoing support, teaching, and monitoring of health, it is the best choice.

33. You know teaching was effective to a cardiac patient and his wife with the following statement:
    A. "I can still have a burger and fries one to two times a week"
    B. "It is okay for my wife to bring in a pizza while I'm here; after all the hospital food is not that good"
    C. **"I should limit my salt intake and increase fiber in my diet"**
    D. "If my husband wants fried shrimp, it's okay because it is seafood"

C: Cardiac patients should be on a sodium-restricted diet. Fried foods and high-fat foods should be very limited and/or excluded from the diet.

34. You are the CNL on a geriatric unit. When walking down the hall, you notice a high-risk fall patient attempting to get out of bed alone. After assisting the patient and ensuring safety, what should you do?
    A. Report the incident to nursing management
    B. Identify the patient's nurse and nursing assistant and confront them with the incident
    C. Develop a new fall prevention policy and post it in the unit conference room for all staff to view
    D. **Obtain the fall statistics and present them at the next unit staff meeting and develop a team to look at revising a fall prevention committee**

D: Using objective data to determine the trends on the unit will allow the CNL to determine a baseline fall rate for the unit. Starting a fall prevention committee will empower frontline staff to determine with evidence-based research which implementations will best meet the needs of their patient population and the staff.

35. As the CNL on a medical/surgical unit, you have noticed a trend over the last 3 months with patients having high blood glucose before lunch and dinner. What is the best way to address this problem?
    A. Investigate whether the blood glucose monitors on the unit are accurate
    B. Provide an educational in-service about diabetes to the staff
    C. Ensure all patients with diabetes receive a consultation with the nutritionist
    D. **Determine what other changes in processes have occurred on the unit in the past 3 months that could influence this trend**

D: While checking the accuracy of blood glucose meters, providing education to staff and patients is important. Other processes on the unit that have changed need to be further evaluated to determine their influence on patient outcomes.

36. After careful review of unit processes, you have determined that the self meal order program was introduced 3 months ago. With this program, patients have the ability to order meals when they are ready to eat rather than eating at predetermined times set by the hospital. This change has altered the timing of medications previously given with meals. What does the CNL do to improve the process?

    A. **Develop an interdisciplinary team, including unit staff, nutritionist, diabetic educator, and meal service team members to investigate the self meal order program**

    B. Have the nurse or nursing assistant order meals with patients; this way the nurse knows what time the patient orders meals

    C. When explaining the self meal order program to patients, instruct patients to notify staff when they order meals

    D. Have the meal service notify the unit secretary when meal orders are placed by patients

A: Having an interdisciplinary team look at the entire process of the self meal order program will provide the team with innovative solutions to the problem.

37. After completing unit audits, you have noticed the nurses are not completing AIR cycles documentation with pain management (AIR: assessment, intervention, reassessment). What should be done to improve documentation?

    A. Tell the unit management which staff are documenting inappropriately

    B. Reeducate staff on the hospital documentation policy

    C. Remind staff of pain documentation during staff meetings and charge report

    D. **Provide staff with a self-audit sheet as a way to review their own documentation during their shifts**

D: Giving staff a checklist will assist them in staying organized during their busy day. This will provide them a way to double check all their documentation before ending a shift. It also empowers staff to take ownership of their work.

38. You are listening to report with a novice nurse. As part of mentoring new staff and supporting clinical decision making, you ask the new nurse which patient she would like to assess first. Which patient should this nurse assess first?

    A. 46-year-old receiving IV antibiotic therapy

    B. **60-year-old s/p liver biopsy**

    C. 56-year-old with pneumonia

    D. 72-year-old hip replacement impatiently waiting for discharge

B: Post-op liver biopsy patients have an increased risk of bleeding and need close monitoring after the procedure. The question does not indicate how recently the biopsy was done and therefore this is the best choice based on the information provided.

39. To help patients maintain healthy skin while in the hospital, all of the following should be considered *except:*
    A. Provide patient with Q2h positioning/turning if patient is unable to self position
    B. Ensure adequate protein intake
    C. Use bed surfaces known to prevent skin complications
    D. **Allow patient to refuse bathing for days if uninterested, as the patient has the right to refuse care**

D: While the patient does have the right to refuse care, a patient who would disengage with personal grooming for multiple days should draw the attention of the staff and CNL. Further investigation into the refusal and disinterest in self-care needs would be required to determine the underlying causes resulting in the patient's behavior and lack of care for self needs.

40. A nurse on the unit comes to you and says that every shift he works day or night he finds at least one of his patients without an identification band in place. He is very concerned about patient safety and feels a harmful mistake could occur in the near future if the practice on the unit is not improved. What do you do as the CNL?
    A. Perform daily audits on all the patients and report results to management
    B. Have the unit secretary make new identification bands for all the patients daily so the charge nurse can place new bands on the patients daily
    C. Research a new style of patient identification bands since the current product does not stay on the patient properly
    D. **Provide support to the nurse on the unit who determines the problem and help him identify areas in the process to improve patient identification**

D: Part of the CNL's role is to provide staff with education, support, and the tools needed to improve practice. This nurse is already concerned about improving a process. As a CNL it is important to foster leadership and ownership instead of providing solutions to problems.

41. Over the past few weeks, nurses on the 30-bed medical unit have been complaining the MD orders related to oxygen do not match what the patient is receiving. Often the patient has more than one oxygen order at the same time. This leads to confusion for nursing and respiratory care staff and could harm the patient. How can the CNL improve the practice?
    A. **Using the informatics team as support, create a hard stop in the computer that does not allow the physician to activate a new oxygen order without discontinuing the previous order**
    B. Tell the nurses they need to remind the doctors to keep orders up to date and have the nurses review orders at rounds with the team
    C. Meet with the unit hospitalist to make a plan to address the problem
    D. Do nothing since CNLs cannot write patient care orders

A: Having the informatics team develop a hard stop in the computer will allow the patient to have only one active oxygen order at a time. It is imperative that nurses and CNLs work with informatics professionals in the design of safe care.

42. The hospital has a goal for patient transfers from ICU to be completed by 12 noon. Your unit has a very low percentage for meeting this hospital goal. How can you best address this problem as the CNL?

    A. Tell the charge nurse to discharge patients in the morning

    B. Ask the manager to staff an extra nurse on day shift to be the discharge nurse

    C. **Use process mapping to determine all the possible factors that contribute to patient discharge and what barriers there are to discharge**

    D. Don't worry about the number; your unit meets the other hospital goals, so it is okay to miss one

C: Process mapping is a tool to provide the team with an objective view of the problem being investigated. This view will help everyone to determine the barriers to transfer. Once the barriers are determined through process mapping, each barrier can be broken down further to determine solutions.

43. You are the CNL at an outpatient care clinic providing care to families in the area. You have noticed it is difficult to get families to bring their children in for their immunizations, and children are often off schedule. How can the clinic best address this issue to meet the needs of their patient populations?

    A. Educate families on immunizations, their purpose, and their children's schedule

    B. Provide reminder phone calls to families the day before a scheduled appointment

    C. If possible, offer extended clinic hours 1 to 2 nights a week, so parents can come in after work

    D. **Use the clinic data to determine why families are not coming to appointments**

D: Before making changes at the clinic, it would be best to look at the data objectively to determine what is causing the problem. Answers A, B, and C assume you know the families' reasons for not coming to appointments.

44. You are the CNL in the day surgery center and have found that many patients come to the center unprepared on the morning of surgery. This delays surgery start times and backs up the operating room schedule for the day. The whole surgery team is frustrated. How can the process be fixed?

    A. Change the first surgery start time and delay it by 20 minutes

    B. **Institute presurgery phone calls 2 to 3 days prior to a patient's scheduled appointment**

    C. Stagger surgery start times more throughout the day

    D. Reschedule patients who come to the center unprepared

B: Having a nurse call the patient before the morning of surgery will allow the patient to ask questions and review what to do the night before and the morning of surgery, to help ensure patients arrive to the center ready and prepared for surgery. This may also help reduce patient anxiety prior to a procedure, thus arriving better prepared.

45. Per the epidemiology report, your unit's hand hygiene scores have steadily decreased over the past 3 months. When reporting these metrics at a staff meeting, most of the staff replies saying, "It's the doctors fault, we always wash our hands." How do you work to change the culture of the unit?
    A. Have secret shoppers monitor the staff and hand out tickets to hand hygiene offenders
    B. Collect hand hygiene metrics related to the unit staff only and use these data to educate staff
    C. Have a hand hygiene campaign to reinvigorate staff
    D. **Investigate the barriers to hand hygiene and collaborate with staff to reduce these barriers**

D: Giving staff warnings, presenting objective data, and highlighting a problem may improve compliance only slightly. Finding out the root cause for noncompliance and collaborating with staff to find viable solutions will change the unit culture over time and empower staff to make positive changes to their work environment.

46. A new nurse on the medical/surgical unit approaches you with concerns about one of her patients. She states the patient has not turned on the lights or television all day and did not order breakfast or lunch. She had to ask the patient what meal they wanted and place the order. This nurse states she is concerned about the change in the patient's behavior. Looking at the patient's chart, you realize this patient is Jewish and it is Saturday. What is your best response to the nurse?
    A. "The patient is sick and needs extra support today"
    B. "The patient needs to be seen by the psychology team for an evaluation"
    C. **"The patient may be following their religious practices and we need to support this"**
    D. "The patient is depressed from being in the hospital"

C: We need to support patients' religious practices whenever possible in the hospital. Considering it is Saturday and this patient is Jewish means the patient is recognizing the Sabbath. This means the patient will not use any electrical devices or ask to use them. The staff would have to ask whether a patient wants the television on or the lights turned on/off, and so on. Patients will also not use the phone or call bell system during the Sabbath. Staff need to be sensitive to patient needs and try to accommodate cultural and spiritual practices whenever possible.

47. When trying to implement a change in the outpatient family clinic, which group of staff should the CNL focus on more?
    A. **Late majority**
    B. Early majority
    C. Laggards
    D. Innovators

A: The innovators and early majority are going to be supportive of change and become champions for the project. The laggards make up a minority portion of the group and will be the last to adopt change. However, the late majority, which makes up a large percentage of the group, is the percentage that will need the most support during a change and they will be resistant.

48. As the CNL on a medical unit, which of the following interventions would you support to reduce the readmission rate on your unit?

   A. Keep patients one extra day to ensure they are prepared for discharge home

   B. Arrange for all patients to have at least 1 week of visiting nursing postdischarge

   C. Review discharge instructions with the patient and one family member

   D. **Begin discharge planning and teaching on the day of admission**

D: Using every opportunity to communicate to and educate the patient and family on their care and planning for discharge will better prepare the patient and family for returning home.

49. You are the CNL on a 32-bed medical–surgical unit. When you walk into the unit, you observe a novice nurse looking extremely busy and stressed. How can you best support her transition on the unit?

   A. Ask the charge nurse to decrease her patient assignment

   B. Give some of her morning medications

   C. Pull the nurse off the unit during her shift

   D. **Meet with this nurse after the shift to discuss organization**

D: As the CNL, you should meet with the novice nurse when she is not scheduled to offer support, guidance, and assistance while she transitions from novice to expert. Newer nurses need help with organization and managing tasks to help support their critical thinking skills.

50. Which type of evidence would you prefer to review and share with a team when trying to support whether an evidence-based intervention should be implemented on your unit?

   A. Meta-analysis

   B. Quasi-experimental

   C. **Experimental**

   D. Qualitative

C: Experimental research is quantitative research, which is a formal, objective, rigorous, and systematic process for generating information about the world. Experimental research is an objective, highly controlled investigation for the purpose of predicting and controlling phenomena in nursing practice.

51. Which group presents the highest challenge in attaining buy-in for a new innovation?

   A. Early innovators

   B. Early adopters

   C. **Late majority**

   D. Laggards

C: Members of the late majority approach any new initiative with a high degree of skepticism and require a large amount of information before adopting change. They will adopt change only in the late stages. Laggards historically will not adopt change.

52. There has been disagreement regarding the suggested adoption of a patient transfer blackout period during change of shift. Staff on the inpatient units favor a 30-minute blackout period, while emergency department staff favor no blackout period. A team of stakeholders from all areas recently agreed on a universal blackout period of 15 minutes during shift change. What type of solution does this represent?
    A. Compromise
    B. **Collaboration**
    C. Accommodation
    D. Confrontation

B: Collaboration involves all parties working together to design optimal outcomes using mutually agreed upon solutions.

53. The CNL can effectively design fiscally efficient patient care using which of the following strategies:
    A. Division of tasks and responsibilities among all team members
    B. **Delegation of responsibilities according to job roles**
    C. Seeking team members' input regarding their strengths and desired responsibilities
    D. Using input from the manager for job assignments

B: The CNL must delegate responsibilities to the appropriate team member according to job description. Each team member should function at the highest level according to licensure. This will help to avoid wasting human resources and will preserve fiscal efficiency.

54. To demonstrate active listening, the CNL would exhibit which behavior:
    A. Avoid making any facial expressions
    B. Preserve at least 3 feet between the parties
    C. **Lean slightly forward**
    D. Folding hands in the lap

C: Learning slightly forward indicates desire to concentrate on the interaction at hand and relays openness and attention to the talker.

55. To confirm a scope of practice question, the CNL should consult which administrative body guidelines:
    A. The Joint Commission
    B. Centers for Medicare and Medicaid Services
    C. Hospital Policy and Procedure Manual
    D. **State Nursing Practice Act**

D: Scope of practice is defined according to each individual state. The CNL must have a full understanding of licensure standards of practice according to role before delegation of tasks.

56. Team coordination skills can help avoid all but
    A. Undefined team member roles
    B. Poor membership involvement
    C. **Member conflict**
    D. Confusion regarding next steps

C: In most working groups, conflict arises at some point. In addition to sound team coordination skills, the CNL must also possess effective conflict management skills.

57. An important element of an effective team meeting is the creation of minutes to be distributed after the meeting. Who is the most appropriate team member to create the minutes?
    A. The meeting facilitator
    B. Any group member
    C. **A preidentified team member**
    D. The meeting scheduler

C: Meeting minutes ideally should be written by the same team member at every meeting. The facilitator should not take minutes, as he or she must devote full attention to running the meeting and observing nonverbal communication of team members. The minute taker, also referred to as the recorder, must listen carefully and may not be able to fully join in the conversation. The recorder may also serve as the timekeeper for the meeting, thus keeping the group on schedule. Recording is a difficult role and is best performed by a defined member with the necessary skills.

58. Which of the following may be a beneficial tool for an interdisciplinary team to use to focus many ideas for improvement of patient satisfaction scores?
    A. Root cause analysis
    B. **Multivoting**
    C. Development of a subcommittee
    D. None of the above; the group should work on all the ideas generated by the group

B: To have effective outcomes, the group should focus on the most significant priorities related to the issue. Multivoting can give members a voice in the process. It is not practical or an effective use of resources to pursue all ideas.

59. Who can function as an important ally to the CNL in engaging frontline staff in a major initiative?
    A. Content expert
    B. **Unit champion**

    C. Initiative sponsor

    D. Senior leadership

B: Unit champions are individuals who work along frontline staff and have earned the respect and trust of their coworkers. Staff will follow their lead. The use of a physician champion is an especially useful strategy for engaging physicians in an initiative. Senior leadership and sponsors must also be engaged, especially financially, but are not as effective at the microsystem level as a unit champion.

60. A team approach utilizing the integration of many different roles working toward common patient and family goals describes the objective of which type of team:

    A. Multidisciplinary team

    B. **Interdisciplinary team**

    C. Patient advocacy team

    D. Care coordination team

B: An interdisciplinary team is composed of many disciplines that all gather together at the same time to work toward a common patient and family goal, such as discharge coordination.

61. Individual consults by many different health disciplines represent which type of approach:

    A. **Multidisciplinary**

    B. Interdisciplinary

    C. Team

    D. Intradisciplinary

A: A multidisciplinary approach is composed of individual consults, occurring independently of each other. Typically the disciplines do not meet to work toward a common goal as in an interdisciplinary approach.

62. In order to generate ideas aimed at designing an implementation plan, a team reviews the topic and members verbalize solution ideas in a random fashion. This is an example of which of the following strategies:

    A. Multivoting

    B. Process mapping

    C. **Brainstorming**

    D. Nominal group technique

C: Brainstorming is creative, interactive, and unstructured, as team members suggest possible ideas in a free-flow format without regard to the details of the suggested solutions.

63. Your unit has worked hard to maintain a very low fall rate. There has now been a sharp increase over the last 2 months. In looking at control chart data related to falls, you see that all of these falls occur on the night shift. What is the most likely reason for this shift?

A. A common cause

B. **A special cause**

C. A coincidence

D. A trend

B: A special cause occurs outside of a stable process and is attributed to a factor that is not commonly part of the process. The CNL would need to investigate whether there are special circumstances that are present on the night shift that have resulted in the increasing number of falls.

64. From which database would the CNL collect the most useful nursing-sensitive indicator metrics?

A. **NDNQI**

B. Hospital Compare

C. TJC

D. NQF

A: The NDNQI (National Database of Nursing Quality Indicators) evaluates unit and hospital-specific nursing-sensitive data. NDNQI also provides benchmarks that can be used for comparison.

65. What is the appropriate ending point of a root cause analysis (RCA)?

A. When several possible reasons for the error have been identified

B. When staff have identified what they think is the reason for the error

C. **When the list of causes is exhausted to no more possible causes**

D. The CNL can identify reasons for occurrence

C: When performing an RCA, the CNL must ask "why to saturation," or until there are no more contributing root causes. This often consists of asking why five or more times.

66. When is an RCA performed?

A. Prior to the initiation of a new treatment to anticipate possible problems

B. During a process to evaluate ongoing problems

C. As part of data analysis to understand why an intervention led to poor results

D. **After a serious safety event has occurred**

D: An RCA is performed as a way to gain insight into the factors that led to a serious safety event. It is a reactive activity with the intention of proactively designing solutions to processes that led to a problem.

67. Your unit has recently been relocated to the new hospital wing. This area is more spacious and modern than the unit's previous environment. Patient satisfaction scores in the area of "physical environment of care" have improved significantly. The added distance that staff must walk to answer call lights has resulted in decreased patient satisfaction scores in the area of "Call bell answered immediately." Based on this, the hospital budget was realigned to build

an additional nurses station at the midpoint of the unit. What is the relationship between these two measures?

A. Confounding measures

B. **Balancing measures**

C. Opposing measures

D. Concurrent measures

B: Balancing measures demonstrate whether improvement in one area is at the expense of another area. When designing initiatives and improvements, it is important to achieve a balance among all areas. Organizational balancing measures are aligned with strategic goals.

68. Your geriatric unit shows the highest average restraint episode duration in the hospital. You have been asked to lead an improvement project to reduce duration. What would be your first step?

A. Obtain national restraint episode duration benchmark data

B. **Conduct a full assessment of your unit, including all restraint-related data and processes**

C. Conduct a literature search to obtain current best practices for geriatric patients in restraints

D. Speak with staff and leadership of other units with lower restraint episode durations

B: A unit assessment should be performed first. This allows the CNL to see current process and how this compares to best practices found in the literature and other units.

69. What is the purpose of a fishbone diagram?

A. **To identify the cause and effect of multiple factors that lead to a result**

B. To identify the root cause of a serious safety event

C. To aid in the development of an improvement project timeline

D. To create the goals and objectives of an improvement project

A: A fishbone diagram, also known as an Ishikawa diagram, is a visual display of the multiple causes and effects of any problem.

70. Nurses on your unit have complained that equipment kept on the unit is not readily available. They have indicated that it often takes a considerable amount of time to locate. You realize that this is a waste of valuable human work resources. An effective process to utilize in solving this problem is the _____ principle.

A. 5P

B. SIPOC

C. FMEA

D. **5S**

D: The 5S (sort, set in order, shine, standardize, and sustain) LEAN technique can be used to organize equipment, resulting in an orderly workplace. "A place for everything and everything in its place."

71. A process improvement project charter or establishment of specific aims can help a project group to avoid which difficulty:

    A. **Scope creep**

    B. Meeting time confusion

    C. Budget constraints

    D. Team communication problems

A: Scope creep occurs when a group identifies an additional problem that may need fixing. A clear project charter defines the goal, objectives, and scope of the original project and will help the team not to divert its attention to other issues.

72. You have been charged with examining the heart failure 30-day readmission rate of your unit. In doing so, it is important for you to examine data from what other sources:

    A. National and state readmission rates

    B. National benchmarks

    C. Readmissions to other units in your hospital

    D. **All of the above**

D: The 30-day readmission rates are a key factor in CMS reimbursement rates to hospitals. A CNL should have a broad perspective of readmission rates across multiple settings. The CNL can then resource share with other areas to gain insight into best practices and pre-existing initiatives at the microsystem, hospital, state, and national levels.

73. One of the nurses on your unit was involved in a medication error. She revealed the error to both you and the nurse manager and documented the error in the online safety event reporting system. You meet with her and begin the process of identifying causes that led to this event, so the risk for future medication errors can be minimized. As evidenced by these actions, what is the culture of your hospital?

    A. A laissez-faire culture

    B. **A just culture**

    C. A punitive culture

    D. A structural culture

B: A just culture recognizes that humans are fallible, and errors may happen in systems that are flawed. A nonpunitive culture fosters patient safety principles, encouraging practitioners to report errors and near misses, which in turn enables organizations to address and correct flawed processes and systems. Errors that result from willfully negligent behavior are not a part of a just culture.

74. You are working with a team to reduce patient waiting time for transport to diagnostic imaging. An effective goal would be to:

A. Decrease waiting time during the evening shift

B. Increase monthly patient satisfaction

C. Improve communication between the ED and the DI departments

D. **Decrease the waiting time for diagnostic imaging by 5%**

D: Improvement goals must be specific and measurable. The team must have clear, measurable results to indicate whether an implementation resulted in improvement.

75. When conducting a literature review, the publication that would provide a comprehensive summary of research on that topic would be:

A. Nonexperimental

B. Experimental

C. Case study

D. **Meta-analysis**

D: A meta-analysis includes an analysis of multiple studies on that topic.

76. When incorporating evidence-based practice interventions into your health care setting, it would be best to:

A. Do what everyone else is doing

B. Do what you think would work in your setting

C. **Choose the interventions you think would work for your setting and perform a rapid cycle test to evaluate the impact**

D. Do everything the literature suggests to improve your chances of a good outcome

C: Incorporating evidence-based practice and then performing rapid cycle tests will give you feedback on whether the changes are working well in your setting.

77. All of the following are steps of evidence-based practice except:

A. Integrating evidence with clinical expertise, patient preferences, and values when making a decision or change

B. Asking the question in a PICO format

C. **Obtaining informed consent from patients involved in the practice change**

D. Critically appraising the evidence

C: Evidence-based practice changes do not require patient consent.

78. You are trying to encourage nurses on your unit to become more active in utilizing research in practice and to learn more about evidence-based practice. What would be a good activity to promote your idea?

A. Leave a few nursing journals on the unit

B. Make a point of discussing research articles you have read with nurses on the unit

C. **Form a journal club on the unit**

D. E-mail the nurses articles to read

C: This will encourage the nurses to read articles relevant to their practice and to evaluate them critically.

79. What type of study would not be included in evidence-based practice if the nurses were looking for quantitative research?
    A. Meta-analysis
    B. Experimental
    C. Quasi-experimental
    D. **Phenomenological**

D: Phenomenological studies are qualitative research that is not directly included in evidence-based practice.

80. In assessing your organization for evidence-based practice environmental readiness, you would evaluate all of the following except:
    A. Do advance practice nurse and educators model evidence-based practice?
    B. **Are the nurses expressing an interest in evidence**-based practice?
    C. Are the librarians available to assist nurses with evidence-based practice research?
    D. Are computers readily accessible to staff?

B: The organization is assessing environmental readiness, not interest.

81. Strategies for advancing evidence-based practice in health care settings include:
    A. Skill-building workshops
    B. Evidence-based practice poster presentations
    C. Evidence-based practice rounds
    D. **All of the above**

D: All of these are good strategies for promoting evidence-based practice.

82. You are considering using a new type of Foley catheter in your setting when the sales representative mentions a study that the manufacturer conducted that showed a reduction of catheter-associated infections with the use of the new device. Which type of study would be most convincing of this new product's potential value:
    A. Case study
    B. **Randomized controlled trial**
    C. Expert opinion
    D. Nonrandomized controlled trial

B: This type of study would provide the highest level of evidence.

83. In an effort to reduce central line infections, you have done some research and found evidence-based guidelines that you would like to implement at your organization. Your next step would be to:
    A. Gather data regarding central line infection rates at your institution
    B. **Convene a team meeting to discuss the problem and impact of central** line infections

C. Run a PDSA of the new guidelines

D. Share what you have found with the manager

B: The team needs to be involved in the whole change process.

84. You have evaluated the fall rate for the previous 12 months on the medical–surgical unit where you work as a CNL. You find that your fall rate is above the national benchmark. Your next step is to:

A. Implement a new fall prevention tool

B. Review the literature

C. **Review current hospital policy and find out what fall prevention strategies are currently being used on the unit**

D. Assemble a team from the unit to brainstorm ideas to reduce the fall rate

C: A CNL needs to know what the current policy and processes are before making changes and improvements.

85. You have reviewed the most recent pressure ulcer prevalence data for your unit. Although your unit's pressure ulcer rates are below national benchmarks, they have been steadily climbing over the past year. Your next step should be to:

A. Make sure you assess all patients' skin daily

B. **Schedule brief in-services for the staff on the unit to review the pressure ulcer prevention policy and strategies**

C. Evaluate the pressure ulcer prevention policy

D. Assess the bed surface on your unit

B: Sometimes simply reviewing policy and strategies with staff will help them remember what they need to do.

86. The manager of the medical unit where you work has just shared some data with you. She is concerned because the 30-day readmission rate for COPD patients is 15%. Your next step should be to:

A. Schedule a meeting with the staff to discuss the problem

B. **Compare your hospital's 30-day readmission rate with other like hospitals on the CMS website**

C. Perform a literature review in preparation for making changes to the current COPD pathway at your hospital

D. Monitor the data over the next 6 months to see if there really is a problem

B: A CNL should find out what this number means before you can act on it.

87. You have done some research and found a new fall prevention tool that you would like to trial on your unit. The tool was recently developed and tested at a large city hospital with a population of open heart patients. You are not sure that this tool can be effectively implemented in your small community hospital. You are questioning the tool's:

A. Relative risk

B. **External validity**

C. Transportability

D. Causal association

B: External validity is the degree to which the results of the original study are applicable to a population other than the one initially targeted.

88. A patient who has been diagnosed with colon cancer remarks that since his diagnosis, many people he knows have mentioned someone they know who has colon cancer. Most of these people live nearby. The patient asks you if colon cancer rates in the area have been increasing recently. The patient is asking about what type of measure:

    A. **Incidence**

    B. Prevalence

    C. Mortality

    D. Correlation

A: This would measure the number of new cases of colon cancer in the area during a specific period.

89. Your hospital has just completed a study comparing outcomes in rehospitalization rates for CHF patients who either received predischarge teaching from an APRN with those who received predischarge teaching from an RN. In the analysis of data, what resulting p-value would indicate that the intervention had a significant result?

    A. **<.05**

    B. <0.8

    C. <.10

    D. <.22

A: A value less than 0.05 is a significant statistical finding in research.

90. You are trying to reduce admission time to your unit from the emergency department. You have completed several PDSA cycles and have reduced the time by 21 minutes. But in the most recent PDSA, the time actually increased by 6 minutes. What stage of the PDSA cycle should the team go to in order to plan the next steps?

    A. Act

    B. Plan

    C. Do

    D. **Study**

D: The information at this stage should tell you where the barriers are.

91. A patient admitted to the hospital in hypertensive crisis is now receiving care at what level of prevention:

    A. Primary

    B. Secondary

    C. **Tertiary**

    D. None of these

C: The patient already has a severe medical problem that now requires treatment; this is tertiary level of prevention focused on maximizing the patient's health, despite the presence of illness.

92. Vaccinations are considered what level of prevention:
    A. **Primary**
    B. Secondary
    C. Tertiary
    D. None of these

A: Vaccinations are preventative and therefore considered primary level of prevention.

93. Patient satisfaction scores on your unit have declined over the last quarter. There are several new nurses on the unit. You suspect that the novice nurses may be contributing to this decline in satisfaction scores. What would be a good strategy to address the issue?
    A. **Schedule a group education session with the new nurses to discuss patient satisfaction**
    B. Have the novice nurse shadow an experienced nurse for the day
    C. While doing patient rounds, apologize for the number of new nurses on the unit
    D. Hang signs around the unit reminding staff that patient satisfaction is the goal

A: This will ensure that the novice nurse gets the correct information regarding patient satisfaction. It will also allow time to discuss specific ways to improve patient satisfaction and at the same time provide a safe environment for the novice nurses to express his or her feelings on the topic.

94. In your role as a CNL, you have implemented some practice changes on your unit that have resulted in an overall reduced LOS for the pneumonia patients. The cost savings will be reflected in which budget:
    A. **Operating budget**
    B. Capital budget
    C. Cash-flow budget
    D. Long-term budget

A: The operating budget reflects the revenue and expenses for the nursing unit. Capital budget refers to larger purchases that may be planned over long periods.

95. The manager on the unit where you work really encourages the staff to learn and grow professionally as individuals and as a group. Several of the staff have earned advanced degrees and moved onto other roles in the hospital. Her goals always seem to be aligned with the organization's vision. This is what type of leadership style:
    A. Charismatic leadership
    B. Relational leadership

C. **Transformational leadership**

D. Transactional leadership

C: Transformational leadership style focuses on change in the organization through a commitment to its vision.

96. The type of care delivery system where the nurse assumes 24-hour responsibility for patient care from admission through discharge is known as:

A. **Primary nursing**

B. Functional nursing

C. Case management

D. Total patient care

A: Primary care is a type of care delivery in which the nurse is responsible for the planning, directing, and evaluating patient care 24 hours a day.

97. Medicaid covers which population:

A. Employed

B. Underinsured

C. Unemployed

D. **Poor and disabled**

D: Medicaid is a publicly funded insurance provided to the poor and disabled in each state.

98. Currently Medicare is moving from a fee-for-service model to a:

A. Managed care model

B. **Pay-for-performance model**

C. Private insurance model

D. Advantage care model

B: Increasingly Medicare is adjusting reimbursement rates to providers on the basis of their patient outcomes.

99. Which most demonstrates advocacy toward a patient?

A. Led interdisciplinary rounds on a group of patients

B. **Consulted a diabetic instructor for a patient who was found to have an HgB A1C of 13.1**

C. Met with the trauma team of physicians to update patient plans of care

D. Conducted an in-service with the nursing staff on how to reduce falls for the unit

B: This is an example of a specific action by the CNL to improve care on a particular patient.

100. To be culturally competent as a clinical nurse leader is best found to be an example of which form of nursing leadership?

A. Lateral integration of care services

B. Horizontal leadership

C. **Advocacy**

D. Vertical leadership

C: An effective advocacy is needed during assessment, intervention, evaluation, and teaching to use cultural competence for communication to be effective.

101. Which clinical nurse leader role from the White Paper best describes advocacy?

    A. Delegating and managing the care team

    B. Using appropriate teaching strategies when teaching clients

    C. **Making sure that patients and families are well informed**

    D. Using information to achieve the best outcomes for patients

C: As clearly defined in the White Paper, the CNL makes sure he or she is informed to be a resource for patients, families, and the interdisciplinary team.

102. Which of the following is a demonstration of how the CNL can be an effective use of self through routine presence?

    A. **Develops a therapeutic alliance**

    B. Uses the most up-to-date technology

    C. Monitors the environment

    D. Provides a comprehensive health assessment

A: By being a constant presence with the patient, the CNL is able to gain better access to the patient.

103. In what way can the CNL serve as an advocate for the patient through other nurses?

    A. Delegate to other members of the profession

    B. **Serve as an advocate for the profession of nursing**

    C. Advocate for the staff to have better hours

    D. Research best practice methods for your unit

B: As an advocate for your profession, you can foster a sense of commitment to learning on your unit and with your staff.

104. Which method of payment accounts for only 5% of the U.S. population?

    A. Out-of-pocket payments

    B. Employment-based private insurance

    C. Government financing

    D. **Individual private insurance**

D: As depicted in health policy books.

105. What is considered to be the highest form of knowledge worker?

    A. Data gatherer

    B. **Knowledge builder**

    C. Knowledge user

    D. Information user

B: Nurses will transition from knowledge users to knowledge builders when they can examine data and trends across patient groups.

106. Which level depicts a nurse with basic computer technology skills?

    A. Informatics innovator

    B. Experienced nurse

    C. **Beginning nurse**

    D. Informatics nurse specialist

C: Beginning nurses have been defined as nurses with basic computer skills such as e-mail, Internet use to locate data, and patient monitoring systems.

107. Which is *not* considered an activity of daily living necessary for coverage by insurance?

    A. Bathing

    B. Dressing

    C. Taking medications

    D. **Going to the park**

D: The other three are necessary for daily life functions.

108. Which group represents the single largest health profession in the United States?

    A. **Registered nurses**

    B. Physicians

    C. Nursing assistants

    D. Clinical case managers

A: As depicted in health policy books.

109. B.F. is a 52-year-old female recently placed with palliative care. She is transferred to another unit with a specific palliative care section. How is this demonstrative of advocacy?

    A. Works between the patients and the health care team to deliver care

    B. **Ensures that the system meets the needs of the population**

    C. Advocates for the professional nurse

    D. Applies ethics toward patient care

B: Makes sure the patient is placed where the most optimal outcomes and care can be delivered.

110. All of the following are found to be an effective use of self except:

    A. Managing group processes

    B. Communicating with other disciplines

C. **Dictating to other staff**

D. Negotiating

C: Delegating is a role, never dictating.

111. While admitting a patient to the unit after a car accident, the patient informs you that she has been off her psych meds Seroquel and Celexa due to the cost and no longer has a doctor. As an advocate, you would talk with the physician in hopes of obtaining what two consults?

    A. Medicine and clinical case manager

    B. **Psychiatry and social worker**

    C. Clinical case manager and social worker

    D. Medicine and psychiatry

B: Without a physician to monitor the results of the patient withdrawing herself from these two medicines, the result could be detrimental. This consult can also help get the patient back with a psychiatrist upon discharge. The social worker would assist with any social issues upon discharge, such as affording medications.

112. The CNL is performing rounds with the physician team on a patient that has a chest tube placed for a collapsed lung. Which is a priority in telling the medical team first?

    A. The patient has continued pain where the chest tube was placed

    B. There is no diet ordered for this patient

    C. **The patient's incentive spirometer results decreased from 1,500 to 750**

    D. The patient complains of a sore throat

C: With a chest tube placed, there is already a decrease in lung capacity; a decrease in the results of incentive spirometer use could be a signal the lung trauma is worsening.

113. Which of these actions can a clinical nurse leader take to help protect a patient admitted for suicide?

    A. Call to have a screen placed on the window

    B. Call dietary to have only plastic utensils delivered on meal trays

    C. Move the patient close to the nursing desk for more frequent monitoring

    D. **Order a psych consult**

D: It is out of the nursing scope of practice to order a physician consults. The CNL may call and ask a physician to do this.

114. A patient is admitted to the unit postoperative fixation of the femur. What is a priority for the clinical nurse leader?

    A. Make sure a diet is ordered post-op

    B. **Make sure the physician addressed or filled out the venous thrombosis embolism or VTE sheet with type and time of anticoagulation**

    C. Make sure the family in the waiting room knows where the patient is

    D. Place the phone near the patient

B: The CNL acts as an advocate for the patient in making sure anticoagulation is addressed on a patient at a severe risk for a DVT or PE.

115. C.W. is a 92-year-old male who is a do-not-resuscitate (DNR). There is no family to visit this patient, and the patient's status has declined over the past 24 hours. The patient's breathing is labored and the physician tells the staff there is nothing else to do. What is an effective use of the CNL?

    A. Spend time talking with staff on their views of the dying process

    B. Call bed management and let them know there will be a bed available soon for a postoperative patient

    C. **Consult pastoral care to come with the patient**

    D. Call dietary and tell them to stop bringing the patient food

C: It is within the scope of practice of nursing to get pastoral care involved.

116. A Korean patient is admitted who speaks little English. An example of culturally competent care is:

    A. Finding a nurse who speaks some Korean

    B. Transferring that patient to a floor that has a Korean-speaking secretary

    C. Calling the patient's family to see if they speak any English

    D. **Obtaining a Korean translator**

D: The translator is the most effective way to deliver culturally competent care, the admission will be complete, the staff will be able to accurately assess the patient, and dietary staff will be able to find out any specific dietary concerns the patient may have.

117. What part of the interdisciplinary team is most important postoperative day 1 from a knee replacement?

    A. **Physical therapy**

    B. Speech therapy

    C. Dietary

    D. Financial counselor

A: It is pivotal for the patient to be getting out of bed and working on mobilization after any extremity surgery.

118. M.L. is a 42-year-old female admitted for domestic violence and being shot by her husband. Which is a priority at this time?

    A. Inform the social worker of the situation

    B. **Place the patient under an alias name with her permission**

    C. Inform the police

    D. Call the domestic violence nurse

B: At this point, the first thing to do is make sure the patient is safe in the hospital and that involves placing her under an alias name, so no one can find her.

119. An example of true advocacy is:
    A. Telling dietary staff if the patient has any concerns with her food
    B. Calling a patient's family to give them updates on a patient's health
    C. **Establishing goals to promote patient health**
    D. Performing handoff communication at change of shift

C: Per a definition in the exam handbook, advocacy is identifying any health problems and working toward their improvement.

120. As a member of the interdisciplinary team, the CNL is effective in all the following except:
    A. Maintaining and updating the plan of care
    B. Collaborating with other members of the team for the care delivery
    C. Delegating to other staff
    D. **Taking charge of all patient care**

D: The CNL is a member of a team and never is in charge; the interdisciplinary team is a process that involves multiple people, not just one.

121. While admitting a patient for COPD, a nurse notices the patient has had two other admissions this month for the same diagnosis and is homeless. A key part of this admission is:
    A. **Consult a social worker on admission**
    B. Notify the physician
    C. Consult a clinical case manager upon discharge
    D. Consult financial counseling

A: As a CNL, it is imperative to notice any reoccurring admissions and patterns—the social worker will be able to start working with the patient on day 1 for supportive services, to help the patient decrease the chance of this happening again.

122. D.M. is admitted for a hip fracture, a fall from standing. As a clinical nurse leader, you would know such a fracture obtained this way is best found from what?
    A. Osteomyelitis
    B. **Osteoporosis**
    C. Anemia
    D. Rheumatoid arthritis

B: A fracture of the hip from a fall from standing is indicative of osteoporosis. It is imperative for clinical nurse leaders to identify such patterns to help the patient get a holistic plan of care.

123. B.L. is a 91-year-old male who was transferred to a skilled nursing facility from an acute care hospital. Upon transfer, the patient's Lasix for CHF was not transferred with the patient. Once the medication error is found and re-started, it is the CNL's job to:

    A. Notify the hospital of the error

    B. Notify the skilled nursing facility of the error

    C. **Go back through all pathways and find where the error in this transfer process occurred**

    D. Notify the family

C: Correcting processes that yield errors and negative outcomes for patients is a critical duty of the CNL.

124. A new graduate RN who recently got out of orientation approaches you, the clinical nurse leader (CNL). One of her patient's physicians wrote an order to place an NG tube. The RN has not done this since nursing school and asks for your help. How do you respond?

    A. Tell her to ask the charge nurse, as this is not one of your CNL roles and you really do not have time at the moment

    B. **Direct her to get the policy and procedure guidelines, review it, assemble the needed supplies, and then you will review it with her and assist her with placing the NG tube**

    C. Direct her to review the policy and procedure guidelines, assemble the needed supplies, and ask an available LPN to assist her with placing it

    D. Review the order, gather the needed supplies, and have her watch you place the NG tube, as she has not done it before as an RN

B: As the clinician team manager, one of your roles is to be a resource for your team, especially for new graduate RNs. From the AACN's White Paper, the CNL designs, implements, and evaluates client care by coordinating, delegating, and supervising the care provided by the health care team, including licensed nurses, technicians, and other health professionals.

125. As you, the CNL, are reviewing one of your patient's charts, you notice that he recently tested positive for methicillin-resistant *Staphylococcus aureus* (MRSA) in his open wound. He has been in the hospital for 2 days, and as far as you can tell, this result has not been addressed. You bring the result to the attention of the primary nurse, who says that the night shift nurse told her about that, but no one has had a chance to "deal with it" since each nurse has six or seven patients. How do you respond?

    A. Tell the nurse you understand how busy she is, and to please make it a priority to "deal with" as soon as possible for patient safety

    B. Tell the nurse you understand how busy she is, and offer to call the physician yourself as well as place the patient on contact precautions

    C. **Ensure the nurse knows why this is a priority, especially since she does have so many other patients, and help her to make time to notify the physician as well as immediately place the patient on contact precautions**

D. Notify the charge nurse so that he may either take the needed steps himself or delegate it to another available nurse

C: MRSA is essential to identify upon admission and implement appropriate precautions so that it does not spread to other patients.

126. You are the CNL on a busy high-risk antepartum unit. One of the nurses comes to you because she is "sick of dealing with a noncompliant patient." The nurse tells you the patient is refusing all of her treatments, including fetal monitoring, vital signs, and insulin administration, and she cannot bear to take care of the patient who does not even care about her baby. What do you do?

    A. Tell the nurse you understand how she feels, but as the nurse, she is going to have to deal with it, at least until the end of her shift. All patients deserve excellent nursing care, even difficult, noncompliant patients

    B. Ask the nurse what has happened between her and the patient, as she was not acting like that previously

    C. Take the issue to the charge nurse and have the nurse's assignment changed so that another nurse may take care of this patient

    D. **Go into the patient's room and ask her if you may talk. Sit down with the patient and try to understand what is going on and why she is refusing all of her treatments**

D: Sometimes patients refuse treatments when they are feeling out of control or have other issues going on. Sitting down and talking with the patient one-on-one can often unwrap many issues.

127. One of your patients, a widow, is reaching end of life. The physician has adamantly suggested to the patient's family to plan for death and to make the decision to remove life support, as he feels it is futile at this point and most likely causing more agony to the patient. The patient has three children, and they cannot agree on a decision. The oldest daughter feels that they should abide by the doctor, as he knows best. The middle child does not agree with "killing" his mother. The youngest child just wants to be with her mother and cannot make a decision. You decide the best thing to do now is hold a patient-care conference. Whom do you invite?

    A. **The family, the team of physicians, the primary nurse, the case manager, the chaplain, an ethics committee member, and the social worker**

    B. The family, the team of physicians, the primary nurse, the nurse manager, the chaplain, the respiratory therapist, and the nutritionist

    C. The team of physicians, the primary nurse, the nurse manager, the case manager, the chaplain, an ethics committee member, and the social worker

    D. The team of physicians, the primary nurse, the chaplain, the respiratory therapist, and the nutritionist

A: The family/patient is a necessity for a patient-care conference; the team of physicians will be able to talk about the patient's prognosis and medical care; the primary nurse can address how the patient is responding/doing on a daily basis; the case manager and social worker can help the family with funeral/end-of-life planning; the chaplain can be a support to the family and even the staff; and an ethics committee member can ensure that an ethical decision is being made.

128. Nurse Alice, whom you work with on a busy antepartum unit, comes to you one Monday morning because she does not agree with one of her patient's medical management. The patient, who is $35\frac{5}{7}$ weeks' gestation, has been NPO (nothing by mouth) since Friday at midnight. She was supposed to have a repeat cesarean section Friday morning for mild preeclampsia and has demonstrated positive lung maturity via an amniocentesis. However, the labor and delivery unit is extremely busy and short staffed due to an outbreak of influenza. The patient is getting upset because she was told she was going to have her baby on Friday and is "sick of being pregnant and is starving." Alice says she talked to the physician on Sunday about it and was told that the patient just needs to be patient. You, the CNL, take these next steps:

   A. Tell Alice you understand how she feels, but since she already spoke with the physician, the team needs to work together and respect the physician's order. You talk with the patient and explain why she needs to continue to be NPO, and hopefully it will not be much longer

   B. **Call the labor and delivery charge nurse to discuss this patient and see when she will be able to get delivered. You are told it will be this evening at the earliest, so you call the physician and get a diet ordered for this morning, and return to NPO status after lunch with IV fluids to start when NPO. You share this plan with Alice and the patient**

   C. Call the labor and delivery charge nurse and demand that this patient be delivered this morning, as she is preeclamptic and has been waiting since Friday

   D. Find out that the patient most likely will not be delivered today, and if so it will be late tonight. You allow the patient to eat breakfast and a light, early lunch, returning to NPO afterward. Alice and the patient agree with and are happy about this plan of care

B: Discussing the patient with the labor and delivery charge nurse will let her know the urgency of getting this patient delivered, and will let you know realistically when that will happen. You can then call the physician with exact timing information, and the physician should agree to allow the patient to eat since delivery will not be within the next 8 hours. Also, once you call the physician and report the situation, he should agree to start IV fluids.

129. You are the CNL on a busy medical–surgical unit. One of your patients, Mr. Thompson, a Type 2 diabetic, has been on your unit for 5 days following a right foot amputation due to necrosis. He has been on IV antibiotics and has now been afebrile for 24 hours. Mr. Thompson, 67 years old, lives alone, but his son lives two miles away and says he will be able to check on his dad at least daily once he is discharged home. In preparation for discharge, you realize Mr. Thompson will need someone to assist him with his dressing changes and to check his vital signs for several days. You think he will also need outpatient physical therapy. You discuss with the physician your

thoughts on discharging Mr. Thompson home with home health. The physician agrees with your plan of care, so you consult the case manager to set up home health and outpatient physical therapy. You also consult with the physical therapist for recommendations on home needs. You assist with making follow-up appointments for Mr. Thompson. Mr. Thompson is able to be discharged home the next day. This is an example of which CNL role?

A. **Lateral integration of care**

B. Risk anticipation

C. Management and use of client-care and information technology

D. Clinical decision making

A: Lateral integration of care involves the delivering and coordination of care using a multidisciplinary approach.

130. Because you are the CNL on a postsurgical unit, staff are regularly bringing you new ideas and questions about current treatment regimens. Today two nurses come to you with conflicting ideas. One nurse, Rachel, says that she will not allow her patients to have anything PO except for clear liquids post-surgery until they are passing flatus. She says that she has worked on this unit for 20 years and that the more experienced doctors support this thought. Tom, a newer nurse of 2 years, says he was taught that patients may eat and drink whatever they want post-op as long as they have positive bowel sounds and are not nauseous. They want to know "who is right." In response, you:

A. Tell them they are both right, depending on the patient, and it is up to the physician's orders

B. Tell them that is a great question, and instruct them to both do research on the topic, bring it back to you, and you will help them take their information forward for a potential practice change

C. Thank them for bringing up such an important question, and tell them you do not know the answer. Guide them to discuss this with the physicians

D. **Assist them in researching this topic in research and evidence-based articles, and evaluate the information. Bring your findings to the unit staff and physicians and come to an agreement on the best practice**

D: As the CNL, a big part of your role is to bring evidence-based practice and research to the bedside. However, you need to get the staff involved and not just do all of the work for them. Staff need to feel ownership.

131. You are the CNL on a busy medical unit. You get a new patient, Mrs. Garcia, admitted through the emergency department (ED) for abdominal pain. Mrs. Garcia is a 37-year-old Spanish-speaking woman. She has her 12-year-old son with her, who has been translating for the medical staff in the ED. Mrs. Garcia is clearly in a lot of pain, but you cannot give her any pain medications until she is admitted into the system. Your next steps are to:

A. Allow the son to translate enough to get Mrs. Garcia admitted so that you may give her some pain medications and then get an interpreter to complete her admission history

B. Ask Mrs. Garcia, through her son, if it is okay with her to use her son as the interpreter. You explain to her this will expedite her pain relief and she agrees

C. Request an interpreter to come as soon as possible and tell Mrs. Garcia through her son that you will make her comfortable as soon as possible. Notify the primary RN who will be caring for her

D. **Explain to Mrs. Garcia that you are unable to give her medicine until she is admitted and that you need an interpreter to admit her. You will give her medicine as soon as possible. You stay with Mrs. Garcia until the interpreter gets there, and try to help relieve her pain with other nonpharmaceutical therapies**

D: Establishes and maintains effective working relationships within an interdisciplinary team to make ethical decisions regarding the application of technologies and the acquisition of data; practice in collaboration with a multicultural workforce.

132. You, the CNL, work on an infectious disease unit in the hospital. Your patients tend to have long lengths of stays, sometimes weeks to months. During your 5Ps assessment, you discovered that the nursing staff is not satisfied with handoff communication. They feel like important information is often left out of report. As a leader of this team, the most appropriate next step would be to:

A. Create a new process based on evidence and implement it

B. **Assess the current communication handoff process**

C. Ask the nursing staff what they think would be the best way to give report

D. Bring this issue up at the next staff meeting

B: Before going any further, you need to collect data and assess the situation. Manage group processes to meet care objectives and complete health care team responsibilities.

133. You, the CNL, are putting an interdisciplinary group together to make improvements to your high falls rate. You are seeking members to be on this team. Carly, an RN, volunteers to be on this team. You and Carly have had many differences in the past and because of personality conflicts have not been able to work well together historically. What should you do?

A. **Thank Carly for volunteering, but politely tell her you will not be needing her for this particular team**

B. Allow Carly to be part of the team—your personal issues should not affect this group's progress

C. Invite Carly to be part of the team, but do not give her any major responsibilities

D. Tell Carly that you think it is best if the two of you just avoid each other

A: When choosing a team, you should avoid people with personal conflicts of interest, if possible.

134. One morning as you, the CNL, are walking into the nurses' lounge, you hear a lot of talk about a nurse who has called out sick that day. The nurses are griping about how this nurse *always* calls out, especially on Fridays. The best response is to:

    A. Sympathize with your team, saying you have no idea how she does not get in trouble or fired. This kind of behavior should not be tolerated

    B. Tell the nurses to stop talking about one of their teammates, especially in front of a new employee

    C. Listen to what the nurses are saying, and notify the manager to address it

    D. **Listen to what the nurses have to say, and then address that it is not our business to discuss someone else's personal life. That nurse's sick days and disciplinary action are up to that nurse and the manager. Ensure they have adequate staffing to make up for the sick call/help to adjust assignments**

D: It is good to show an empathetic ear, but it is not helpful for a team to speak badly about one of the teammates. Adequate staffing is a big concern for the team, so ensure that this is addressed.

135. You are the CNL on a postpartum unit. You have noticed that lately you have had an increased number of patients readmitted with wound infections. You know that the most appropriate next step is to:

    A. Perform a failure mode and effects analysis

    B. Ask the doctors why their patients are getting so many infections lately

    C. **Perform a root cause analysis**

    D. Consult the wound-ostomy care nurses

C: An RCA addresses a systems issue. It is a broad, retrospective qualitative process that looks past the individual to enable development of an overall action plan.

136. As the CNL on a medical–surgical unit, you are asked to participate in a root cause analysis of a group of sentinel events that have occurred recently throughout the hospital. Your team determines that a lack of effective communication in emergent situations is the root problem. Now what?

    A. **Lead the team in researching evidence-based practice improvements to implement a better way of communicating during emergencies**

    B. Submit your findings to the administration that assigned you this task

    C. Share the findings with the units that had these sentinel events and instruct them to come up with better, research-based communication techniques

    D. Take the findings directly to the individuals involved in the sentinel events and show them what they need to improve to prevent these adverse outcomes

A: Once you discover what the problem is, a solution needs to be created. This is something that should be nonpunitive and benefit the whole hospital. Focusing on individuals will not be beneficial to the big picture.

137. A medical equipment representative approaches you to incorporate his new product into your unit supplies. He tells you that this new device has been proven to be the best device in its arena to prevent DVTs. Preventing DVTs is one of your goals as the CNL on this medical–surgical unit. The price is only slightly higher than the current equipment you use now, but he says the research shows you will save money in the long run by preventing more DVTs. How do you go about getting this new device?

    A. Since you do not have any purchasing power as the CNL, you direct him to the director of the purchasing department

    B. You have the representative speak with your manager, since your manager must approve all items purchased for your unit

    C. You thank him for the information, but pass on the offer since it costs more than the equipment you currently use, and as a CNL you are only looking for cost-effective ventures

    D. **You perform your own research on the device and compare it with the equipment you have now. If it proves to be as good as the representative says it is, you will take it forward to administration**

D: Gathers, analyzes, and synthesizes data related to risk reduction and patient safety.

138. What is the best way for the CNL to analyze systems and outcome datasets to anticipate individual client risk and improve quality care?

    A. Perform a root cause analysis of all postoperative patients who have been readmitted to your unit within the last year

    B. **Perform a failure mode and effects analysis on all congestive heart failure patients on your unit within the last year**

    C. Implement the Systems Theory to evaluate individual risks to each patient population on your unit

    D. Utilize the Complexity Theory to make the needed changes to the defective systems

B: A FMEA is proactive and anticipates potential risks rather than looking back on events that have happened that need to be changed.

139. You work in the emergency department at a major public hospital. You have noticed that you see the same diabetic patients regularly. They are indigents and do not have primary care physicians. They never check their blood sugars at home because they do not have a glucometer, so by the time they get to the emergency department their blood sugars are well into the 300s and 400s. Usually the plan of care involves treating the blood sugars, instructing them to follow up at the clinic, and giving them a snack for the road. What would be a positive change in the plan of care from the CNL perspective?

    A. **Set up a program to give free glucometers to these patients who do not have one and schedule the follow-up appointment for them before they leave the emergency department, sending them home with information**

B. Admit the patients to the hospital so they can get instruction on diabetes care, including the diet, exercise, insulin administration, and blood glucose monitoring

C. Instruct the patients on where to purchase an inexpensive glucometer, and instruct them on the importance of checking their blood sugar regularly and making and keeping follow-up appointments

D. Incorporate diet teaching into their visit. Stress the importance of a diabetes-friendly diet, and send them home with a packet of information and a healthy snack

A: Understands economies of care, cost-effectiveness, resource utilization, effecting change in systems.

140. Of the following choices, what is the best way that you, the CNL, could have an environmentally positive impact?

A. Incorporate the importance of the environment into your teaching with each of your patients

B. **Institute a recycling program into your hospital**

C. When teaching patients and families, make sure they know how to properly dispose of their medical waste

D. Have patients start calling their physicians instead of going to their appointments to save on gas and time

B: Every hospital probably uses an extraordinary amount of products that could be recycled.

141. You are caring for Mrs. Jackson, a patient with congestive heart failure, on a cardiac unit. As you are looking through Mrs. Jackson's chart, you notice her last blood pressure was 188/110, following a blood pressure of 176/106. You see an order for labetalol 20 mg IV × 1 now written on her chart. What do you do now?

A. Find the primary nurse and make sure she has given the labetalol

B. Get an order for a second dose of the labetalol, as this first dose clearly has not been effective and Mrs. Jackson's blood pressure is rising

C. Verify Mrs. Jackson's allergies and the order and ensure the medication is on the unit ready to be given

D. **Get the order discontinued and make sure it has not been given**

D: Beta-blockers are contraindicated in patients with CHF.

142. You are caring for Sara, a 76-year-old grandmother recovering from heart failure. You know that she is ready to go home because:

A. Her ECG is normal, her pulse oximetry is normal, and she has a supportive family to help care for her at home

B. She tells you she is ready to go home

C. **You observe her ambulating in the hallway, free from dyspnea**

    D. She is free from dyspnea and fatigue, she has a follow-up appointment set up for the following Monday morning, her daughter said she can drive her to the appointment

C: HF symptoms are often not well evaluated, as clients remain relatively inactive while in the hospital. Activities such as walking in the hall provide an opportunity for objective evaluation of dyspnea, fatigue, and gait issues.

143. As the CNL, you know that one of the first steps in building a team is to:

    A. **Build trust**

    B. Assign roles to each member

    C. Designate a mission of the team

    D. Determine meeting times and locations

A: Building trust among different disciplines is a key first step to opening the lines of communication on a team.

144. You are working with your team to modify the unit's budget. You know that the best way to create a budget is:

    A. Looking at the previous budget's variance

    B. Requesting a large capital budget

    C. Being in line with your budget goal

    D. **Utilizing a case mix**

D: Case mix is the best way to create a budget. It looks at human and material costs and environmental resources.

145. You know that regulatory agencies' purpose is to:

    A. Stress out hospital employees

    B. **Decrease fragmentation and medical errors resulting in deaths**

    C. Give the public a source of standards for health care facilities

    D. Make the public feel safe and give them guidelines to follow with lawsuits

B: This is the definition.

146. A new health policy is being voted on in Congress. Your professional organization supports this policy and is recruiting nurses to go to Washington, DC, to help promote their view and to have a bigger voice. You do not support this policy. Your manager wants you to go as a leader and represent your unit. What should you do?

    A. You should go, as you need to stick together with your professional organization and yield to your manager

    B. **Learn more about the policy and why your organization supports it**

    C. You should politely decline, as you do not agree with the policy

    D. You should go, but rally against the policy since you do not agree with it. This is America and you are exercising your freedom of speech

B: You should know how your professional organization stands—we need to support each other and have one voice as nurses.

147. You want to do some research for a potential policy change. All of the following are excellent resources, except:

    A. Centers for Disease Control

    B. **Wikipedia**

    C. American Diabetes Association

    D. WebMD

B: This is NOT a validated site—anyone can post to this site.

148. As a CNL, what is your number one priority?

    A. Cost-effectiveness of care

    B. Improving quality of care

    C. **Patient safety**

    D. Decreasing fragmentation of care

C: This is directly from the White Paper.

149. Leah, a CNL on an obstetrical high-risk unit, looked at the evidence regarding women taking folic acid during pregnancy. Because it shows evidence to prevent neural tube defects in the fetus, she recommends this be included on the order set for antepartum patients. This is an example of which of the following:

    A. **Health promotion**

    B. Health literacy

    C. Qualitative review

    D. Quantitative analysis

A: Health promotion requires knowledge about health risks and methods to prevent or reduce these risks in individuals and populations.

150. Sam is a homeless 59-year-old male admitted with CHF. He arrives alone and crying. His vitals are BP = 173/96, HR = 83, O_2 = 86%, and temperature = 98.9°F. During your assessment, you notice multiple bruises and lacerations. His clothes are torn and soiled. According to Maslow's Hierarchy of Needs, what should you do first?

    A. Inquire about his bruises and lacerations

    B. Call the social worker regarding shelter placement

    C. Ask why he is crying

    D. **Apply oxygen**

D: According to Maslow's Hierarchy of Needs, physiological needs have to be met first, then safety, love/belonging, esteem and, finally, self-actualization.

151. Which of the following would not correlate with a major goal of Healthy People 2010?
    A. Providing free clinics for underprivileged children
    B. Educating a 76-year-old on smoking cessation
    C. **Implementing a unit to place all positive HIV patients**
    D. Designing a nutritious meal plan for school systems

C: Two major goals for Healthy People 2010 are to increase quality and years of healthy life and to eliminate health disparities. Although HIV is a focus area for Healthy People 2010, there is no rationale/evidence to have a specific unit in which to place these patients.

152. Tim is a 31-year-old admitted for pneumonia. During his hospitalization, you discovered he smokes cigarettes 1 ppd. You provided handouts on smoking cessation and gave him a helpline number. At discharge you made a follow-up appointment with his PCP for his pneumonia and smoking cessation. What did you forget to do?
    A. Ask
    B. **Advise**
    C. Assist
    D. Arrange

B: It is always important to advise people to stop smoking on each visit.

153. Marie's capstone project for her CNL immersion experience focused on wound infections and readmission rates. She conducted a literature review on the best way to provide education to surgical patients, reduce surgical infections, and prevent readmissions. On the basis of literature review and evidence-based practice, she developed a protocol for this patient population. What key principle did Marie use by incorporating this protocol?
    A. Team coordination
    B. **Risk reduction and prevention management**
    C. Lateral integration of care
    D. Information management

B: Marie uses evidence to keep an illness or injury from occurring early in its course and preventing further deterioration by focusing on health promotion, disease prevention, risk reduction, and prevention management.

154. Tim, a CNL in the clinic setting, begins seeing a lot more Hispanic patients with high blood pressure and/or diabetes and many with a lack of knowledge on nutrition. They often say someone in their family has the same problems. He knows the best way to educate them is to:
    A. Set aside extra time at each appointment to focus on education
    B. Set up educational posters at a local Hispanic supermarket
    C. **Set up a health fair with bilingual educators at a local highly populated park in a Hispanic neighborhood**

   D. Make up handouts to be given to patients at their appointments to take home

C: A health fair would reach the most people to educate and they feel comfortable in their own setting. Many clinics do not have extra time to make appointments longer, and many people do not even go to the clinic, so a health fair would reach the largest amount of people for this setting.

155. Marcia, a CNL, reviews the diet with a newly diagnosed gestational diabetic. She inquires about the patient's previous diet and habits, and after spending much time with the patient and asking questions, she discovers the patient eats a lot of fast food. She says she rarely has time to cook and has four kids who are always on the go. What should Marcia do?

   A. **Look up the nutritional information on the patient's favorite fast food places and pick out good food choices together with which she can be compliant**

   B. Tell her it does not really matter what she eats because she only has gestational diabetes

   C. Tell her she cannot eat fast food and give her another list of what she can eat

   D. Consult the dietician again to review her meal plan

 A: The patient confided in you and stated she is going to eat fast food. In order to help her be compliant with her meal plan and diet, it is best to help her make good food choices at the places she will be eating. It is important for the patient to follow a diabetic diet with gestational diabetes not only for her own health, but also for the well-being of the fetus.

156. A 6-year-old boy named Braden is a patient in your microsystem. He is terrified of the shots he has to get twice a day for the next 3 weeks. It is the most therapeutic medication and route for his illness. He becomes hysterical every time the medication is due and has to be held down by two people while the nurse gives the injection. They will not have three people at home to do this. Working on discharge planning, what should you do?

   A. Plan on Braden being in the hospital for the next 3 weeks to receive his injections

   B. Obtain restraints for the parents to use at home in order to give the injection

   C. Talk with the physician to prescribe a pill instead

   D. **Work with the child specialist and sit down with Braden to find out what scares him about the injections**

D: Working with the interdisciplinary team to provide the patient the best treatment is ideal. Encouraging the child to become involved in his care and letting him help enables him to cooperate and feel more secure.

157. A CNL on an orthopedic floor notices the legs on several of the walkers are not secure. She immediately calls medical equipment to replace the walkers on the floor and puts defective stickers on the current walkers. This is an example of:

A. Health promotion

B. **Injury prevention**

C. Health care informatics

D. Delegation

B: Providing safe care is one of the primary goals of the CNL, and this scenario prevented injury by ensuring safe equipment.

158. Jen is an obese patient admitted with COPD and CHTN. Part of her social history is that she smokes 2 ppd. Her CNL, Erika, makes a goal for her to decrease by one cigarette a day until there are no more by August 1. This goal will not work because:

A. There is not a measurable outcome

B. Jen should decrease by two cigarettes a day

C. The patient has COPD

D. **Jen should help make the goal**

D: In order for a goal to be effective and the patient to be compliant, it should be mutually set by the CNL and patient.

159. Elizabeth performed a CNL capstone project on group shift report. First she conducted a literature review and then developed new guidelines based on the research in the literature review. She measured the amount of time the report took prior to and after the change. This is an example of what type of research?

A. **Evidence-based practice**

B. Randomized control trial

C. Cohort

D. Ethnography

A: Looking at research and implementing changes based on the basis of findings and best practices is an example of evidence-based practice.

160. All of the following are components of evidence-based practice and clinical decision making except:

A. Clinical expertise

B. Information about patient preferences and values

C. **Research utilization**

D. Evidence from research and theories

C: Research utilization uses knowledge typically based on only one study, whereas EBP looks at evidence from research, evidence-based theories, opinion leaders/expert panels, evidence from patient assessment and history, clinical expertise, and information about patient preferences and values.

161. Pam, a CNL on a surgical unit, posted new evidence-based guidelines on preventing constipation in post-op patients. Pam notices an experienced nurse is

not following these guidelines correctly. She realizes this nurse is demonstrating what behavior?

A. Avoidance

B. Angry there are more changes

C. Lack of nursing competence

D. **Lack of knowledge**

D: One of the biggest barriers to health care providers failing to provide evidence-based care is lack of knowledge/familiarity with the guidelines and not having information on why the change is more effective.

162. Angela, a CNL, reviews RCTs on care for preterm labor patients. She discovers bedrest has not been proven to prolong pregnancy for preterm labor patients. This is typically ordered for all preterm labor patients at her facility. She posts her findings for the staff to review and gives an in-service to the nurses. Angela goes to the physicians to get the orders changed for her group of patients. What should Angela have done before implementing this change?

A. Look at case studies

B. **Meet with the interdisciplinary team to discuss protocols before initiating change**

C. Meet with the nurse manager to discuss the research

D. Look at more qualitative studies to get more information

B: Before making a big change, it is important to collaborate with an interdisciplinary team to get input from all disciplines to achieve better outcomes.

163. A patient care nurse, Kristin, comes to you about a new idea she has to provide better patient care. You agree this is a great idea. You should:

A. Research the latest evidence on this topic

B. Set up a meeting with the interdisciplinary team to discuss

C. Start implementing the change

D. **Encourage Kristin to take on this project**

D: As a leader, we should encourage others to get involved and help them be successful by providing support and knowledge using evidence-based practice.

164. Julie, a CNL, hears that another hospital does hourly rounding and thinks this is a great idea to reduce falls on her unit. She meets with her interdisciplinary team and they decide to try this on their unit. She informs the rest of the staff and makes a start date. What did Julie forget to do?

A. **Look at the latest evidence/literature review**

B. Ask her nurse manager

C. Ask other units if they do hourly rounding

D. Get data from the other hospital

A: When making a change, it is important to look at the EBP by performing a literature review and then decide whether there is sufficient evidence to make the change or whether there is not much literature on the topic to collect data to see if the change is effective.

165. According to the PICOT method to make a search for your clinical question, the "P" stands for:

    A. Processes

    B. **Population**

    C. Patterns

    D. Practice

B: The "P" in PICOT stands for the population/patients in the clinical question.

166. Carey, a CNL, thinks utilizing volunteers in a microsystem will benefit the staff and the patients. She performs a literature review and does not find much literature evaluating volunteers being effective in a health care setting. She decides to go ahead and implement a volunteer program and collects data to see whether this is an effective change. Should Carey have implemented this?

    A. No, there was no evidence volunteers would be beneficial

    B. No, she should have waited until there were data on this topic

    C. **Yes, if there is no literature on a topic, data should be collected to evaluate the change to see whether it is effective**

    D. Yes, it is always good to try something new

C: If sufficient literature/evidence is not found for a particular group, it can still be implemented if done correctly and if data are collected to see whether the change should continue or not.

167. You are trying to get literature on using music to relieve pain. One research article uses methods you forget how to interpret. You should:

    A. Not use this article

    B. Google the methods to try and figure it out

    C. Look at the conclusion and just use that information

    D. **Ask a mentor to assist you, so you understand the data**

D: It might be a valid study, so it is important to ask for assistance with understanding the data. Having mentors is important to maintain through your career.

168. What is the first essential key to implementing a change in a microsystem?

    A. **A clear vision of what outcomes are to be accomplished**

    B. A strategic plan

    C. Persistence on the change implementation to be successful

    D. Belief the change will be a success

A: A clear vision of what is to be accomplished by the change is the first element to a successful outcome. The others come after the vision is made.

169. Cassidy, a CNL at an outpatient setting, starts seeing an increase of Japanese patients. This is a culture she does not know much about and does not have very much educational materials to give to patients in this language. She goes online to valid websites and learns more about culture and their health care practices. She also discovers a site within her health care system that translates information and has handouts in 12 different languages. Cassidy demonstrated knowledge of:

    A. Team coordination

    B. Injury reduction

    C. **Health care informatics**

    D. Health care policy

C: Health care informatics applies using technology to improve patient care.

170. Many handouts are given to all the patients on admission to the hospital. The CNL notices many patients leave them or throw them away. She decides to make binders for all the rooms with laminated copies of the information and lets each patient know they can get a copy to take home if wanted. This CNL exhibited what concept?

    A. Health care informatics

    B. **Fiscal responsibility**

    C. Team coordination

    D. Health promotion

B: A lot of paper and ink was being wasted. This saved a lot of money and will continue to do so over time.

171. Chloe, a CNL, walks into a patient's room and notices she has labored respirations and is pale. She immediately takes her vitals and calls the patient care nurse. Her vitals are BP = 183/101, HR = 121, R = 28, T = 98.1, O_2 = 90%. What should Chloe do?

    A. Call the doctor

    B. Lay the patient down and recheck the VS in 30 minutes

    C. Give labetalol 20 mg IVP

    D. **Instruct the patient care nurse to call the doctor**

D: Delegate to the nurse to call the physician for further orders.

172. A 5Ps assessment was completed by each CNL in the hospital. As a CNL, you know this is an assessment of the:

    A. **Microsystem**

    B. Mesosystem

    C. Macrosystem

    D. Health care system

A: A 5Ps assessment is an analysis of the microsystem. It consists of analyzing the purpose, patients, professionals, processes, and patterns of the microsystem.

173. A patient asks the CNL about the regulations on abortion in North Carolina. What should the CNL do?

   A. Tell the patient you cannot answer that because it is an ethical situation

   B. Let the doctor know the patient is asking about abortion

   C. Inform the patient care nurse

   D. **Look up the regulations in North Carolina and share them with the patient**

D: Being able to look up policies and regulations is an important role of the CNL, along with educating patients. Giving the policy does not cross any ethical barriers, it is only providing facts.

174. A nurse approaches you and expresses her knowledge deficit regarding the difference between signs and symptoms of left- and right-sided heart failure. You explain the physiology between the two types of heart failure and identify which of the following as a primary symptom of right-sided heart failure?

   A. Shortness of breath on exertion

   B. Heart murmur and distended veins

   C. **Peripheral edema**

   D. Cool extremities and weak peripheral pulses

C: Peripheral edema. Right-sided heart failure leads to congestion of systemic capillaries. This generates excess fluid accumulation in the body and usually affects the dependent parts of the body first.

175. As a CNL you know that the most important nursing intervention to monitor a patient with CHF includes which of the following?

   A. Assessing the patient's knowledge of the disease

   B. Encouraging coughing and deep breathing

   C. Encouraging frequent ambulation

   D. **Monitoring fluid intake and output**

D: Monitoring fluid intake and output. In heart failure, the compensatory mechanisms cause the retention of fluid and sodium.

176. A nurse notifies you that her patient is complaining of chest pain. As you enter the room, the patient becomes unresponsive. Upon verification that a pulse is absent, the cardiac monitor reveals the patient is in ventricular fibrillation. The nurse begins CPR. As a CNL, you anticipate the need for which treatment next?

   A. Amiodarone (Cordarone)

   B. Labetolol (Normodyne)

   C. **Defibrillation**

   D. Cardiac catheterization

C: Defibrillation is the most effective treatment for ventricular fibrillation.

177. Your patient was recently diagnosed with non–small-cell cancer to the lung. Postradiation she reports to the nurse that she has a sore throat. The nurse approaches you indicating that he is unaware of what to do. You explain to the nurse that mucositis is a common side effect for patients receiving radiation treatment. What will you instruct the nurse to do next?

    A. **Assess the patient's oral mucosa for swelling and redness with ulcerations**

    B. Call the physician and obtain an order for an antiseptic mouthwash

    C. Instruct the patient to rinse her mouth before and after meals with a solution of salt and sodium bicarbonate

    D. Use a soft-bristled toothbrush to clean her teeth and tongue

A: Assess the patient's oral mucosa for swelling and redness with ulcerations. Swelling and redness with ulcerations in the oral mucosa are consistent with mucositis.

178. You are providing discharge instructions to a young patient with sickle cell anemia. What statement made by the patient would concern you most for the potential of this patient readmitting to the hospital?

    A. "I am scared about my pain being kept under control"

    B. **"I will need to find someone to take me to my hematology follow up appointment"**

    C. "My mother helps me manage my pain medicine"

    D. "I get tired throughout the day and often have to take naps"

B: "I will need to find someone to take me to my hematology follow-up appointment." Studies have shown that no outpatient hematology follow-up appointment within 30 days of hospitalization is the greatest risk factor for hospital readmission.

179. As a CNL you are educating a patient with type 1 diabetes mellitus about the potential advantages of an insulin pump. The patient has been frequently re-admitted with labile blood sugars although she has followed her prescribed insulin regimen of Lantus and Humalog. What is most important to emphasize on the benefits of an insulin pump?

    A. An insulin pump allows you to decrease the number of injections throughout the day

    B. An insulin pump will provide intermittent doses of insulin in response to the patient's blood sugar

    C. An insulin pump has the capability to read your blood sugars throughout the patients' waking hours

    D. **An insulin pump provides continuous doses of insulin around the clock as a basal rate that can be adjusted**

D: The pump provides continuous doses of insulin around the clock as a basal rate that can be adjusted. Lantus provides a consistent basal rate that does not respond to the body's needs for increased basal demands throughout the day. An insulin pump will provide the capability of increasing basal rates dependent on that patient's needs throughout the day.

180. You are caring for a patient who has suffered a cerebrovascular accident. The patient's daughter approaches you expressing that the patient has been frequently crying during her visits. What would be the best explanation to help the daughter cope with her mother's emotions?

    A. "I will call the doctor and get medication ordered for depression"

    B. **"Emotional responses may be unpredictable after a stroke"**

    C. "Your mother is dealing with her hospitalization and diagnosis appropriately"

    D. "Your mother may need an increased amount of family support during this difficult time"

B: "Emotional responses may be unpredictable after a stroke." Patients who have had a cerebrovascular accident may have difficulty controlling their emotions, which may be exaggerated or unrelated to surrounding events.

181. A nurse has called you into a room with a patient who is newly admitted to your unit with a diagnosis of urinary tract infection. The patient is 86 years old, and his vital signs reveal a temperature of 97.8°C, respiratory rate of 24, heart rate of 115, and blood pressure of 75/48. The nurse has called the doctor and has received orders to bolus that patient with IVF that the patient is currently receiving. The patient is becoming increasingly confused. What is the *most appropriate* response to delegate to the nurse while you stay with the patient?

    A. Recheck the vital signs in 15 minutes to ensure the blood pressure is rising

    B. Call the patient's family to obtain a full medical history

    C. **Ask the nurse to call the physician and notify him of the need to evaluate the patient for a higher level of care**

    D. Give the patient a prn dose of Ativan to help with the patient's confusion

C: Ask the nurse to call the physician and notify him of the need to evaluate the patient for a higher level of care. The patient is displaying signs of sepsis although temperature is normal. Temperature is an unreliable sign of infection in the elderly; however, increased respirations and heart rate, decreased blood pressure, and change in mental status indicate infection.

182. You are working in a unit that has recently seen an influx of patients with substance-related disorders. The nurses on the unit are complaining that frequently these patients are "drug seeking" and often signing out against medical advice in order to receive drugs elsewhere. What is an intervention that a CNL may implement to improve the treatment for this patient population?

    A. Educate the staff on not labeling the patients as "drug seekers" because they often require higher doses of pain medications to achieve an acceptable level of comfort

B. Provide an in-service to the staff about patients' withdrawal symptoms

C. Follow each patient that comes in with a diagnosis of a substance-related disorder in order to identify trends in mistreatment

D. **Research on whether the hospital uses an evidence-based tool that may help with the assessment of patients for alcohol addiction and/ or withdrawal**

D: Research on whether the hospital uses an evidence-based assessment tool that may help with the assessment of patients for alcohol addiction and/or withdrawal. Patients' withdrawal symptoms must be acknowledged and treated appropriately. Failure to do so may lead to noncompliance with medical and nursing care and/ or patient elopement.

183. You are reviewing a patient's morning laboratory values. The patient's hemoglobin has dropped from 12.5 to 7.3. The nurse has called the physician and received orders for two units of packed red blood cells to be transfused. The patient was admitted for diabetic ketoacidosis. What is the next step you should perform?

A. Research whether the patient has ever had a history of any anemia or gastrointestinal bleeding

B. **Assess the patient for any signs and/or symptoms of bleeding**

C. Call the physician and inform him to redraw the labs

D. Review the rest of the patient's laboratory values

B: Assess the patient for any signs and/or symptoms of bleeding. If the significant decrease in hemoglobin is unexpected and laboratory error is suspected, the clinician must first assess the patient to ensure no signs and/or symptoms of bleeding are present.

184. You are helping a new nurse with the admission of a patient with the diagnosis of COPD exacerbation. You explain the differences between the two types of COPD. Together you review the findings that you would expect to assess on a patient with chronic bronchitis versus emphysema. Which of the following would not be an expected finding on a patient with chronic bronchitis?

A. Wheezing and bronchi upon lung field auscultation

B. **Dry cough with little sputum production**

C. Cyanotic

D. Hypercapnia and respiratory acidosis

B: Dry cough with little sputum production. A patient with chronic bronchitis will have a chronic cough with production of large amounts of thick, tenacious mucus.

185. Which of the following is an example of knowledge management?

A. Forming a multidisciplinary team to evaluate your patient's plan of care

B. Provide counseling for patients and families on smoking cessation

C. **Presenting to your unit's staff a comparison of your institution and unit fall rates against national benchmarks**

D. Participating in a community event that focuses on cholesterol screening

C: Presenting to your unit's staff a comparison of your institution and unit fall rates to national benchmarks. Knowledge management includes the CNL using institutional and unit data for comparison against national benchmarks.

186. Your unit has recently been participating in a study to evaluate the use of new, more affordable gloves. You have noticed that many of the nurses are complaining that the gloves are cheap and tearing easily. You present this to your unit manager and discuss the risk of infection. What is this an example of?

    A. Patient advocacy

    B. Evidence-based practice

    C. Team coordination

    D. **Knowledge management**

D: Knowledge management includes anticipating risks when new technology, equipment, treatment regimens, or medication therapies are introduced.

187. Your unit has recently had an increase in fall rates. When you compare what other units in your department are doing, you identify that each unit is using a different fall risk assessment tool. You research each tool and identify which one has the strongest evidence-based research in preventing patient falls. This tool is later standardized throughout the hospital. What is this an example of?

    A. **Applying tools for risk analysis**

    B. Patient advocacy

    C. Gathering, analyzing, and synthesizing data related to risk reduction and patient safety

    D. Demonstrating accountability for the delivery of high-quality care

A: Researching and presenting evidence-based data to apply tools for prevention of falls (risk analysis).

188. As the CNL, you have identified that postsurgical pneumonia has been a frequent occurrence within your unit. Your manager approaches you and identifies that each occurrence of postsurgical pneumonia costs the unit $5,000. You develop a respiratory program that includes frequent incentive spirometer use, ambulation at least three times a day, if warranted, and frequent mouth care. You are able to reduce the unit's occurrences of postsurgical pneumonia by 75%. What is this an example of?

    A. Conceptual analysis and implementation of the CNL role

    B. **Knowledge management**

    C. Effective use of self

    D. Horizontal leadership

B: Knowledge management improves clinical and cost outcomes.

189. You have noticed that on your unit many elderly patients are unable to return home with their family members due to loss/decrease of their functional abilities. You research and implement a tool that scores a patient's functional ability when they enter the hospital and once upon discharge. You use these data to share with staff and create ideas to improve maintenance of an elderly patient's functional ability. What is this an example of?

    A. **Interpreting and using quantitative data**

    B. Interpreting and using qualitative data

    C. Risk analysis

    D. Using evidence to identify and modify interventions to meet specific client needs

A: Quantitative research collects information in the form of numbers.

190. You are providing discharge education to a patient who was diagnosed with Parkinson's disease. The patient is being discharged with a home health nurse and physical therapist. Which of the following statements made by the patient's wife identifies a need for more education?

    A. "I am afraid my husband will fall"

    B. "I am uncertain that I will be able to provide the right care for my husband"

    C. **"My husband enjoys watching TV for long periods of time"**

    D. "I may ask my daughter to stay with us for the next couple of weeks"

C: My husband enjoys watching TV for long periods of time. Pneumonia is the most frequent cause of death in patients with Parkinson's disease.

191. You are discharging a young patient diagnosed with a urinary tract infection. To help prevent future urinary tract infections, you instruct the patient to do the following:

    A. Urinate forcefully to clear bacteria from the tract

    B. Urinate before sexual intercourse to limit transmission

    C. **Wear cotton underwear to prevent moisture**

    D. Pat dry after urinating to prevent infection

C: Wear cotton underwear to prevent moisture. Cotton absorbs moisture and pulls it away from the skin. Bacteria thrive in moist environments.

192. Which of the following is an example of transcultural nursing?

    A. Maintaining eye contact with an Asian family

    B. Reporting to the physician that you are unsure your American Indian patient understands his plan of care because he stares at the floor when you talk to him

    C. A male nurse giving his Hispanic female patient a hug

    D. **Alerting the physician to write for a pork-free diet for your Islamic patient**

D: Alerting the MD to write for a pork-free diet for your Islamic patient. The goal of transcultural nursing is to improve and to provide culturally congruent care to people that is beneficial, will fit with, and will be useful to the client, family, or group healthy lifeways (Leininger, 1991b).

193. You are caring for a patient with CHF. He has just completed a transfusion of 2u of PRBCs. Upon entering the room, he complains of shortness of breath. His O$_2$ saturations are 85% on 2 L and he is breathing 28 respirations a minute. What drug do you anticipate administering?

    A. Nitroglycerin SL

    B. **Lasix IV**

    C. Albuterol HHN

    D. Prednisone PO

B: Patient is most likely in pulmonary edema. Lasix is a loop diuretic.

194. Your manager has approached you regarding her need to decrease the unit's budget. Which of the following would have the greatest impact on decreasing the unit's budget?

    A. **Exploring why staff is not leaving on time and creating overtime**

    B. Eliminating unused supplies on the unit

    C. Increasing nurse to patient ratio

    D. Deciding not to update the unit's computers

A: Exploring why staff is not leaving on time and creating overtime. Nurses' salaries are very costly; to help decrease a unit's budget, get rid of contract RNs and/or overtime.

195. Which accrediting body is an independent, nonprofit organization that works outside of government to provide unbiased and authoritative advice to decision makers and the public?

    A. Centers for Medicare and Medicaid Services (CMS)

    B. **Institute of Medicine (IOM)**

    C. Institute for Safe Medication Practices (ISMP)

    D. Division of Health Service Regulation (DHSR)

B: The Institute of Medicine is an independent, nonprofit organization that works outside of government to provide unbiased and authoritative advice to decision makers and the public.

196. Which of the following is not part of the PDSA change model?

    A. Plan

    B. **Assess**

    C. Do

    D. Study

B: The PDSA change model consists of plan, do, study, and act.

ANSWERS AND RATIONALE **327**

197. You have recently encountered many people in your community who have been sick from drinking park water. As a CNL, which of the following actions would have the greatest impact for your community?

    A. Inform your local news station

    B. **Participate in a petition to send to legislators**

    C. Research whether this has become a national problem

    D. Do nothing

B: Collaborate with the community to appear in front of legislators to promote and preserve healthy communities. As a CNL, you are responsible to influence regulatory, legislative, and public policy in private and public arenas to promote and preserve healthy communities.

198. Which accreditation body is responsible for overseeing medical, mental health, and adult care facilities; emergency medical services; and local jails?

    A. Institute of Medicine (IOM)

    B. The Joint Commission (TJC)

    C. **Division of Health Service Regulation (DHSR)**

    D. Centers for Medicare and Medicaid Services (CMS)

C: DHSR is responsible for overseeing medical, mental health, and adult care facilities; emergency medical services; and local jails.

199. A 65-year-old man with a history of chest palpitations was seen by his cardiologist for new onset palpitations and put on a beta blocker and told to return for a follow-up in 1 week after taking a stress test. The beta blocker's action includes:

    A. Increasing the consistency of the heart rate

    B. Decreasing the ability of the heart muscle to contract

    C. Decreasing the chance of dysrythmia

    D. **Increasing contractility and decreasing heart rate**

D: This is the mechanism of action of all β-blocker medications.

200. When assessing a patient for a diagnosis of pneumonia, it is more difficult to make a proper diagnosis in the absence of the following symptom:

    A. **Cough**

    B. Cyanosis

    C. Tachycardia

    D. Bradycardia

A: Cough is one of the paramount symptoms used to help diagnose pneumonia.

201. In order to complete a thorough assessment of a 55-year-old male beginning an exercise program, the CNL should include the following in the instructions:

    A. Begin an exercise program of a minimum of 60 minutes of vigorous exercise each day

    B. **Keep a daily written log of exercise and include the type of exercise, time of exercise, and the intensity of the exercise**

    C. Avoid drinking more than 8 oz of water per day when exercising

    D. Side effects are common when beginning exercising and should be ignored

B: When starting a new exercise regimen, it is important to keep a log of the specific exercise, amount of time, and intensity to determine what the patient can tolerate at baseline before increasing the exercise plan.

202. An 88-year-old lady suffers a stroke in the nursing home and develops pneumonia and is transferred to the hospital. She continues to decline, is having trouble breathing, and becomes unconscious with little hope of recovery or quality of life. She has no family and no health care proxy, living will, or directions about whether she wants to be intubated or not. The physician wants to intubate the patient. The staff nurse strongly believes the patient would not want to be intubated, as she had cared for the lady before she became unconscious. What is the BEST thing for the CNL to do first:

    A. Take a vote among the staff nurses

    B. **Call for an ethics consultation**

    C. Ask the social worker to make a recommendation or decision

    D. Do a literature review on quality of life of elderly patients with pneumonia

B: When a patient has not declared his or her wishes and there is no family or documentation and there is a dispute, then there is an ethical issue and the best choice is to ask for an ethics consultation.

Case Study 1

You are a CNL in a critical care unit. You have recently been asked to join a task force to address specific clinical outcomes. The first priority of the group is to address critically ill patients intubated for more than 24 hours who are at high risk of developing ventilator-associated pneumonia (VAP). Other risk factors for VAP include decreased level of consciousness, supine positioning with a head of bed less than 30°, gastric distension, trauma, and a COPD diagnosis.

1. Ventilator-associated pneumonia (VAP) in mechanically ventilated patients is a complication that can be prevented. Your ICU has an opportunity to improve. Choose the best response that illustrates the incidence of VAP in your unit.

    A. **Trend analysis of ICU-acquired pneumonia for the last fiscal year**

    B. Average length of stay in the ICU

    C. The latest research

    D. All of the above

A: This action demonstrates the systems analyst and risk anticipator role of the CNL.

2. Reviewing and evaluating the current patient care guidelines and protocols for all intubated patients demonstrates which CNL role function:

   A. Member of the profession

   B. Team manager

   C. Advocate

   D. **Systems analyst**

D: As a systems analyst, review of a system to critically evaluate and anticipate risks to patient safety is a CNL role function that is necessary to improve health care outcomes.

3. Understanding of the ICU as a clinical microsystem includes an exploration of its:

   A. Processes, patients, and paperwork

   B. Paperwork, purpose, and professionals

   C. Professionals, patterns, and paperwork

   D. **Purpose, patients, processes, patterns, and professionals**

D: A microsystem's assessment often utilizes a 5P assessment: patients, professionals, processes, patterns, and purpose.

4. Process mapping is a method of creating a diagram showing the steps and the flow of the intubated patient's care process. Flowcharting:

   A. Identifies unwanted variation, rework, and waste

   B. Engages the interdisciplinary team

   C. Replaces words with a picture

   D. **All of the above**

D: Flowcharting has many benefits for improvement groups looking to greater understand a process.

5. The standard of care for all intubated patients now includes a 30° head of bed position and oral care with chlorhexidine every 4 hours. After two quarters of practice, the incidence of VAP can be best trended using:

   A. Root cause analysis

   B. An audit by the nurse manager

   C. **A run chart**

   D. A pie chart

C: A run chart is an easily utilized tool to study variation and data over time.

Case Study 2

Jenny, an 18-year-old, was admitted through the ED to your general medical unit during the night. Her admitting diagnosis is asthma exacerbation. Six months ago she was transferred from receiving care at the hospital pediatric clinic to the adult women's health clinic. This is her second admission in 3 months.

1. What are important components of your initial nursing assessment?

    A. Her ED course of treatment, medication history, living situation

    B. Her medication history, lab work, living situation

    C. Medications, labs, family, clinic appointment history, smoking history

    D. **Her ED course of treatment, present vital signs, medication history, living situation, social history, smoking status**

D: The CNL assessment should include physical information as well as social factors in an attempt to identify factors that have led to two admissions within 3 months of each other.

2. Jenny's clinic history shows a history of appointment noncompliance and failure to fill her prescriptions. When Jenny does take her medication, she tells you that she uses a steroidal inhaler once or twice a day if she feels she needs it. She does not take a rescue inhaler (bronchodilator) unless she has very bad wheezing because she complains it makes her "jittery." You recognize that:

    A. This is the correct sequence for her medications

    B. She is taking both medications incorrectly. She needs medication administration instructions

    C. **You need to assess Jenny's knowledge regarding the mechanism of actions and administration of her medications prior to any further action**

    D. You should ask the physician to prescribe other medications

C: Before providing medication instructions, the CNL should assess the patient's knowledge level about the medications. This includes asking the patient why the medications have been prescribed and how they can be used to best treat symptoms.

3. Jenny lives with her mother and two younger siblings. She is a nonsmoker, but her mother smokes one to two cigarettes per day. Jenny's mom states she only smokes outside the house. There are also two cats in the home. You feel it is important to:

    A. Tell Jenny's mother that it is irresponsible to smoke in the house, as it may make Jenny's symptoms worse, and provide informational pamphlets about smoking cessation programs

    B. Suggest that the cats be removed from the home and offer to facilitate communication with pet adoption agencies

    C. **Speak with Jenny and her mother together and explain the role that allergens, such as smoke and cat hair, may have in exacerbating asthmatic symptoms**

    D. Inform the family to keep cats and smoke outside of the house

C: An important step in asthma control is the limitation of outside allergens. The patient and family must understand this relationship. The CNL as an educator may provide the patient and family with this information and work with them to identify potential triggers and work toward solutions to remove them from the home environment.

4. Beginning with your first visit, you begin to prepare Jenny for discharge. You feel that her needs would be best served by conducting an interdisciplinary meeting to discuss her discharge plan and future care. You invite the following people to this meeting:

    A. Pulmonologist, social worker, dietician

    B. **Pulmonologist, PMD, former pediatrician, Jenny, Jenny's mother, school nurse**

    C. Pulmonologist, PMD, Jenny, dietician

    D. PMD, Jenny, Jenny's mother, social worker

B: An important advocate in Jenny's ongoing care is the school nurse. Additionally, although she has transitioned from a pediatric clinic, her pediatrician can add valuable insight into her former plan of care.

5. As a CNL, you know that a key part of Jenny's ongoing care after discharge that would help improve her outcome is:

    A. A medication reconciliation record

    B. **An asthma plan**

    C. A peak flow diary

    D. Discharge instructions

B: Adherence to an asthma plan that is mutually agreed upon by the patient and health care provider has been shown to be the best defense against asthma exacerbations. An asthma plan should include instructions for daily treatment and ways to recognize and handle worsening symptoms. A peak flow diary is one part of an asthma plan.

6. Prior to discharge, the CNL should pay particular attention to:

    A. **Vaccination status**

    B. Diet plan

    C. Exercise plan

    D. Labwork

A: The most common precipitator of asthma exacerbation is viral infection. Jenny should be up to date on all immunizations, including flu and pneumonia vaccines prior to discharge. If she cannot receive them during the hospitalization, the CNL should ensure there is a plan to receive them from the PMD at a later date.

Case Study 3

You are a CNL on a medical–surgical unit in a community hospital. A few of the nurses from the unit come to you because they are concerned about a recent increase in falls on the unit. They tell you that they believe that the increase is due to insufficient staffing on the unit. They would like you to help them investigate this topic.

1. What should be your first step?

    A. Compare your unit's fall rate to similar like-sized hospitals nationwide

    B. **Look at your current rates for this unit and see if there has been an increase in the fall rate over the last year, as the nurses suspect**

    C. Compare your fall rates to other units in the hospital to see if they are higher or lower

    D. Look at staffing ratios over the last year to see if they have changed

B: The nurses have come to you with some observations and you need to confirm that they are in fact correct before you proceed.

You find that the fall rate on your unit has in fact been increasing over the past 6 months. More troubling is that the number of patient injuries due to falls has also increased. You decide to form a unit-based subcommittee to look into the issue further.

2. Who should be the initial members on the committee? (Check all that apply)

    A. **Physical therapist**

    B. **Nurses**

    C. Housekeeper

    D. **Nurse manager**

    E. **Nurses' aides**

    F. Secretary

    G. Physicians

    H. **Coordinator of patient safety**

    I. Risk manager

A, B, D, E, and H: All of these people can have valuable input and insight into what is happening on the unit and help with developing and implementing changes on the unit. Additional members may be asked to join as the group evolves.

3. What information should the committee evaluate in the initial phase of this project? (Choose all that apply)

    A. What types of injuries the patients are sustaining when they fall

    B. **The current fall policy**

    C. **Chart audits of documentation related to falls and safety assessments**

    D. **The current fall prevention tool**

    E. Current research on the topic

    F. **Staffing ratios on the unit**

    G. **Current fall prevention strategies on the unit**

B, C, D, F, and G: These items are most relevant to the current policies and practices regarding the identified issues. It is critical for the group to clearly understand what is currently in place and adherence to present practices before moving toward change.

You find that staffing ratios have not changed on the unit. There have been several days when the unit has been short staffed, owing to staff resignations, but there has not been a higher fall rate on those days as compared with days when the unit is well staffed. New staff have been hired for the unit and will be starting over the next few weeks.

There is a fall prevention policy in place and a fall prevention tool that is to be filled out each shift by the nursing staff. The problem seems to be lack of documentation and consistent implementation of fall prevention strategies by the nursing staff.

4. What would be the best way to find out what the barriers are for the nursing staff with documentation and implementation of fall prevention strategies?

   A. Create a written survey and ask all of the nurses and nurses' aides on the unit to complete it

   B. Brainstorm with the other members of the committee on ways to improve documentation among the staff

   C. **Get a group of nurses and nurses' aides together, representing each shift and go through the fall prevention tool with them item by item to find out where the barriers are**

   D. Go around the unit and question the staff who have had a patient fall over the past 6 months about what they think led to the fall

C: This will probably allow you to gather the most comprehensive information, as it includes representatives from all shifts. The group format may also allow you to gather more information, as talking among each other about the issue may allow for valuable discussion.

After meeting with a group of nurses and nurses' aides, you learn that the responsibilities for each group were not clear, and that led to fall prevention strategies not being consistently implemented on patients who were identified as being at risk for falling.

5. What should the subcommittee's next step be?

   A. Make sure that the nurses understand that they are solely responsible for fall prevention on the unit

   B. Look for a new fall prevention tool to implement and revise the current policy. Then provide education for the staff regarding the new tool

   C. See if they are having the same problem on other units in the hospital

   D. **Develop an educational tool based on the current fall prevention policy and tool. Provide education to all of the staff, so they understand their own and each other's role in fall prevention**

D: The commitee found no deficiencies with current policy and tools. The issue was with inconsistent implementation of fall prevention strategies. Staff need education on role responsibility in fall prevention.

Case Study 4

You are a CNL on an oncology unit. A nurse comes to you to share concerns about Mrs. Lopez, an 84-year-old patient admitted for shortness of breath. The patient was diagnosed 6 months ago with small cell lung cancer treated with chemotherapy and radiation therapy. On admission to the hospital, the patient had evidence of significant metastatic disease. The patient is being treated with morphine and oxygen, but remains significantly short of breath. The physician meets with the patient and family to share the plan for radiation treatment in an attempt to reduce the size of the current tumors. When the physician and family leave, the patient shares that she no longer wants aggressive treatments, but prefers to be comfortable and would like to go home, if possible.

1. Which of the following is an appropriate intervention for the nurse to suggest to the concerned nurse to do first?

   A. Report the patient's wishes to the physician

   B. Take the family aside and tell them what the patient shared

   C. Call an immediate family meeting with all members of the patient's health care team to discuss the matter

   D. **Ask the patient if she would like to see the palliative care nurse and discuss options regarding her wishes for care**

D: Palliative care is a field of nursing that is unique in its approach, focus, and goals of patient interaction. This approach to care concerns patients whose disease is not responsive to curative treatment, where control of pain, symptoms, psychological, and spiritual distress is paramount. The patient is clearly hesitant to express her true wishes to her physician and family and the discussion and knowledge gained through a meeting with a palliative care expert may better equip her to share her feelings. The nurse and CNL must advocate for the patient and answer D best exemplifies meeting the needs of the patient at this particular time.

2. Mrs. Lopez shares with her physician and family that she does not plan to have the suggested radiation and would like a plan for a safe discharge with the support of hospice. All involved are supportive of this plan except for one daughter, who is very opposed to withdrawing treatment. Mrs. Lopez is concerned that the conflict among her children will impact her wishes when she can no longer make her own decisions. The best recommendation to Mrs. Lopez would include:

   A. Have the physician speak to all of Mrs. Lopez's children to explain the prognosis

   B. Contact the Pastoral Care department to speak to the daughter who is resisting the current plan

   C. **Support the necessary steps to help Mrs. Lopez create an advanced directive**

   D. Support the necessary steps to develop the patient's do-not-resuscitate orders for her hospital stay

C: Advanced directives are legal documents, such as a living will, durable power of attorney, and health care proxy. These documents allow people to convey their decisions about end-of-life care. Advanced directives are a way for patients to communicate their wishes to family friends and health care professionals. The use of these documents can help avoid confusion, turmoil, guilt, and promote a person's choices for care. Once developed, Mrs. Lopez should share these documents with her family.

3. The events of the past 48 hours have been very stressful on Mrs. Lopez and her family. The CNL recognizes this emotional distress and offers to have a certified therapeutic touch volunteer come and visit the patient. This action is best described as:

   A. Inappropriate, given the patient's circumstances

   B. **Appropriate to the holistic needs of the patient**

   C. A standard practice for hospitalized patients

   D. An example of a quality improvement initiative focused on increasing patient satisfaction for the long-term purpose of increased financial reimbursement

B: Complementary alternative medicine (CAM) has a role in the traditional treatment of patients with medical conditions. The CNL should be aware of CAM interventions, some of which involve vitamins, minerals, or herbal supplements.

4. On day 4 of the admission, Mrs. Lopez is ready for discharge home with home care services and hospice care. The discharge process represents what opportunities regarding assuring a safe transfer of care in all of the following?

   A. Risk anticipation—through medication reconciliation and education, because Mrs. Lopez is being discharged on a high-risk medication (morphine)

   B. Knowledge management—as information about Mrs. Lopez is communicated to her hospice nurse in a written plan as well as oral communication

   C. Advocacy—as the nurse should ensure that a copy of any advance directive is provided to the homecare agency and confirmed through verbal communication

   D. Tertiary health promotion through the continuation of physical therapy to maximize physical mobility and minimize preventable complication of her condition

   E. **All of the above**

E: All of the choices represent opportunities for CNLs to provide safe, effective care at upon discharge. Transitions from one area of care in the health care system to another are at high risk for miscommunications, errors, and patient safety issues.

Case Study 5

Walter is a 63-year-old African American who was readmitted to the telemetry unit of your hospital after being home for just 8 days. He has previously been diagnosed with stage 2 left heart failure secondary to a septal myocardial infarction (MI) that occurred 2 years ago. He has a 40-pack smoking history but quit at the time of the MI. Walter has had to retire from his job as a postal service employee and lives with his wife who continues to work full time. On this admission, Walter had the following data collected in the Emergency Department:

Blood pressure: 150/90	Respiratory rate: 28
Heart rate: 124 bpm	BMI: 29
Arterial blood gas:	
pH	7.48
PaO_2	78%
$PaCO_2$	28 mm Hg
HCO_3	24 mEq/L
Sao_2	88%

1. Based on the results of the ABG, your preliminary classification of the patient would be:

   A. Respiratory acidosis

   B. **Respiratory alkalosis**

   C. Metabolic acidosis

   D. Metabolic alkalosis

B: Respiratory alkalosis. The increased pH and decreased Paco2 indicate an uncompensated respiratory alkalosis.

2. Walter is preparing for discharge on day 3 of hospitalization. The CNL chooses the following next step in discharge preparation:

   A. A discussion with Walter's wife regarding their home situation

   B. A team meeting with those involved in Walter's care with inclusion of the outpatient team members

   C. A session of patient education focused on teach-back techniques to assure knowledge

   D. **A conversation with Walter regarding what factors he felt contributed to his readmission**

D: For a holistic assessment of the patient experience and a true sense of contributing factors, this intervention is most appropriate. All other interventions mentioned may be utilized at some point.

3. Based on priorities of care for those with heart failure, which intervention should the CNL ensure is part of Walter's discharge plan?

   A. **Scheduling of a follow-up appointment with the primary care provider within 7 days**

   B. Smoking cessation

C. Cardiac rehabilitation

D. Visiting nurse services

A: Outcomes in the field of heart failure indicated improved coordination of care when patients are seen soon after discharge.

4. In preparation for discharge, the CNL ensures that the patient understands the medication plan for home and provides a written plan to the patient. The patient is being discharged on metoprolol. The CNL understands this drug is used for which of the following purposes:

A. To reduce myocardial oxygen consumption

B. To reduce platelet aggregation and risk of coronary occlusion

C. **To reduce cardiac workload and oxygen demands of the heart**

D. To reduce plasma aldosterone concentrations

C: β-blockers are often used in heart failure but must be started slow, or they may worsen symptoms. It is imperative that patients understand the possible side effects of medication and what symptoms to report to their providers. Medication mismanagement and associated issues often cause hospital readmissions.

Case Study 6

You are receiving a 24-year-old patient from the intensive care unit (ICU). The patient has been in an ICU for 1 week. He was admitted due to a motor vehicle accident in which he had to have surgical repair of his femur and right hip. His medical history is significant for smoking (cigarettes) and occasionally drinking alcohol. Vital signs are stable and the patient is alert and oriented × 4. When you are reviewing his plan of care, he indicates that he has not been out of bed although he has been cleared by the surgical trauma physician.

1. Which of the following complications would you be most concerned about following this patient's surgery?

A. Sepsis

B. Bowel obstruction

C. **Acute respiratory failure**

D. DVT

C: Typical post-op complications of atelectasis, pneumonia, and pulmonary edema are common among patients who are bed bound for an extended period.

2. The patient states that he does not understand why he would be at risk for pulmonary complications. You explain to the patient that pulmonary complications such as infection, aspiration, bronchospasm, respiratory failure, pleural effusion, and atelectasis are common after surgery. You indicate that all of the following are risk factors for developing postoperative pulmonary complications *except*:

    A. Hemoglobin level <10 g/dL

    B. Emergency procedure

    C. **Respiratory infection during the previous year**

    D. Older age

C: Respiratory infection during the previous year. A respiratory infection that occurred previously would not put this patient at risk for developing postoperative pulmonary complications.

3. The patient acknowledges the importance of mobility to prevent these complications. What would be the next most important intervention to help further reduce that patient's chances for developing pulmonary complications?

    A. Smoking cessation education

    B. **Appropriate pain management**

    C. Nutrition

    D. Chest physical therapy

B: Pain management. Inappropriate use of narcotics may cause respiratory depression; however, appropriate pain management is vital for patient recovery and ensuring a patient will participate in mobility exercises.

4. Your patient begins to complain of leg pain. When you assess his leg, he points to his thigh. His pulses are +1, where previously they have been +3. You notify the physician and he orders a Doppler ultrasound, which is positive for a DVT. What other complications are you most concerned about this patient developing?

    A. **Pulmonary embolus**

    B. Loss of blood flow to the patient's extremity

    C. Edema

    D. Immobility

A: After hip surgery, thrombi often form in the veins of the thigh. These clots are more likely to lead to pulmonary embolus.

5. Your patient suffers a pulmonary embolus, which leads to his requiring mechanical ventilation. The patient returns to ICU. As a clinical nurse leader, what would be the most appropriate intervention after caring for this patient?

    A. Perform a root cause analysis

    B. **Forming a multidisciplinary team to review the patient's plan of care and gather whether anything could have been done to prevent this from occurring**

    C. Review the case with your nurse manager

    D. Review evidence-based practice and research on caring for and preventing pulmonary complications postoperatively

B: Formation of a multidisciplinary team to review the patient's plan of care and gather whether anything could have been done to prevent this from happening.

It is very important as a CNL to include your multidisciplinary team members in assessing whether a patient's plan of care is successful or not.

Case Study 7

You are the CNL on an obstetrical unit. You receive a patient, Sharon T, from the doctor's office, admitted with mild preeclampsia at 28 weeks' gestation.

1. Over the next 24 hours, you should review all of the following except:

    A. Pregnancy history, allergies, medical history

    B. **Birth plan, sleep history, hobbies, exercise routine**

    C. Alcohol, drug, and tobacco use; social history; diet

    D. Medications prior to admission, immunization status

B: The patient is early in her pregnancy with only mild preeclampsia; thus a birth plan is not imperative information right now. Her sleep history, hobbies, and exercise routine do not impact her plan of care for the first 24 hours.

The next morning you walk into Sharon's room and find her to be withdrawn with a flat affect. You sit down and start talking with her, and she tells you that she and her husband recently started their own business so they do not have medical insurance, and her husband has to work 16 hours a day just to keep up with the business. She is worried about how she will pay for this hospitalization, and who is going to take care of their 3-year-old daughter while she is in the hospital. She also did not sleep well last night because hospital staff was in and out of her room all night.

2. As the CNL, what are some appropriate interventions that you can perform?

    A. Consult the physical therapist

    B. Give the patient an application for Medicare

    C. **Consult the social worker and case manager**

    D. Write an order to keep all staff out of her room between 2300 and 0600

C: The social worker can help with financial planning/coverage options; the case manager can help insurance/billing questions; bundling care will decrease Sharon's interruptions and allow her more resting time.

Sharon is very grateful for your interventions and feels much better about her situation. She has now been on your unit for 2 ½ weeks and has developed gestational diabetes and severe preeclampsia. The doctors have told her that she will have to remain in the hospital on bedrest with bathroom privileges for the duration of her pregnancy. Sharon is not happy about this, but knows it is the best thing for her and her baby and is compliant.

3. As the CNL who is managing her plan of care, you will be sure to include in her plan of care all of the following except:

    A. Daily rounding with her care team, and weekly interdisciplinary team meetings

    B. **Instructions on how to self-administer insulin, and daily walks outside**

    C. Physical therapy consult, visits with her family

    D. Utilization of antithromboembolism pump/antithromboembolism therapy

B: As the CNL, you need to be involved in her plan of care, which means rounding with the care team. At least weekly interdisciplinary meetings are recommended by TJC; PT will assess for bedrest and give exercises; visits with her family will help her mental health; nutritionist for preeclampsia and diabetic diet; diabetes educator for newly diagnosed gestational diabetes; and antithromboembolism therapy for prolonged bedrest. All other choices are not appropriate at this time.

Two weeks later, Sharon's vital signs and labs start going downhill and she is having subjective symptoms of preeclampsia. She is 32 ½ weeks pregnant, and the doctors have decided that it is time to move toward delivery. As it is not urgent at this time, they will allow Sharon to attempt a vaginal delivery.

    4. As the CNL, what should you make sure happens prior to delivery?

    A. Steroid administration

    B. Blood glucose control

    C. **Neonatologist consult**

    D. Sharon's birth plan of no medications be upheld

C: Sharon needs to know what to expect when her baby is born, which will help to reduce her anxiety and improve her labor outcomes. She should have already received steroids; blood glucose control, although important, is out of your hands now; she will definitely need medications for her blood pressure, so she needs to have a discussion about this and not uphold her birth plan.

The next day you go to check on Sharon. She had a successful vaginal delivery of a baby girl at 0249. The baby went to the NICU. Sharon is still in labor and delivery on magnesium sulfate. She will be transferred once her acuity level decreases enough not to have one-on-one nursing care. Her vital signs are stable, but her blood pressure is still elevated. Her labs are beginning to trend back to normal. Sharon thanks you for all your care.

    5. What would your next priority be?

    A. **Begin discharge teaching**

    B. Have the transport team take Sharon to the NICU to see her baby

    C. Consult the social worker

    D. Consult child life

A: Discharge teaching needs to be started early, so the patient has plenty of time to hear and retain information and ask questions.

Case Study 8

Erika is a Caucasian 72-year-old female being admitted by her primary care physician for uncontrolled DM Type II.

1. What other information do you need right now upon admission?

    A. **FSBG**

    B. Mental status

    C. Does she live alone?

    D. Does she have a glucometer?

A: Although all these things are important to know, the FSBG is the first thing to obtain to know how to treat the patient on admission. The other three can come at a later time.

Her FSBG is 327 on admission. The primary care nurse gives her insulin on the basis of the physician's orders. You introduce yourself to Erika and start gathering information. You ask the patient whether she is taking her medication at home. Erika tells you, "I take my medicine all the time. I have no idea why my blood sugar is so high! It's never even close to that at home!"

2. What do you want to know next while gathering information?

    A. Does she have a glucometer?

    B. Falls risk score

    C. **HgbA1c**

    D. Mental status

C: Again, these are all things that are important to obtain at some point during the hospitalization, but the most important of those is the HgbA1c. The patient is admitted for uncontrolled diabetes; the main way to find out how uncontrolled it really is, is by checking what her HgbA1c is Erika's HgbA1c is 10.2.

3. From this HgbA1c, you know:

    A. It is normal

    B. **It is high**

    C. Erika is taking her medication

    D. It is inconclusive

B: A HgbA1c above 6 is considered abnormal. A HgbA1c correlates with blood sugars averaging about 240 mg/dl for at least the past 3 months.

You realize Erika's diabetes is not well controlled. You look up her home medications to see what regimen she is supposed to be taking and consult the diabetes educator per the physician's orders.

4. What should you do next?

    A. **Get a dietician consult to review her knowledge about diabetic diets and develop a meal plan**

    B. Call her son, whom she lives with, to develop a POC

    C. Call her PCP and see if she is compliant with her appointments and medication regimen

    D. Tell her she cannot eat any potatoes, rice, or refined sugars at all

A: Working with the interdisciplinary team is an important role of the CNL. It is important to know how much knowledge the patient has and also to work with them to come up with a meal plan they can actually follow.

After the diabetes educator and dietician have seen the patient, you discover the patient did not have very much money and was having trouble buying the right foods. She was also having severe diarrhea from the metformin and was very embarrassed after she had a few accidents in public. You contact the social worker to come help the patient work on getting the right foods and you make a list of healthy foods that are not very expensive to help the patient make better food choices.

5. What else should you do?

A. Call her son to go get her metformin from the pharmacy

B. Tell the patient the metformin is important and to just wear some Depends

C. Discontinue the metformin and start glyburide

D. **Call her PCP to discuss her side effect from taking the metformin and to develop a POC**

D: An important part of being a CNL is being a patient advocate and also working in close, trusting relationships with physicians. Letting her PCP know why she is not compliant and coming up with a new POC is needed in order for the patient to be compliant when at home.

Index